To My Savior and the Creator of All:
Thank You for The Good News, and the blessings that You bestow upon me daily as I travel through life. I pray that all come to realize the only Way, the Truth, and the Life.

To My Family:
Lisa, Devin, and Reagan, you inspire me to be a better husband and father, though I know I am wanting in many ways. Please keep in mind that I love you and my love for you is eternal, regardless of distance or time.

PREFACE

Diagnostic medical sonography has rightfully been recognized as a necessary imaging modality in the practice of modern medicine. An obvious example of this truth can readily be observed daily in the medical specialties of Gynecology and Obstetrics. The impact that sonography has established in female patient care is truly extraordinary. As an inexpensive, reliable, and nonionizing diagnostic examination for the female pelvis—gravid or not—sonography is truly unparalleled. While the practice of sonography on the nongravid patient can be, at times, straightforward and potentially certain in the diagnosis of disease, obstetric sonography provides unique challenges for those practitioners charged with the duty to operate the equipment accurately, quickly, and analytically, while at the same time essentially assessing a moving target—the fetus. It is during these challenging exams, that one begins to recognize that a sonographic imaging protocol is necessary, and that this protocol must be organized, succinct, and investigative. This book has been created for those with minimal sonographic experience because it will optimistically provide an image-guided protocol to assist in the organization of sonographic practice. Thus, sonography students and medical students will appreciate the unique format and structure provided, while it may also serve the advanced practitioner as a reference guide and a quick review of normal sonographic anatomy and common pathology. Accordingly, the primary objective of *Pocket Anatomy & Protocols for Obstetrics & Gynecology Ultrasound* is to provide the user with a readily handy resource that assists with clinical assessment, protocol establishment, and the identification of normal and some abnormal sonographic anatomy of the nongravid and gravid female patient.

Pocket Anatomy & Protocols for Obstetrics & Gynecology Ultrasound

Pocket Anatomy & Protocols for Obstetrics & Gynecology Ultrasound

Steven M. Penny, RT (R), RDMS (AB, PS, OB/GYN)
Director of Sonography Programs
Johnston Community College
Smithfield, North Carolina

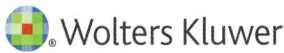
 Wolters Kluwer

Philadelphia • Baltimore • New York • London
Buenos Aires • Hong Kong • Sydney • Tokyo

Acquisitions Editor: Matt Hauber
Development Editor: Eric McDermott
Editorial Coordinator: Remington Fernando
Editorial Assistant: Kristen Kardoley
Marketing Manager: Kirsten Watrud
Production Project Manager: Kirstin Johnson
Manager, Graphic Arts & Design: Stephen Druding
Manufacturing Coordinator: Lisa Bowling
Prepress Vendor: Aptara, Inc.

First edition

Copyright © 2025 Wolters Kluwer

All rights reserved. This book is protected by copyright. No part of this book may be reproduced or transmitted in any form or by any means, including as photocopies or scanned-in or other electronic copies, or utilized by any information storage and retrieval system without written permission from the copyright owner, except for brief quotations embodied in critical articles and reviews. Materials appearing in this book prepared by individuals as part of their official duties as U.S. government employees are not covered by the above-mentioned copyright. To request permission, please contact Wolters Kluwer at Two Commerce Square, 2001 Market Street, Philadelphia, PA 19103, via email at permissions@lww.com, or via our website at shop.lww.com (products and services).

9 8 7 6 5 4 3 2 1

Printed in Mexico

Library of Congress Cataloging-in-Publication Data

Names: Penny, Steven M., author.
Title: Pocket anatomy & protocols for obstetrics & gynecology ultrasound / Steven M. Penny.
Other titles: Pocket anatomy and protocols for obstetrics & gynecology ultrasound
Description: First edition. | Philadelphia, PA : Wolters Kluwer, [2025] |
 Includes bibliographical references and index. | Summary: "The primary audience for this pocket book will be individuals training in or practicing, OBGYN sonography. Sonography programs last between 2 and 4 years and are offered at community colleges, 4 year colleges and career schools. There are 393 programs in the US (8,000 Sonography students). Students typically come to the sonography program with either bachelors or higher level training in a healthcare field or with experience as a radiation technologist. Secondarily, this pocket-sized book will provide a quick clinical reference for practitioners in vascular sonography. According to the US Bureau of Labor Statistics, the US has 78,640 practicing sonographers. The presentation of the material will be based on Pocket Anatomy & Protocols for Abdominal Ultrasound. It is image-based with distinct summary tables for specific organ measurements and protocol guidelines as well. Content will be presented in a bullet format. The layout will be both succinct and distinct. Diagrams will used as appropriate and only essential tables will be provided with information regarding normal organ dimensions and echogenicities (the ability to bounce an echo signal). All diagrams, sonographic images, and illustrations that are provided in the text will be modern imaging and drawings. There exists a need for a concise clinical pocket-sized protocol book for students. The audience for this book can move beyond the sonography student and aid practicing sonographers and medical radiology residents during imaging rotations as well. The series will encompass obstetrics & gynecology, vascular, adult echocardiography, and musculoskeletal"– Provided by publisher.
Identifiers: LCCN 2024038668 (print) | LCCN 2024038669 (ebook) | ISBN 9781975218614 (paperback) | ISBN 9781975218621 (epub)
Subjects: MESH: Ultrasonography, Prenatal–methods | Pelvis–diagnostic imaging | Handbook
Classification: LCC RG527.5.U48 (print) | LCC RG527.5.U48 (ebook) | NLM WQ 39 | DDC 618.2/07543–dc23/eng/20240923
LC record available at https://lccn.loc.gov/2024038668
LC ebook record available at https://lccn.loc.gov/2024038669

This work is provided "as is," and the publisher disclaims any and all warranties, express or implied, including any warranties as to accuracy, comprehensiveness, or currency of the content of this work.

This work is no substitute for individual patient assessment based upon healthcare professionals' examination of each patient and consideration of, among other things, age, weight, gender, current or prior medical conditions, medication history, laboratory data and other factors unique to the patient. The publisher does not provide medical advice or guidance and this work is merely a reference tool. Healthcare professionals, and not the publisher, are solely responsible for the use of this work including all medical judgments and for any resulting diagnosis and treatments.

Given continuous, rapid advances in medical science and health information, independent professional verification of medical diagnoses, indications, appropriate pharmaceutical selections and dosages, and treatment options should be made and healthcare professionals should consult a variety of sources. When prescribing medication, healthcare professionals are advised to consult the product information sheet (the manufacturer's package insert) accompanying each drug to verify, among other things, conditions of use, warnings and side effects and identify any changes in dosage schedule or contraindications, particularly if the medication to be administered is new, infrequently used or has a narrow therapeutic range. To the maximum extent permitted under applicable law, no responsibility is assumed by the publisher for any injury and/or damage to persons or property, as a matter of products liability, negligence law or otherwise, or from any reference to or use by any person of this work.

shop.lww.com

HOW TO USE THIS POCKET BOOK

The composition of this book is marginally different than the abdominal equivalent in the series—*Pocket Anatomy & Protocols for Abdominal Ultrasound*—which was published in 2020. Whereas that book was constructed in organ-specific chapters, this book is examination-specific, based on recommendations made by presiding sonographic organizations, such as the American Institute of Ultrasound in Medicine (AIUM). The first part of the book is related to Gynecologic Sonography, while the second part is Obstetric Sonography. Nonetheless, each chapter, though small, is information and image-packed, with clinical practice in mind. Before the examination begins, this book can serve as a review of imaging requirements, clinical questions, sonographic anatomy, and protocol suggestions. During the examination, one can return to its pages for reference materials, such as normal measurements, pathology, and image correlation. The following suggested steps are also provided to offer a means whereby one can maximize the utilization of this—outwardly, deceptively diminutive, but inwardly rich—resource appropriately in the clinical setting.

STEP #1: POCKET IT!

The book is sized perfectly to be placed in the pocket of a scrub top or pant. It could also occupy only a small spot on a shelf or even be placed upon the ultrasound machine to remain nearby for quick access. Even if you have one of the other pocket books in the series, all together they will only take up a tiny space.

STEP #2: REVIEW NORMAL ANATOMY AND PHYSIOLOGY

While this book is not admittedly a thoroughly detailed textbook concerning all anatomy, physiology, or pathology, it does contain enough information to provide a quick recap of the most beneficial information in these areas.

STEP #3: REVIEW PATIENT PREPARATION AND SUGGESTED EQUIPMENT

This resource provides some patient preparation information and positioning techniques that may be useful. Also, equipment suggestions have been made, including what transducer might serve the user best and how to optimize each imaging study.

Prior to the start of the examination, ensure that your patient is best served by maintaining your machine in the best working order and keeping it cleaned appropriately in order to deter patient exposure to nosocomial infections.

STEP #4: REVIEW NORMAL SONOGRAPHIC ANATOMY

Briefly review normal sonographic anatomy. Though you will hopefully carry this book with you, a proactive quick anatomic review over normal sonographic anatomy and the appearance of variances in structures would be beneficial.

STEP #5: REVIEW THE SUGGESTED PROTOCOL

The AIUM, in conjunction with other medical organizations, works to establish indications and recommendations for sonographic imaging. In each chapter, AIUM-specific recommendations for individual examinations are offered. With these recommendations in mind, a fundamental, and yet flexible, protocol has been provided in each examination-specific chapter. Protocols do vary per institution, and thus the recommended protocol is malleable, providing a primary groundwork, upon which additions or subtractions can be made by the practitioner in conjunction with previously established routines and advances in future technology.

STEP #6: CLINICAL INVESTIGATION

A vital role of the sonographer is the obligation to obtain an adequate clinical history. In each of the examination-specific chapters, several clinical history questions are offered. If many of these questions are answered effectually before the examination commences, the sonographer can be aided to provide a more focused examination. However, one must realize that with obstetric sonography, clinical findings can be vague at best, and thus an exceptional test is presented in these circumstances. Unfortunately, the obstetric sonographer must learn to expect the unexpected, but where clinical history and data are obtained and truly applicable to the case at hand, it can at times dramatically aid in determining the correct diagnosis.

STEP #7: PERFORMING THE EXAMINATION

Refer to the pages of this book throughout the examination when needed for sonographic anatomy, proper measuring techniques and normal measurements, scanning tips, and a section titled "where else to look."

STEP #8: ESSENTIAL PATHOLOGY FOCUS AND UNIQUE CHAPTERS

Essential pathology is provided within several of the chapters. Furthermore, Chapter 4 provides an overview of sonohysterography and three-dimensional sonography, while the two final chapters of the book include multiple gestations and common chromosomal abnormalities.

FINAL WORDS

Diagnostic medical sonography is an ever-changing and advancing imaging modality. Our impact upon patient care, as those who practice within the field, can be life-altering. In fact, it should be. The goal of this book is to assist you as you strive to provide the best possible patient care that you can afford. Remember, your patients deserve your optimum effort at all times. Thank you for choosing to use *Pocket Anatomy & Protocols for Obstetrics & Gynecology Ultrasound* as a resource. My prayer is that this book positively impacts your skills as a practitioner and as a result serves you and your patients well.

Steven M. Penny

ACKNOWLEDGMENTS

I would like to thank everyone involved in this pocket series thus far, which began with the idea for my first miniature book titled *Pocket Anatomy & Protocols for Abdominal Ultrasound* published in 2020. Those who played a major role in this project are my Acquisitions Editor Nicole Dernoski, my Development Editor Eric McDermott, and my Editorial Coordinator Remington Fernando. I would also like to thank Matt Hauber, my newest Acquisition Editor. There are many unnamed, and to me even unknown, individuals at Wolters Kluwer whom I would like to thank because I know that ultimately this is a group project with many working parts.

I would also like to express gratitude to my coworkers and the administration at Johnston Community College who encourage me daily and provide an atmosphere for learning and the opportunity for me to contribute to my profession in this distinctive manner. These individuals include Dr. Marc David, Ann Jackson, Catherine Rominski, Brittany Barefoot, and Alison Arnn.

Finally, once again I feel obligated to acknowledge all of my past and current students for ensuring that I am provided a regular challenge to keep learning, not only for them, but for the benefit of their future patients.

CONTENTS

PREFACE vi •
ACKNOWLEDGMENTS x

Section 1: Gynecologic Sonography 1

1: Gynecologic Sonography Overview 1

2: Adult Female Pelvic Sonography 30

3: Pediatric Female Pelvic Sonography 76

4: Sonohysterography and Three-Dimensional Gynecologic Sonography 105

Section 2: Obstetric Sonography 123

5: Overview of Obstetric Sonography 123

6: Standard First-Trimester Sonography 158

7: Detailed First-Trimester Sonography 201

8: Standard Second- or Third-Trimester Sonography 245

9: Detailed Second- or Third-Trimester Sonography and Multiple Gestations 292

10: Chromosomal Abnormalities and Neural Tube Defects 320

INDEX 345

Gynecologic Sonography — SECTION 1

CHAPTER 1

Gynecologic Sonography Overview

INTRODUCTION

This concise chapter will provide information about many indications and recommendations offered by the American Institute of Ultrasound in Medicine (AIUM) and other institutions for the practice of sonography in gynecology. General sonographic terminology, patient positioning, and common sonographic artifacts are also offered. This chapter furthermore provides a summary of relevant laboratory findings and a reminder to practice proper body mechanics while performing sonographic examinations to reduce the likelihood of work-related musculoskeletal disorders (WRMSDs).

AIUM INDICATIONS FOR A SONOGRAM OF THE FEMALE PELVIS[1]

- Evaluation of pelvic pain
- Evaluation of pelvic masses
- Evaluation of endocrine abnormalities, including polycystic ovaries
- Evaluation of dysmenorrhea (painful menses)
- Evaluation of amenorrhea (absent menses)
- Evaluation of abnormal uterine bleeding
- Evaluation of postmenopausal bleeding
- Evaluation of delayed menses
- Follow-up of a previously detected abnormality
- Evaluation, monitoring, and/or treatment of patients with infertility

- Evaluation when there is a limited clinical examination of the pelvis
- Evaluation for signs or symptoms of pelvic infection
- Further characterization of a pelvic abnormality noted on another imaging study
- Evaluation of congenital uterine, gonadal, and lower genital tract anomalies
- Evaluation of excessive bleeding, pain, or signs of infection after pelvic surgery, delivery, or abortion
- Localization of an intrauterine device
- Screening for malignancy in high-risk patients
- Evaluation of incontinence or pelvic organ prolapse
- Guidance for interventional or surgical procedures
- Preoperative and postoperative evaluation of pelvic structures

AIUM INDICATIONS FOR SONOHYSTEROGRAPHY

- Abnormal uterine bleeding
- Uterine cavity evaluation, especially relating to uterine leiomyomas, polyps, synechiae, and cesarean scar niches
- Abnormalities detected on transvaginal sonography, including focal or diffuse endometrial or intracavitary abnormalities
- Congenital or acquired abnormalities of the uterus in relation to infertility
- Recurrent pregnancy loss
- Suboptimal visualization of the endometrium by standard sonography

AIUM INDICATIONS FOR HYSTEROSALPINGO-CONTRAST-SONOGRAPHY[2]

- Determination of tubal patency in patients desiring fertility
- Confirmation of tubal occlusion after sterilization procedures

EQUIPMENT SELECTION AND QUALITY CONTROL[3]

- Ultrasound equipment inherently varies between institutions.
- It is the institution's obligation to offer high-quality sonographic examinations, and therefore these providers should supply equipment that balances cost-effectiveness with state-of-the-art features for their sonographic practitioners to utilize.

Chapter 1. Gynecologic Sonography

- Both the institution and sonographic practitioner should be aware of the potential musculoskeletal injuries that can result from improper equipment or poor scanning practices and should work together to prevent such injuries.
- Ultrasound machines should be capable of standard real-time imaging, have color, power, and spectral Doppler applications, and be capable of providing adequate diagnostic imaging for interpretation by a qualified interpreting physician. These physicians should meet the specified AIUM Training Guidelines in accordance with AIUM accreditation policies.
- Sonographers performing these examinations should be appropriately credentialed in the specialty area in accordance with AIUM accreditation policies.
- Physicians not performing the examination should provide supervision as defined by Federal regulations.
- The female pelvis should be examined sonographically with a real-time scanner, preferably a 3.5-MHz or higher curved linear array or sector transducer for transabdominal imaging (Fig. 1-1).
    - This technique provides a global view of the complete pelvic region.
    - Unfortunately, one limitation of the transabdominal technique is that the resolution of the pelvic structures is dependent upon several factors, including the patient's body habitus and the position of the uterus. For example, if the patient is obese, resolution will be inhibited. Furthermore, if the uterus is retroverted, the endometrium may not be clearly visualized.
- An endocavity transducer, also known in gynecologic imaging as either a transvaginal or an endovaginal transducer, should also be used if acceptable and tolerated by the patient. The transvaginal transducer is typically 5 MHz or higher (Fig. 1-2).
    - The transvaginal technique provides a more detailed view of the uterus, ovaries, and other pelvic structures.
    - Two limitations of the transvaginal technique are that it does indeed require patient acceptance and tolerance, and the imaging penetration of the transducer is not as far reaching as the transabdominal technique. Consequently, some anatomy or possibly even pathology may lie out of the transvaginal field of view and thus may be overlooked.

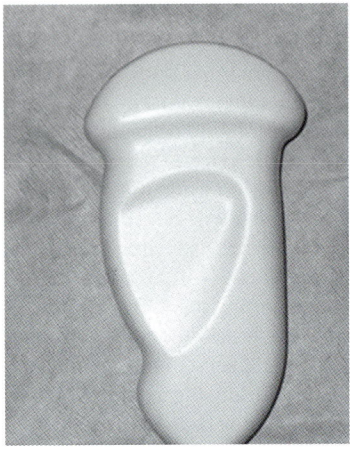

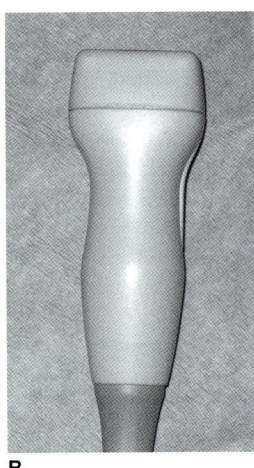

Figure 1-1. Transducers for transabdominal pelvic imaging. A. Curvilinear array. Curvilinear, curved, or convex array transducer. Used commonly in transabdominal examinations. B. Linear phased array transducer may be used occasionally. (**A.** Reprinted with permission from Rose JS, Bair AE. Fundamentals of ultrasound. In: Cosby KS, Kendall JL, eds. *Practical Guide to Emergency Ultrasound*. Lippincott Williams & Wilkins; 2006. Figure 3.16. **B.** Reprinted with permission from Rose JS, Bair AE. Fundamentals of ultrasound. In: Cosby KS, Kendall JL, eds. *Practical Guide to Emergency Ultrasound*. Lippincott Williams & Wilkins; 2006. Figure 3.18.)

Chapter 1. Gynecologic Sonography

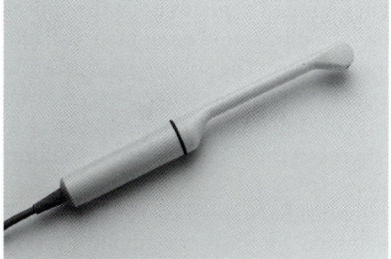

Figure 1-2. Transducer for transvaginal pelvic imaging. Transvaginal transducers provide outstanding resolution of pelvic structures.
(Reprinted with permission from Prince BD. Instrumentation. In: Sanders RC, Hall-Terracciano B, eds. *Clinical Sonography: A Practical Guide*. 5th ed. Wolters Kluwer; 2016. Figure 2-14.)

- Occasionally, a linear transducer may be employed as an adjunct to the examination if superficial structures need to be evaluated **(Fig. 1-3)**. For example, if an ovary or mass is located superficially, a linear transducer may aid the sonographer by providing higher resolution. A linear transducer is also utilized for appendix imaging.

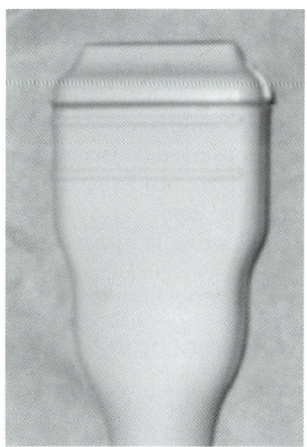

Figure 1-3. Linear sequenced array transducer. High-frequency linear transducers may be utilized for the analysis of superficial structures. (Reprinted with permission from Rose JS, Bair AE. Fundamentals of ultrasound. In: Cosby KS, Kendall JL, eds. *Practical Guide to Emergency Ultrasound*. Lippincott Williams & Wilkins; 2006. Figure 3.17.)

- The frequency applied depends upon the approach as well. Furthermore, the ultrasound equipment will offer differing operating frequencies. The sonographic practitioner should ensure that the highest frequency is always utilized, appreciating the fact that as operating frequency increases, there is a trade-off between resolution and beam penetration.
- Other supplies needed to perform sonohysterography or hysterosalpingo-contrast-sonography will vary per institution. These supplies may include syringes, sterile saline, catheters, and other aseptic technique equipment (see Chapter 4).
- Quality control and improvement, safety, infection control, patient education, and equipment performance monitoring should be developed and implemented in accordance with the AIUM Standards and Guidelines for the Accreditation of Ultrasound Practices found at https://www.aium.org/accreditation/accreditation.aspx

THE ALARA PRINCIPLE[1]

- Sonography should be practiced by trained health care practitioners.
- The ALARA (as low as reasonably achievable) principle pertains to patient exposure to diagnostic ultrasound.
- According to the AIUM, "the potential benefits and risks of each examination should be considered. The ALARA principle should be observed for factors that affect the acoustical output and by considering the transducer dwell time and total scanning time."
- Sonographers should strive for image optimization, while simultaneously minimizing patient exposure to ultrasound energy to practice the ALARA principle.

SONOGRAPHIC TERMINOLOGY[4]

- Common sonographic descriptive terms are provided in **Table 1-1**.

COMMON ARTIFACTS[5]

- Ultrasound artifacts abound during sonographic imaging, with several of them providing useful diagnostic information **(Table 1-2)**.

Chapter 1. Gynecologic Sonography

Table 1-1. SONOGRAPHIC TERMS AND A BRIEF EXPLANATION

SONOGRAPHIC DESCRIPTIVE TERM	EXPLANATION
Anechoic	Without echoes
Complex	Consists of both solid and cystic components
Echogenic	Structure that produces echoes; often used as a comparative term
Heterogeneous	Of differing composition
Homogeneous	Of uniform composition
Hyperechoic	Having many echoes
Hypoechoic	Having few echoes
Isoechoic	Having the same echogenicity

Table 1-2. COMMON ULTRASOUND ARTIFACTS

ARTIFACT	DESCRIPTION
Acoustic shadowing (Fig. 1-4)	Occurs when sound encounters a high attenuator
Comet tail (Fig. 1-5)	Type of reverberation artifact caused by small structures
Dirty shadowing (Fig. 1-6)	Acoustic shadowing containing reverberation artifact
Edge shadowing (Fig. 1-7)	Sound refracts off round surfaces
Mirror Image (Fig. 1-8)	Occurs when sound reflects off a strong reflector and creates a duplicate of the anatomy which can be seen deeper in the image
Posterior acoustic enhancement (through transmission) (Fig. 1-9)	Occurs when sound encounters a weak attenuator
Refraction (Fig. 1-10)	Causes the duplication of anatomy because of the sound beam striking an interface at nonperpendicular angles
Reverberation (Fig. 1-11)	Bouncing of the sound beam between two or more interfaces
Ring-down (Fig. 1-12)	Caused by sound interacting with small air bubbles causing the bubbles to vibrate

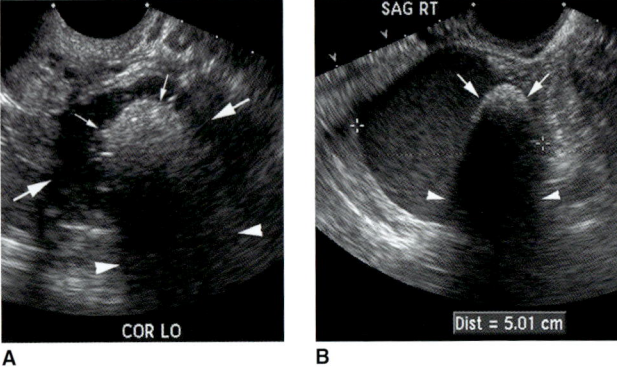

Figure 1-4. Acoustic shadowing from an ovarian mass. **A.** A coronal image of the female pelvis demonstrating a complex ovarian mass (*between large arrows*) with several typical sonographic characteristics of a dermoid, including the dermoid plug (*small arrows*) and the posterior acoustic shadowing (*between arrowheads*) from the plug. **B.** In the sagittal plane, this dermoid [*between calipers* (+)] contains a solid (*arrows*) shadowing (*between arrowheads*) structure within its borders. (Reprinted with permission from Doubilet PM, Benson CB. *Atlas of Ultrasound in Obstetrics and Gynecology: A Multimedia Reference.* 2nd ed. Wolters Kluwer Health/Lippincott Williams & Wilkins; 2012. Figure 28.3.4.)

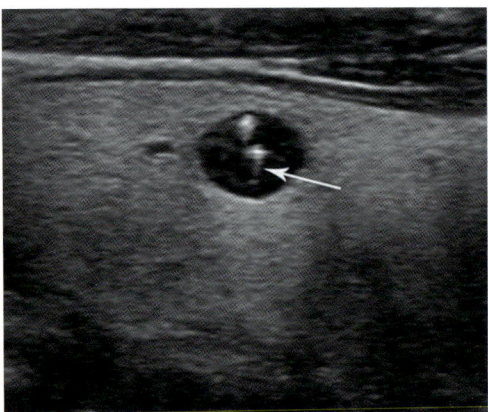

Figure 1-5. Comet tail artifact. A sharply defined cystic lesion shows floating punctate echogenic foci with a tapering tail (*arrow*). (Reprinted with permission from Brant WE. Chest, thyroid, parathyroid, and neonatal brain ultrasound. In: Brant WE, Helms CA, eds. *Fundamentals of Diagnostic Radiology.* 4th ed. Wolters Kluwer Health/Lippincott Williams & Wilkins; 2012. Figure 38.13.)

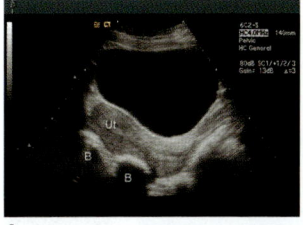 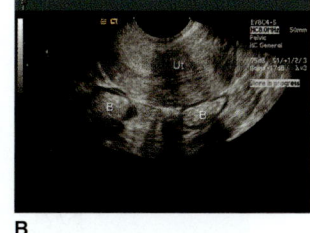

Figure 1-6. Dirty shadowing. A. Dirty shadowing (*B*) is noted emanating from an air-filled bowel posterior to the uterus (*Ut*). **B.** Endovaginal image of the uterus (*Ut*) reveals bowel (*B*) posterior to the uterus. (**A, B.** Reprinted with permission from Kupesic S. Normal anatomy of the female pelvis. In: Stephenson SR, Dmitrieva J, eds. *Diagnostic Medical Sonography: Obstetrics & Gynecology*. 4th ed. Wolters Kluwer; 2018. Figure 5-54.)

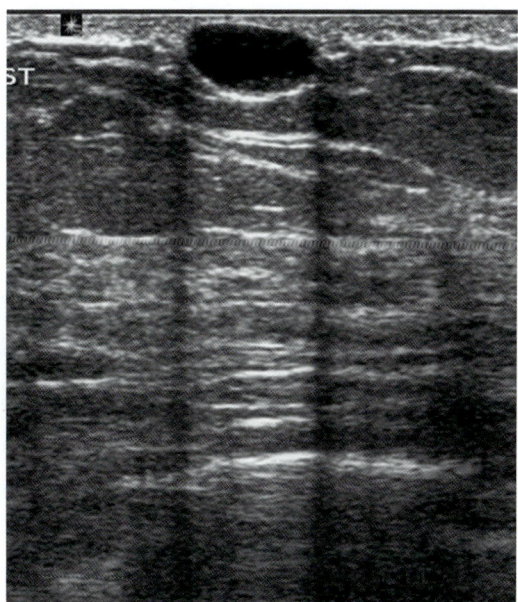

Figure 1-7. Edge shadowing. Distinct shadowing can be seen emanating from the edge of this cyst. (Reprinted with permission from Fornage BD. Breast sonography. In: Shirkhoda A, ed. *Variants and Pitfalls in Body Imaging: Thoracic, Abdominal and Women's Imaging*. 2nd ed. Wolters Kluwer Health/Lippincott Williams & Wilkins; 2011. Figure 30.3A.)

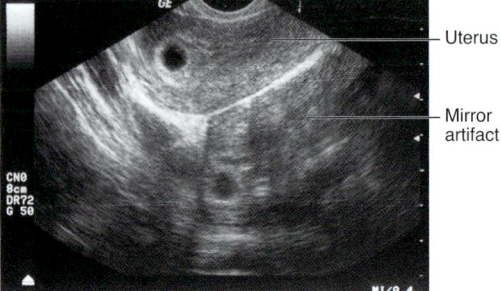

Figure 1-8. Mirror image artifact. Identical images of the uterus are seen side by side. (Reprinted with permission from Kelley K, Rose JS, Bair AE. Fundamentals of ultrasound. In: Cosby KS, Kendall JL, eds. *Practical Guide to Emergency Ultrasound*. 2nd ed. Wolters Kluwer Health/Lippincott Williams & Wilkins; 2014. Figure 2.11B.)

BASICS OF DOPPLER SONOGRAPHY IN GYNECOLOGIC SONOGRAPHY

- Color Doppler (CD) and power Doppler (PD)
  - CD allocates varying colors to traveling red blood cells depending upon their velocity and the direction of their flow relative to the location of the transducer.
  - For most ultrasound machines, flow toward the transducer is allocated red, while flow away from the transducer is allocated blue **(Fig. 1-13)**.

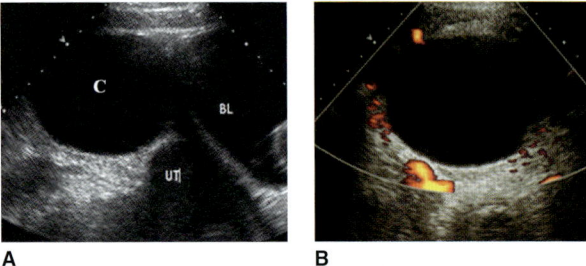

Figure 1-9. Ovarian cyst with acoustic enhancement. A. Acoustic enhancement is noted posterior to this ovarian cyst (*C*). The cyst is located adjacent to the uterus (*UT*) and urinary bladder (*BL*). B. This Doppler color image demonstrates no flow within the ovarian cyst. (Reprinted with permission from Siegel MJ. Female pelvis. In: Siegel MJ, ed. *Pediatric Sonography*. 4th ed. Wolters Kluwer Health/Lippincott Williams & Wilkins; 2011. Figure 13.11.)

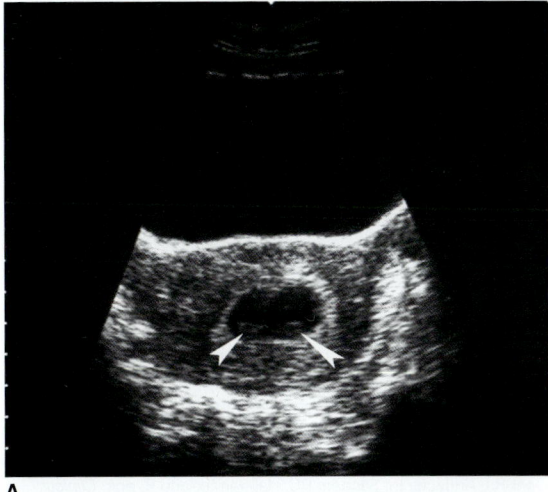

A

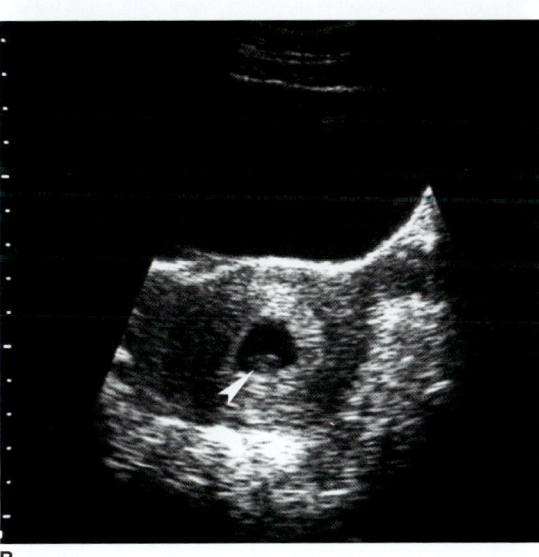

B

Figure 1-10. Refraction. Refraction caused the appearance of two gestational sacs (image A *arrowheads*) when there was truly only one (image B *arrowhead*). (Reprinted with permission from Middleton WD, Robinson KA, Siegel MJ. Ultrasound artifacts. In: Siegel MJ, ed. *Pediatric Sonography*. 5th ed. Wolters Kluwer; 2019. Figure 2-9.)

Chapter 1. Gynecologic Sonography

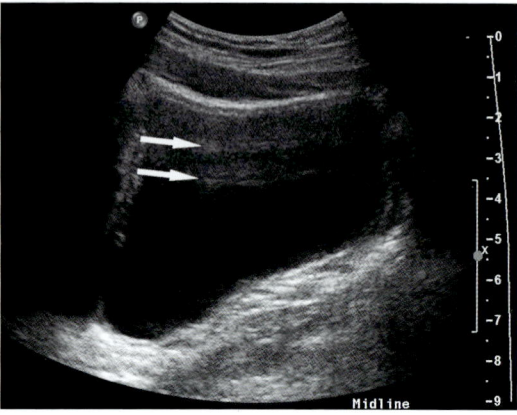

Figure 1-11. Reverberation. Reverberation artifact echoes (*arrows*) are seen in the near field of a urine-filled bladder. (Reprinted with permission from Gent RJ. Artifacts. In: Sanders RC, Hall-Terracciano B, eds. *Clinical Sonography: A Practical Guide*. 5th ed. Wolters Kluwer; 2016. Figure 6-9A.)

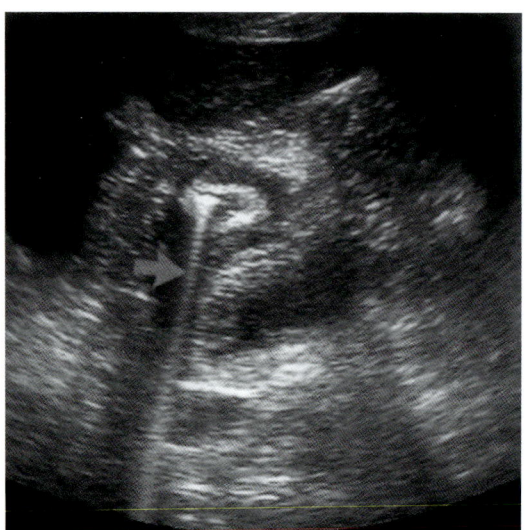

Figure 1-12. Ring-down artifact. Longitudinal image of the gastric antrum shows a prominent ring-down artifact (*arrow*) caused by air bubbles in the stomach. (Reprinted with permission from Brant WE. *The Core Curriculum: Ultrasound*. Lippincott Williams & Wilkins; 2001:16.)

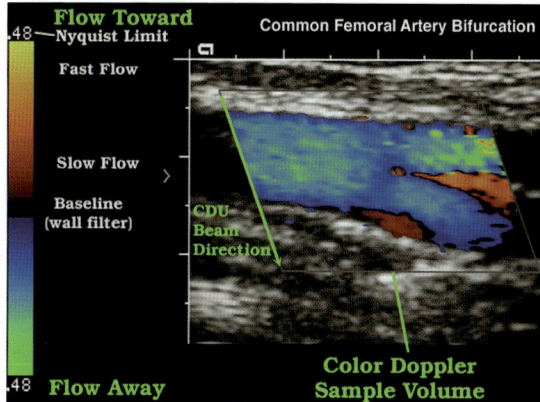

Figure 1-13. Color Doppler. The color map on the left side of the image shows *red* as the dominant color above the baseline indicating flow relatively toward the color Doppler beam direction. *Blue* is the dominant color below the color map baseline indicating flow relatively away from the color Doppler beam direction. (Reprinted with permission from Brant WE, Dougherty RS. Vascular ultrasound. In: Brant WE, Helms CA, eds. *Fundamentals of Diagnostic Radiology*. 4th ed. Wolters Kluwer Health/Lippincott Williams & Wilkins; 2012. Figure 39.8.)

- Faster speeds are typically depicted with brighter colors and slower velocities are depicted with darker colors.
- Optimal CD imaging is obtained with oblique imaging, whereas a perpendicular orientation will be void of color.
- In gynecologic imaging, CD is often utilized to depict flow direction within the ovaries, uterus, or specific vascular structures and to identify flow within identified masses.
  - Increased CD within an organ or structure may be indicative of hyperemia and can be a sign of inflammation or infection.
- PD is a more sensitive form of CD **(Fig. 1-14)**.
  - PD exploits the amplitude of the Doppler signal.
  - PD does not typically provide flow direction.
  - PD is useful in providing evidence of flow in smaller or low-flow vessels.
  - Excessive motion can inhibit the effective use of PD.
- Pulsed-wave Doppler (PW)
  - PW is utilized to analyze the flow characteristics of a specific vascular structure, with the ability to evaluate a specific area within that vessel.

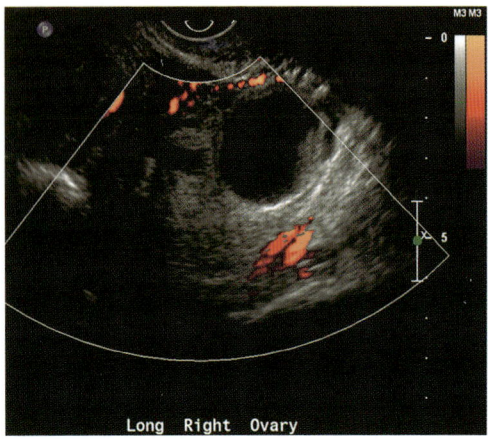

Figure 1-14. Power Doppler. This transvaginal image reveals torsion of the ovary. The ovary is enlarged, with no demonstrable internal flow with power Doppler. (Reprinted with permission from Dunnick NR, Newhouse JH, Cohan RH, Maturen KE. *Genitourinary Radiology.* 6th ed. Wolters Kluwer; 2018. Figure 17.11B.)

- The pulsed sound is placed in a sample gate, thus providing Doppler information from the specific selected point within the chosen vessel.
- PW can provide flow direction.
  - Flow toward the transducer is often displayed above the baseline, while flow away from the transducer is often displayed below the baseline.
  - Be sure to evaluate whether the flow direction control has been inverted before making a final diagnostic conclusion.
- Flow patterns can also be analyzed with PW. Veins typically have a continuous rhythmic flow pattern in diastole and systole.
  - Arteries typically have an alternating pitch, with high peaks in systole and lower crest in systole.
- Resistive patterns can be depicted with PW.
  - Vessels can be described as having a low-resistive pattern or high-resistive pattern.
    - Low-resistive patterns are depicted by a biphasic systolic peak and a comparatively high level of diastolic flow **(Fig. 1-15)**.
    - High-resistive patterns are depicted by a high systolic peak and low level of diastolic flow **(Fig. 1-16)**.

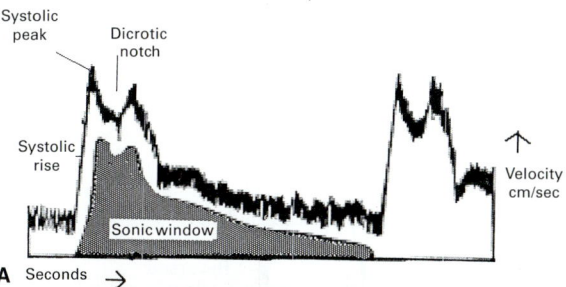

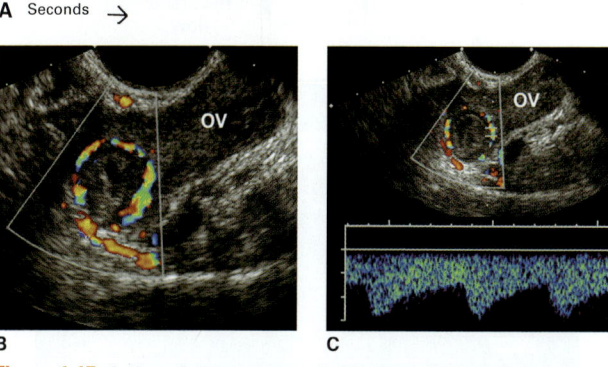

Figure 1-15. Low-resistance pattern. A. Diagram of an arterial spectral waveform in a low-resistance bed. Note the relatively high diastolic flow. (**A.** Reprinted with permission from Prince BD. Doppler and color flow principles. In: Sanders RC, Hall-Terracciano B, eds. *Clinical Sonography: A Practical Guide*. 5th ed. Wolters Kluwer; 2016. Figure 4-6A.) **B. Color Doppler** demonstrates that a mass found in the adnexa has prominent blood flow surrounding it. **C.** Spectral Doppler waveform from the periphery of the mass demonstrates a large amount of blood flow at end-diastole, indicative of low-impedance flow. (**B, C.** Reprinted with permission from Doubilet PM, Benson CB, Benacerraf BR. *Atlas of Ultrasound in Obstetrics and Gynecology: A Multimedia Reference*. 3rd ed. Wolters Kluwer; 2019. Figure 32.1.6B-C.)

- Continuous-wave Doppler (CW)
  - CW is a technique in which the sound beam is continuously emitted from one crystal, while a second crystal receives the returning signal.
  - CW is not typically utilized in gynecologic imaging.
- M-mode
  - M-mode, or motion mode, is often utilized in obstetric sonography.
  - This is further discussed in Section 2, Chapter 5.

High-Resistance Wave

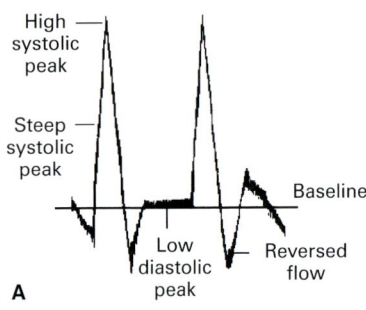

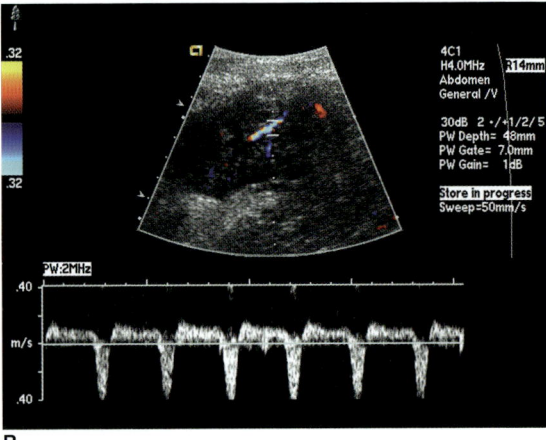

Figure 1-16. High-resistance pattern. A. Diagram of an arterial spectral waveform in a high-resistance bed. B. Pulsed Doppler sonogram from a high-resistance system. (Reprinted with permission from Prince BD. Doppler and color flow principles. In: Sanders RC, Hall-Terracciano B, eds. *Clinical Sonography: A Practical Guide*. 5th ed. Wolters Kluwer; 2016. Figure 4-5.)

GENERAL CLINICAL HISTORY QUERIES

- Why did your doctor order this sonogram? *Though some patients may be poor historians, others may be capable of providing much beneficial information regarding their current and past clinical records.*
- When was the first day of your last menstrual cycle? *Some patients may be able to provide you with an exact date when*

menses began. *This is relevant for correlating the sonographic appearance of the endometrium and the cycle. This date should be entered into the obstetric calculation package within the machine or placed on an image containing the thickness measurement of the endometrium.*
- Is there any chance that you could be pregnant? *This is an obvious question for females of reproductive years. If the answer is yes, then subsequent obstetric questions should ensue (e.g., Have you performed a pregnancy test?), and the examination would be altered to meet obstetric sonogram standards.*
- Have you had any changes in your menstrual cycle? *This question is relevant if the patient complains of irregular menstrual cycles. More details should be gathered regarding specific changes (e.g., increase or decrease in flow, spotting, duration, etc.).*
- Gravidity and parity score? *Gravidity refers to the number of pregnancies, parity refers to the number of pregnancies that led to birth at or beyond 20 weeks gestational age or of an infant weighing more than 500 grams. Some institutions may utilize TPAL (term, preterm, abortions, and living children) to further describe the patient's history.*
- Where is your pain **(Fig. 1-17)**? *If possible, have the patient point—with one finger—to the most painful region. Assessing the area of the complaint prior to a pelvic sonogram can provide some beneficial insight. Figure 1-17 provides a clinical algorithm for pelvic pain and Table 1-3 provides some key laboratory findings for various pelvic pathologies.*
- How long have you had pain? *This question can reveal a chronic or acute situation (see Fig. 1-17).*
- Are you experiencing any nausea or vomiting? *Nausea and vomiting can be associated with many pelvic issues. If possible, inquire as to how often vomiting has occurred.*
- Are you diabetic or have high blood pressure? *Diabetics and those suffering from high blood pressure can have related clinical issues. This is a good question to assess the overall health of the patient as well.*
- Have you had any recent weight loss? *Unexplained weight loss is a worrisome clinical history complaint that has been associated with some forms of cancer. Inquire as to how much weight loss has occurred and over how much time as well.*
- Have you had any relevant surgeries (specific to the pelvis)? *This question is helpful in providing a surgical history to*

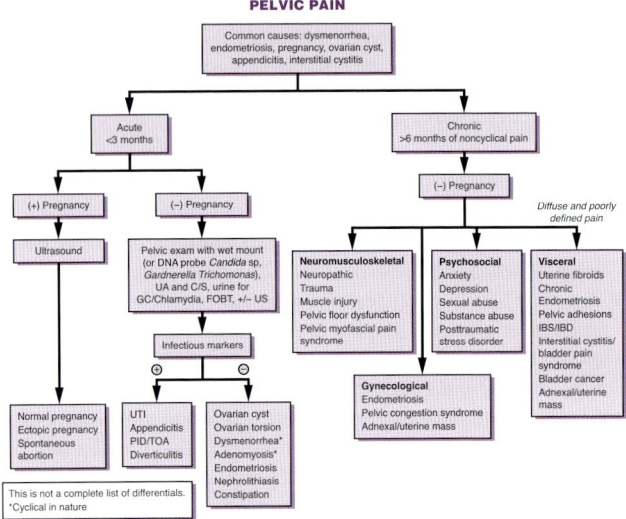

Figure 1-17. Pelvic pain and possible causes. (Reprinted with permission from Domino FJ, Baldor RA, Barry KA, Golding J, Stephens MB, eds. *The 5-Minute Clinical Consult 2024*. 32nd ed. Wolters Kluwer; 2024:A-90.)

establish the possible absence of organs, such as an ovary, or the existence of known deviations from normal anatomy that may be encountered during the sonographic examination.

- Have you had any other imaging tests for this issue? *Knowing if the patient has had another imaging exam can be helpful in determining if pathology has already been identified. Computed tomography (CT), magnetic resonance imaging (MRI), and radiography reports should be examined prior to the sonogram.*
- Are you taking any medications (especially birth control pills or fertility drugs)? *Some medications may alter the menstrual cycle and thus the sonographic appearance of the endometrium. Fertility medications can also affect the menstrual cycle and the sonographic appearance of the endometrium and ovaries.*
- Are you using any form of birth control (for females in childbearing years)? *As stated earlier, birth control pills and other forms of birth control may affect the sonographic*

appearance of pelvic organs. It would also be helpful to know if the patient has an intrauterine device.
- History of increased abdominal girth, bloating, pelvic fullness? *This could be associated with ascites or possibly ovarian carcinoma.*
- History of constipation or bowel issues? *Large pelvic masses can lead to lower gastrointestinal symptoms.*

SUMMARY OF RELEVANT LABORATORY VALUES AND KEY PELVIC FINDINGS (TABLE 1-3)[5]

Table 1-3 POSSIBLE LABORATORY FINDINGS AND POTENTIAL PELVIC PATHOLOGIES

LABORATORY FINDING	KEY PELVIC FINDINGS
+ Bacteriuria	Urinary tract infection
↑ Lactate dehydrogenase	Possible ovarian mass
↑ Blood urea nitrogen (BUN)	Possible kidney stone(s) causing pelvic pain and urinary tract obstruction
↑ CA-125	Endometriosis, leiomyoma, ovarian carcinoma, pelvic inflammatory disease
↑ Creatinine (Cr or Creat)	Possible kidney stone(s) causing pelvic pain and/or urinary tract obstruction
↑ Human chorionic gonadotropin (β-hCG)	Pregnancy or possible ovarian tumor (nongravid)
↑ Partial thromboplastin time (PTT)	Anticoagulation therapy and hereditary coagulopathies
+ Proteinuria	Urinary tract infection, dehydration, inflammation
+ Sexually Transmitted Diseases (e.g., chlamydia, gonorrhea, syphilis)	Pelvic inflammatory disease or other pelvic infection
↑ White blood cell (WBC)	Endometritis, pelvic inflammatory disease, or other infections
↓ Hematocrit	Hemorrhage resulting from ruptured ectopic pregnancy or other internal causes of bleeding

PATIENT PREPARATION AND POSITIONING FOR GYNECOLOGIC SONOGRAPHY[5]

- Patient preparation
  - Transabdominal female pelvic sonogram
    - The patient's urinary bladder can be distended to displace the bowel and to provide an acoustic window for the visualization of the uterus, ovaries, and adnexa **(Fig. 1-18)**.
    - Some authors suggest having the patient drink at least enough liquid (possibly 32 ounces of water) to distend the urinary bladder to the point where the entire fundus of the uterus is clearly visualized.
    - The bladder should not be excessively distended. If this occurs, the patient may need to partially empty her bladder.
    - If the patient has a Foley catheter in place, and the transabdominal technique has been deemed crucial for diagnostic purposes, filling the urinary bladder with sterile saline may be employed **(Fig. 1-19)**. This is termed bladder retrofilling. *Note retrofilling the urinary bladder in this manner is a protocol decision that is initiated by the institution, ordering physician, or interpreting*

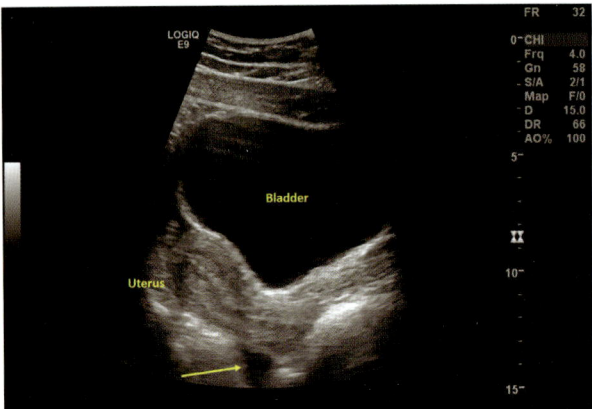

Figure 1-18. Proper filling of the urinary bladder for a transabdominal sonogram. Note that in this sagittal midline image of the female pelvis, the fundal portion of the uterus can be clearly identified because the urinary bladder (*Bladder*) is distended sufficiently. A small amount of posterior cul-de-sac fluid is noted as well (*arrow*). (Reprinted with permission from Huntley BJF, Goldshmid FM, Huntley ESL. Does the patient have a viable intrauterine pregnancy? In: Bornemann PH, ed. *Ultrasound for Primary Care*. Wolters Kluwer; 2021. Figure 27-5.)

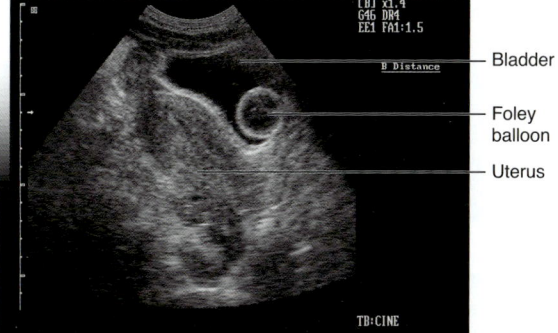

Figure 1-19. Retro-filling the urinary bladder for sonography. The bladder displaces bowel gas and provides an acoustic window to the uterus. **(Note the inflated Foley balloon in the bladder.)** (Reprinted with permission from Kelley K, Rose JS, Bair AE. Fundamentals of ultrasound. In: Cosby KS, Kendall JL, eds. *Practical Guide to Emergency Ultrasound.* 2nd ed. Wolters Kluwer Health/Lippincott Williams & Wilkins; 2014. Figure 2.6.)

> *physician. The practitioner should be instructed on how to perform this task correctly and safely.*

- If an abnormality of the urinary bladder is noted, it should be reported as well.
  - Transvaginal female pelvic examination
    - The patient's urinary bladder should be empty for a transvaginal pelvic sonogram.
    - Preparation of transvaginal transducers between patients requires routine mandatory high-level disinfection and the use of a high-quality single-use transducer cover during each examination. (See **Infection Control and Equipment Maintenance**.)
    - The patient, the sonographer, or the physician may introduce the vaginal transducer, preferably under real-time monitoring.
    - Consideration of having a chaperone present should be in accordance with local policy.
    - Transvaginal sonograms should be performed prior to contrast imaging examinations of the female pelvis if possible.
- Patient positioning
  - Transabdominal female pelvic sonogram
    - The patient is typically placed in the supine position **(Fig. 1-20)**.

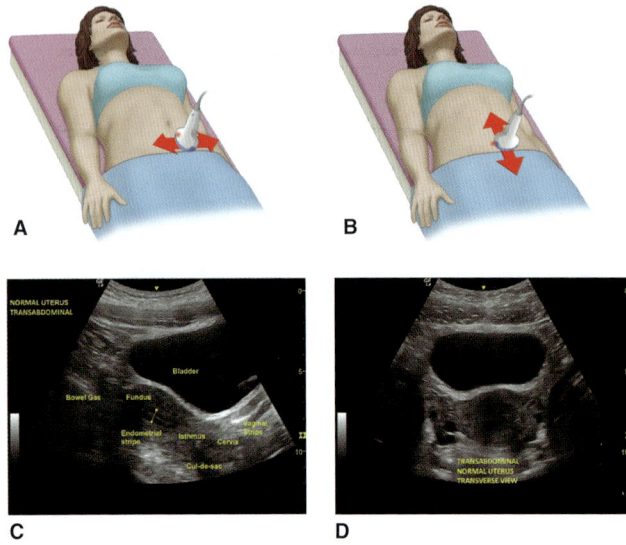

Figure 1-20. Transabdominal pelvic scanning. Note the locations of the index or notch in the drawings (*red dot*). A. Patient positioning with probe in the sagittal plane. Fan through the structures in the direction of the red arrows using the urinary bladder as an acoustic window (side-to-side). B. Patient positioning with probe in the transverse plane. Fan through the structures in the direction of the red arrows (superior to inferior). C. Transabdominal sagittal view of normal anteverted uterus. D. Transverse view of normal uterus (right ovary also visible). (Reprinted with permission from Shen-Wagner J, Castleberry L. Is the patient's intrauterine device in the proper location? In: Bornemann PH, ed. *Ultrasound for Primary Care.* Wolters Kluwer; 2021. Figure 34-2.)

- Transvaginal female pelvic sonogram
  - The patient is typically placed in the lithotomy position **(Fig. 1-21)**.
  - The patient may be placed in the supine position with the hips elevated up from the examining table with the use of a positioning pad as well.

LABELING OF SONOGRAPHIC EXAMINATIONS[6]

- All sonographic images, whether still-frame images or video, should include the following:
  - Patient's name and other identifying information (e.g., medical record number)

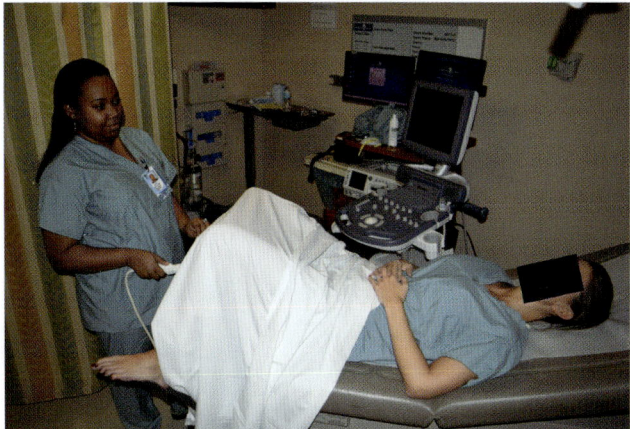

Figure 1-21. Lithotomy positioning for a transvaginal sonogram.
(Reprinted with permission from Castleberry L, Shen-Wagner J. How thick is the patient's endometrial stripe? In: Bornemann PH, ed. *Ultrasound for Primary Care*. Wolters Kluwer; 2021. Figure 31-1.)

- Facility's identification information
- Date and time of the examination
- Output display standard (thermal index and mechanical index)
- Label the anatomic location and which side of the body, when appropriate
- Image orientation when appropriate

INFECTION CONTROL AND EQUIPMENT MAINTENANCE[7]

- Infection control
  - Institutional guidelines should be in place for transducer disinfection to reduce the risk of iatrogenic and nosocomial infections.
  - Always follow your facility's established protocol for infection control.
  - The following is a summation of the AIUM's *Guidelines for Cleaning and Preparing External- and Internal-Use Ultrasound Transducers and Equipment Between Patients as well as Safe Handling and Use of Ultrasound Coupling Gel.*
    - Transabdominal transducers
      - Preparation of transabdominal transducers between patients requires a low-level disinfection process **(Fig. 1-22)**.

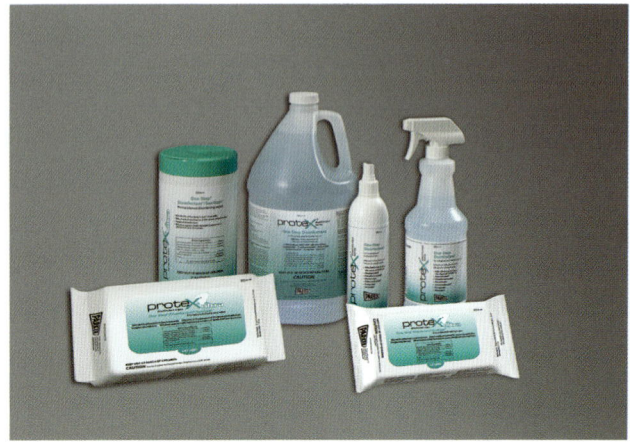

Figure 1-22. Transducer disinfectant. Commercially available disinfectant sprays and wipes for ultrasound transducers. Check with the manufacturer's cleaning recommendations before using. (Courtesy of Parker Laboratories, Inc., Fairfield, NJ.)

- Nonsterile gel is used.
- No transducer cover is required unless there is contaminated intact skin or nonintact skin, in which case both a cover and sterile gel are recommended.
- Transvaginal transducers
  - Barriers (probe covers) used for transvaginal transducers must be single-use transducer covers that meet the sterility requirements of the procedure **(Fig. 1-23)**.
  - Use sterile or bacteriostatic gel.
  - Consult the manufacturer's instructions for disinfecting devices.
  - After the procedure, perform high-level disinfection. Commercially available wall or table-top disinfectant units are available for transvaginal transducers **(Fig. 1-24)**.
  - A complete list of Food and Drug Administration (FDA)-cleared liquid sterilants and high-level disinfectants is available online.
  - Rinse to remove disinfectant.
- Equipment maintenance
  - Regular interval inspection of equipment and transducers (connector, cable, housing, acoustic lens) is recommended

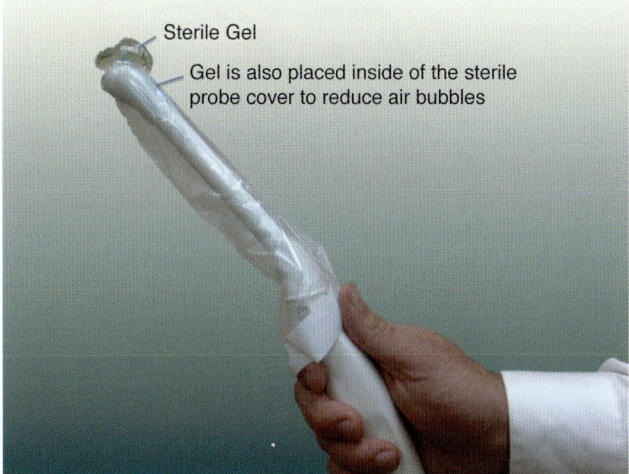

Figure 1-23. Example of how to drape a transvaginal transducer. Note, ultrasound gel is placed inside of the probe cover to prevent air artifact, while sterile gel is placed on the outside of the cover. (Reprinted with permission from Shen-Wagner J, Castleberry L. Is the patient's intrauterine device in the proper location? In: Bornemann PH, ed. *Ultrasound for Primary Care*. Wolters Kluwer; 2021. Figure 34-4.)

to ensure performance. Imaging with a tissue mimicking phantom may help reveal imaging degradation.
- A record of quality assurance activities must be maintained and kept current. The ultrasound equipment must meet all state and federal guidelines and testing must be maintained in good operating condition and undergo routine quality assurance at least once a year or more frequently if problems arise.
- Always report machine or equipment malfunction to facility management and remove such equipment from use.

ERGONOMICS[8]
- Ergonomics is the scientific study of creating tools and equipment that help humans adapt to the work environment.
- The use of proper ergonomics includes having the proper room design and adjustable equipment to reduce the risk of WRMSDs.

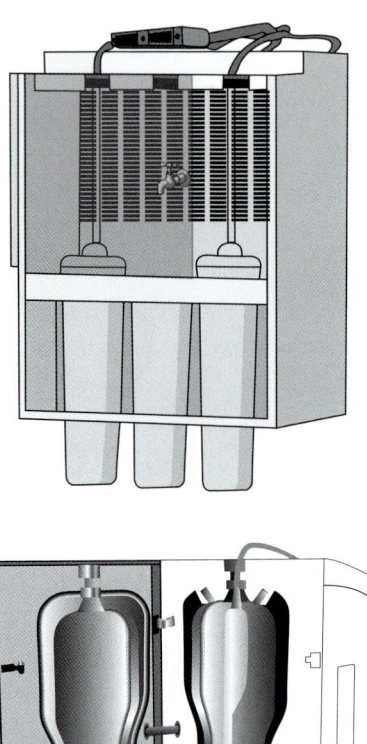

Figure 1-24. There are several means whereby a transducer can be disinfected, including a wall unit (upper image) and tabletop unit (lower image). (Reprinted with permission from Penny SM. *Introduction to Sonography and Patient Care*. 2nd ed. Wolters Kluwer; 2021. Figure 12-25.)

- Though a thorough explanation of WRMSDs is beyond the scope of this text, below are a few of the best practices:
  - Take regular breaks or microbreaks between examinations. Relax muscles throughout the day.
  - Minimize sustained bending, twisting, reaching, lifting, pressure, and awkward positions.

- Focus on using all your fingers and the palm, a light grip, and apply minimal or no pressure to the probe.
- Keep your wrist in a neutral position with limited flexion and extension.
- Use correct body mechanics when moving the patient.
- Place the patient as close to you as possible to reduce shoulder abduction (<30°). The scanning arm should be in a relaxed position, close to the body with minimal flexion.
- Use a cable brace or support device for the cable.
- The neck should be straight, and neck extension should be avoided.
- Use a height-adjustable scanning table and ultrasound equipment.
- Stand to scan occasionally and vary scanning positions to work different muscles.

FEMALE PELVIC COMPUTED TOMOGRAPHY AND MAGNETIC RESONANCE IMAGING ANATOMY

- Sonographers should have some appreciation of normal female pelvic anatomy noted in a CT and MRI study (**Figs. 1-25** and **1-26**).

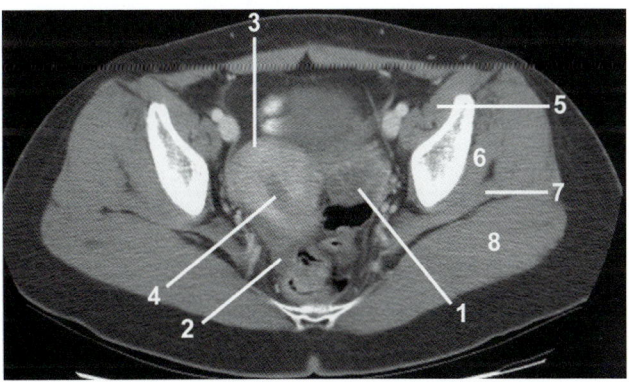

Figure 1-25. CT anatomy of the female pelvis. Transverse axial labels include the following: (*1*) Left ovary; (*2*) Physiologic fluid in pelvis (normal in menstruating-age female); (*3*) Uterine fundus; (*4*) Endometrial cavity; (*5*) Iliopsoas muscle; (*6*) Gluteus minimus muscle; (*7*) Gluteus medius muscle; (*8*) Gluteus maximus muscle. (Reprinted with permission from Rubin P, Hansen JT. *TNM Staging Atlas with Oncoanatomy*. 2nd ed. Wolters Kluwer Health/Lippincott Williams & Wilkins; 2012. Figure 42.7A.)

28   **Chapter 1.** Gynecologic Sonography Overview

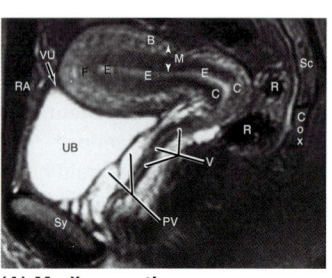
(A) Median section

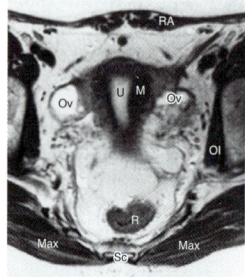
(B) Transverse section

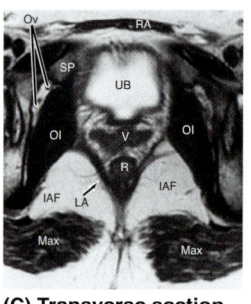
(C) Transverse section

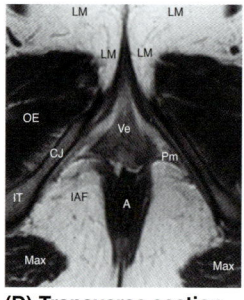
(D) Transverse section

Key					
A	Anus	LM	Labium majus	RA	Rectus abdominis
B	Body of uterus	M	Myometrium	Sc	Sacrum
C	Cervix of uterus	Max	Gluteus maximus	SP	Superior ramus of pubis
CJ	Ischiopubic ramus	OE	Obturator externus	Sy	Pubic symphysis
Cox	Coccyx	OI	Obturator internus	U	Uterus
E	Endometrium	Ov	Ovary	UB	Urinary bladder
F	Fundus of uterus	Pm	Perineal membrane	V	Vagina
IAF	Ischio-anal fossa	PV	Perivaginal veins	Ve	Vestibule of vagina
IT	Ischial tuberosity	R	Rectum	VU	Vesico-uterine pouch
LA	Levator ani				

Figure 1-26. MRI images of the female pelvis and perineum. (Reprinted with permission from Moore KL, Agur AMR, Dalley AF II. *Essential Clinical Anatomy*. 5th ed. Wolters Kluwer Health; 2015. Figure 3.57.)

REFERENCES

1. *AIUM Practice Parameter for the Performance of an Ultrasound Examination of the Female Pelvis*. Accessed on September 14, 2023. https://www.aium.org/docs/default-source/resources/guidelines/femalepelvis.pdf?sfvrsn=f5d0c38b_1
2. *AIUM Practice Parameters for the Performance of Sonohysterography and Hysterosalpingo-Contrast Sonography*. Accessed on September 14, 2023. https://www.aium.org/docs/default-source/resources/guidelines/sonohysterography.pdf?sfvrsn=423541da_1

3. Norton ME, Scoutt LM, Feldstein VA. *Callen's Ultrasonography in Obstetrics and Gynecology.* 6th ed. Elsevier; 2017:805-882.
4. Penny SM. *Introduction to Sonography and Patient Care.* 2nd ed. Wolters Kluwer; 2016:58.
5. Penny SM. *Examination Review for Ultrasound: Abdomen & Obstetrics and Gynecology.* 3rd ed. Wolters Kluwer; 2022:11-19 & Section II.
6. *AIUM Practice Parameter for Documentation of an Ultrasound Examination.* Accessed on September 24, 2023. https://www.aium.org/docs/default-source/resources/guidelines/aium-practice-parameter-for-documentation-of-an-ultrasound-examination.pdf?sfvrsn=3135b66_3
7. *Guidelines for Cleaning and Preparing External- and Internal- Use Ultrasound Transducers and Equipment Between Patients as Well as Safe Handling and Use of Ultrasound Coupling Gel.* Accessed September 24, 2023. https://www.aium.org/resources/official-statements/view/guidelines-for-cleaning-and-preparing-external-and-internal-use-ultrasound-transducers-and-equipment-between-patients-as-well-as-safe-handling-and-use-of-ultrasound-coupling-gel
8. AIUM practice principles for work-related musculoskeletal disorder. *J Ultrasound Med.* 2023;42:1139-1157.

CHAPTER 2

Adult Female Pelvic Sonography

INTRODUCTION

This chapter will provide both schematics of the female pelvis and sonographic anatomy. Furthermore, the physiology of the menstrual cycle and the correlation between the normal ovarian and endometrial cycles will be offered. Image orientation, scanning tips, some vital pathology, and an overview of the Ovarian-Adnexal Reporting & Data System (O-RADS), created by the American College of Radiology, will be included. Lastly, several images of pelvic pathology demonstrated on computed tomography and magnetic resonance imaging are located at the chapter's conclusion.

AIUM RECOMMENDATIONS FOR SONOGRAPHY OF THE FEMALE PELVIS[1]

- Uterus
  - The uterine size, shape, and orientation should be analyzed.
  - Measurement of the uterus should be acquired.
    - The uterine length is evaluated and obtained with electronic calipers in the sagittal view.
      - The length is measured as a straight line from the fundus to the external os of the cervix by using the outer-to-outer technique.
      - The length can also be measured by measuring from the fundal region along the endometrial lining and endocervical canal using the outer-to-outer technique.
    - The uterine (depth) anteroposterior (AP) dimension is also evaluated and obtained with electronic calipers in the sagittal view.

- The calipers are placed from the anterior to posterior walls perpendicular to the length measurement.
- The maximum width is measured in the transverse or coronal view.
- A uterine volume can be obtained in the same manner as above, though the cervix should not be included.
- The various layers of the uterine wall should be evaluated, which include the myometrium and endometrium.
  - Abnormalities of the myometrium and endometrium should be documented, including contour changes, echogenicity, masses, and cysts.
    - Myometrium
      - The anterior myometrial thickness of the uterus should also be compared for symmetry with the posterior wall.
        - The myometrium should be homogeneous, though small blood vessels may be noted. Color Doppler can be used to prove the presence of vessels.
        - There should be no heterogeneous regions, cystic spaces, or hypoechoic masses.
        - Posterior wall thickening may be indicative of adenomyosis.
    - Endometrium
      - The endometrium should be analyzed for focal abnormalities, echogenicity, and the presence of fluid or masses within the uterine cavity.
      - The endometrial thickness should be obtained.
        - The thickest part of the endometrium should be measured perpendicular to its longitudinal plane in the AP diameter from the anterior echogenic border to the posterior echogenic border (basal layer to basal layer), using the outer-to-outer technique.
        - The adjacent hypoechoic myometrium is not included in this measurement.
        - Intracavitary fluid is not included in this measurement. If fluid is present, the two separate endometrial layers should be measured and added together to obtain the true thickness of the endometrium.

- If the patient has an intrauterine device (IUD), the location of the device should be documented.
- The cervix and vagina should be examined.
  - Abnormalities of the cervix and vagina, including masses or cysts, should be evaluated, and measured.
- The size, which is obtained in two dimensions, and the location of clinically relevant lesions should be documented. Not all uterine fibroids necessarily must be measured. Some patients may have numerous fibroids. It may be useful to measure the largest two or three fibroids and use a numbering system.
- Three-dimensional sonography can be helpful in many circumstances including:
  - Further analysis of the relationship of masses within the endometrial cavity
  - Uterine congenital anomalies
  - Thickened and/or heterogeneous endometrium
  - Location and orientation of an IUD
  - Integrity of the pelvic floor
- Sonohysterography can be used to evaluate a poorly identified endometrium, assess for intracavitary abnormalities, and be used for patients complaining of abnormal uterine bleeding or who have an abnormally thickened endometrium.
- Ovaries and adnexa
  - Ovaries
    - Ovarian size may be determined by measuring the ovary in three dimensions (longitudinal, transverse, and AP diameter).
    - The views should be in two orthogonal planes (e.g., sagittal and transverse).
    - Any ovarian abnormalities should be documented.
    - If the ovaries are not visualized, this should be noted. They may not be seen when small or if they lack follicular development, as is often the case with pubertal or postmenopausal patients.
  - Adnexa
    - The adnexa, right and left, should be evaluated for abnormalities or evidence of dilated fallopian tubes.
    - The abnormality should be noted in relation to the ovaries and uterus and the sonographic appearance and size should be provided.

- The description of the abnormality should be documented as to whether it is cystic, solid, simple, or complex.
  - Further analysis for septations (thick or thin), solid components, mural nodules, excrescences, papillary components, and vascular characteristics should be offered.
- Doppler sonography, including the use of spectral, color, and/or power, may be useful to evaluate the vascular characteristics of pelvic masses.
- Cul-de-sac
  - An evaluation of fluid within the posterior cul-de-sac should be performed.
  - The cul-de-sac should also be evaluated for masses and those masses should be measured and their position, shape, and sonographic characteristics should be obtained.
  - The location of the mass should be compared to the relationship between the ovaries and uterus.
  - Slight probe pressure may be used to distinguish the relationship between pelvic structures and adjacent masses.
- The ALARA (As Low as Reasonably Achievable) principle should be observed for factors that affect the acoustic output by considering the transducer dwell time and total scanning time.

ESSENTIAL ANATOMY AND PHYSIOLOGY OF THE FEMALE PELVIS[2]

- Uterus
  - Uterine anatomy **(Fig. 2-1)**
    - The uterus is bordered anteriorly by the urinary bladder and posteriorly by the rectum. It is typically located in the midline, though much variance in position exists.
      - The patient's functional midline may vary dramatically from her actual midline.
      - The transducer may need to be manipulated from the midsagittal plane to achieve an image of the functional midline.
    - The typical uterus is shaped like an upside-down pear.
    - The uterus is a hollow organ, whose cavity is contiguous with the fallopian tubes superiorly and bilaterally, and the cervix and vagina inferiorly.

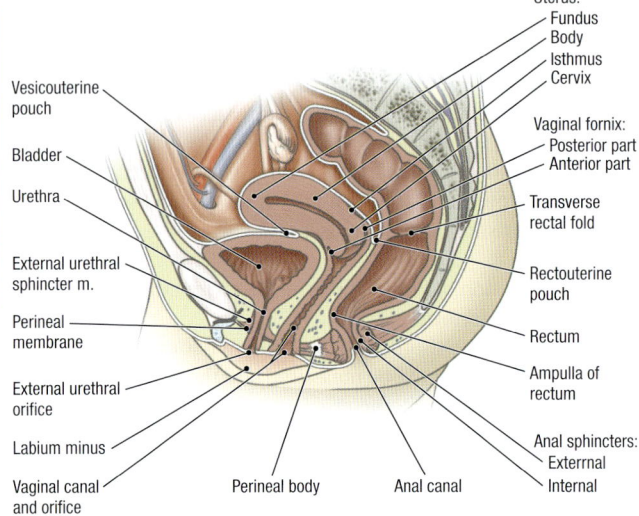

Figure 2-1. Female pelvic anatomy median section. (Reprinted with permission from Tank PW, Grant JCB. *Grant's Dissector*. 15th ed. Wolters Kluwer Health/Lippincott Williams & Wilkins; 2013. Figure 5.34.)

- The uterus can be divided into the following sections:
  - Cervix
    - The rigid part of the uterus that is located superior to the vagina.
    - It consists of an internal os, cervical canal, and external os.
  - Uterine isthmus
    - Referred to as the lower uterine segment during pregnancy.
    - It is located between the body and cervix.
  - Uterine body
    - The body is the largest section of the uterus.
    - It is also referred to as the corpus.
  - Uterine fundus
    - The fundus is the superior and widest section of the uterus.
    - It is the location of the bilateral attachment regions for the fallopian tubes, referred to as cornua (uterine horns).

Chapter 2. Adult Female Pelvic Sonography   35

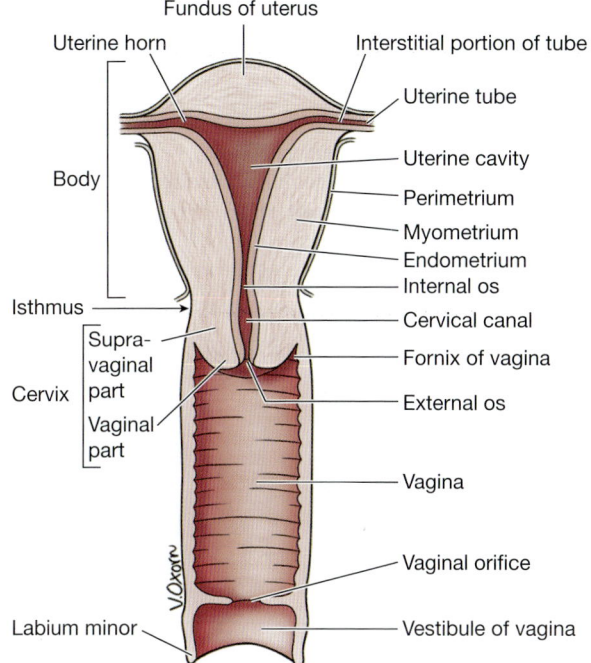

Figure 2-2. Coronal uterine anatomy (Reprinted with permission from Moore KL, Agur AMR. *Essential Clinical Anatomy.* 2nd ed. Lippincott Williams & Wilkins; 2002. Figure 4.17A.)

- The layers of the uterus include **(Fig. 2-2)**:
  ○ Perimetrium
    – The perimetrium is the outer layer of the uterus.
    – It is also referred to as the serosal layer.
  ○ Myometrium
    – The myometrium is the muscular portion of the uterus.
    – It comprises the bulk of the uterine tissue.
  ○ Endometrium
    – The endometrium is the lining of the uterus that is located adjacent to the uterine cavity.
    – It consists of the outer paired basal layers and inner paired functional layers (see Overview of the Menstrual Cycle in this chapter).

- The functional layer varies in thickness throughout the menstrual cycle secondary to the stimulation of estrogen and progesterone that is produced by the ovaries.
- The basal layer only varies in thickness slightly throughout the menstrual cycle.
- Uterine variants and congenital anomalies
  - Variants in uterine position (Fig. 2-3)
    ○ Anteversion
      - Anteversion is considered the most common position of the uterus.

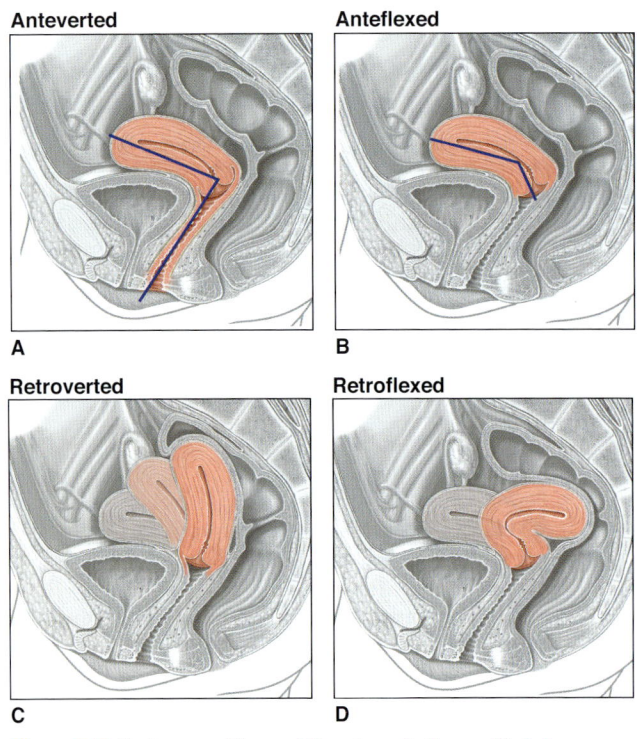

Figure 2-3. Various positions of the uterus in the sagittal plane. A. Anteverted. B. Anteflexed. C. Retroverted. D. Retroflexed. (Adapted with permission from Pansky B, Gest TR. *Lippincott's Concise Illustrated Anatomy: Thorax, Abdomen & Pelvis*. Vol 2. Wolters Kluwer Health/Lippincott Williams & Wilkins; 2013. Figure 3.8.)

- Anteflexion
  - Anteflexion is when the uterine body folds forward, possibly contacting the cervix.
- Retroversion
  - Retroversion is when the uterine body tilts posteriorly, without a bend where the cervix meets the body.
- Retroflexion
  - Retroflexion is when the uterine body tilts posteriorly and contacts the cervix.
- Levoverted
  - Levoversion is the left lateral position of uterus.
- Dextroverted
  - Dextroversion is the right lateral position of uterus.

- Congenital uterine anomalies **(Fig. 2-4)**
  - Bicornuate uterus
    - Bicornuate is the most common uterine variant.
    - It has two endometrial cavities with one cervix.
  - Septate uterus
    - Septate can be either complete or partial (subseptate).
    - There are two separate uterine cavities separated by a thin layer of tissue either partially (subseptate) or completely (complete).
  - Uterus didelphys
    - Didelphys is the complete duplication of the vagina, cervix, and uterus.
    - It can have one large vagina with no septum (uterus duplex bicornis) as well.
  - Unicornuate uterus
    - Unicornuate is when the uterus has only one horn.

- Vagina
  - Vaginal anatomy
    - The vagina is a hollow tube, that superiorly comes in contact and envelopes the cervix, while inferiorly it provides an opening.
    - The vagina consists of structures referred to as vaginal fornices (singular fornix).
      - There are four vaginal fornices—a right and left lateral fornix, anterior fornix, and posterior fornix.

- Ovaries
  - The ovaries are paired endocrine organs **(Fig. 2-5)**.

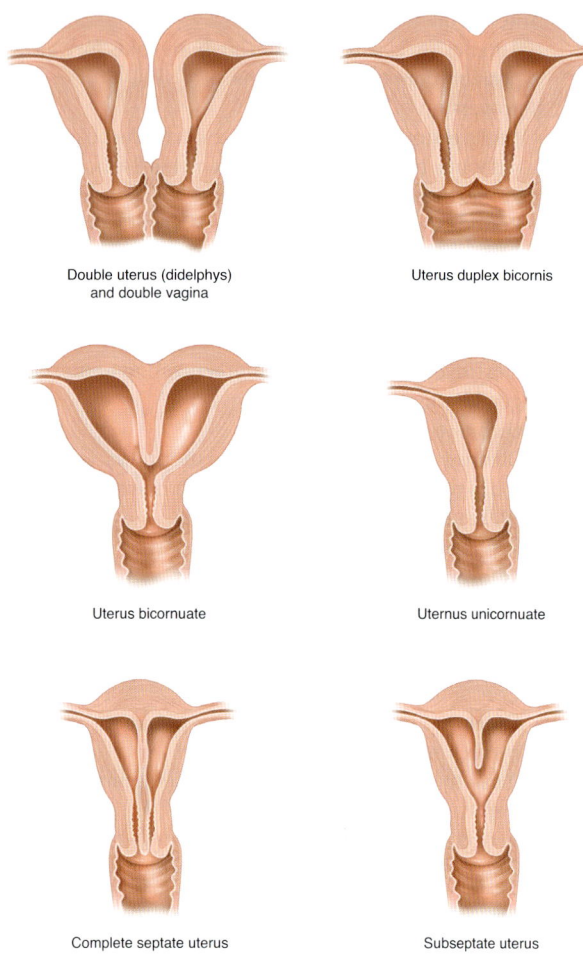

Figure 2-4. Congenital uterine anomalies. (Reprinted with permission from Hutson F. Congenital anomalies of the female genital system. In: Stephenson SR, Dmitrieva J, eds. *Diagnostic Medical Sonography: Obstetrics & Gynecology*. 4th ed. Wolters Kluwer; 2018. Figure 3-6.)

- The ovaries are typically located anywhere within the true pelvis **(Fig. 2-6)**.
  - The ovarian fossa is located posterior to the ureter and internal iliac artery and superior to the external iliac artery.

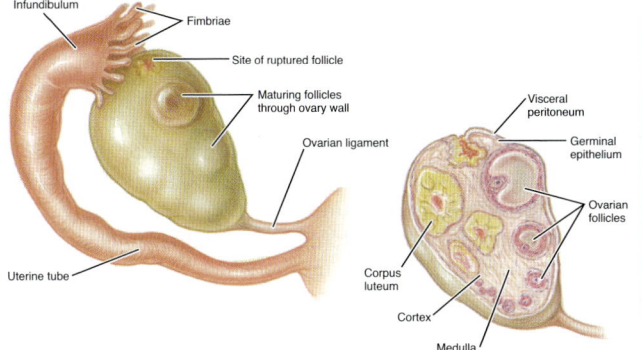

Figure 2-5. Ovarian anatomy. (Reprinted with permission from Wingerd BD. *The Human Body: Concepts of Anatomy and Physiology*. 3rd ed. Wolters Kluwer Health/Lippincott Williams & Wilkins; 2014. Figure 17.9.)

- They are not typically located between the bladder and the uterus, which is the area of the anterior cul-de-sac.
- The ovaries are mobile, and can thus be displaced by a distended bladder, bowel, pelvic mass, or pregnancy.
- The ovaries produce estrogen and progesterone throughout the menstrual cycle (see Overview of Menstrual Cycle in this chapter).

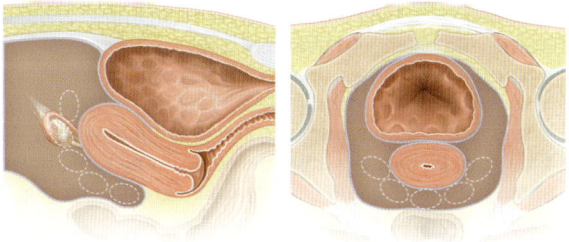

Figure 2-6. Positions of the ovary. A. Sagittal. B. Transverse. The ovary may be found in the posterior aspect of the pelvis or above the fundus of the uterus, in the adnexal spaces, or in the posterior cul-de-sac, but not in the anterior cul-de-sac or between the urinary bladder and the uterus. (Reprinted with permission from Kupesic SP, Turner T. Normal anatomy of the female pelvis. In: Stephenson SR, ed. *Diagnostic Medical Sonography: Obstetrics & Gynecology*. 3rd ed. Wolters Kluwer Health/Lippincott Williams & Wilkins; 2012. Figure 5-50A-B.)

- The ovary has an inner medulla and an outer cortex.
  - The medulla contains the ovarian vasculature and lymphatics.
  - The cortex contains the functional elements of the ovary and is the site of oogenesis.
- Throughout the first half of the menstrual cycle, the ovary contains follicles, which are small fluid-filled cysts that may contain a developing ovum.
- One follicle becomes a dominant or Graffian follicle.
- Around day 14, ovulation occurs, which is the rupture of the dominant follicle, releasing a small amount of fluid and an ovum into the peritoneum.
  - This fluid typically collects in the posterior cul-de-sac.
- The corpus luteum develops on the ovary after ovulation.
- Each ovary has a dual blood supply.
  - Blood is supplied to the ovary via the ovarian artery from the aorta and the ovarian artery branch of the uterine artery.
- Each ovary is drained by an ovarian vein.
  - The right ovarian vein drains into the inferior vena cava.
  - The left ovarian vein drains into the left renal vein.
- Other adnexal structures
  - The adnexa are the regions located posterior to the broad ligaments and adjacent to the uterus bilaterally.
  - The adnexa include the ovaries, fallopian tubes, ligaments, bowel, and pelvic vasculature.
    - The fallopian tubes, though not always imaged sonographically, consist of an interstitial (intramural) segment, isthmus, ampulla, and infundibulum (Fig. 2-7).
  - Fluid may be located within the adnexa, and when noted, should be imaged, and described sonographically (e.g., simple, complex, etc.).
  - When fluid is present in the pelvis, some ligaments, especially the broad ligaments, may be identified sonographically.

OVERVIEW OF THE MENSTRUAL CYCLE

- The first menstrual cycle is referred to as menarche, which typically starts by the age of 12, but can occur before or after this age.
- The menstrual cycle begins with the first day of menstrual bleeding.

Chapter 2. Adult Female Pelvic Sonography

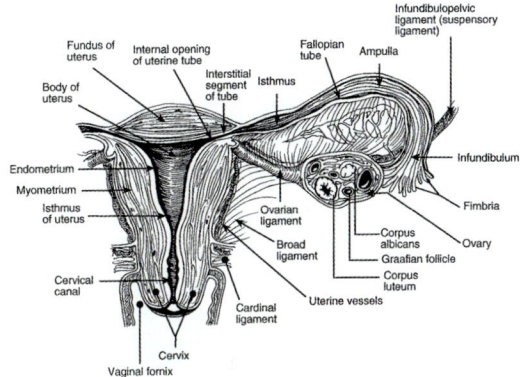

Figure 2-7. Fallopian tube anatomy. (Reprinted with permission from Beckmann CRB, Ling FW, Smith RP, Barzansky BM, Herbert WN, Laube DW. *Obstetrics and Gynecology*. 5th ed. Lippincott Williams & Wilkins; 2006. Figure 3.10.)

- The typical cycle lasts 28 days, with ovulation occurring around day 14.
- Common menstrual cycle terms can be found in **Table 2-1**.
- Phases of the menstrual cycle **(Fig. 2-8)**
  - Ovarian cycle
    - Follicular phase (days 1 to 14)

Table 2-1 COMMON MENSTRUAL CYCLE TERMS[2]

MENSTRUAL CYCLE TERM	DESCRIPTION
Amenorrhea	Absence of menstruation
Dysmenorrhea	Painful or difficult menstruation
Menarche	First menstrual cycle
Menorrhagia	Abnormally heavy and prolonged menstruation
Metrorrhagia	Intermenstrual bleeding
Menometrorrhagia	Excessive or prolonged bleeding at irregular intervals
Mittelschmerz	Pain at the time of ovulation

Adapted with permission from Penny SM. *Examination Review for Ultrasound: Abdomen & Obstetrics and Gynecology*. 3rd ed. Wolters Kluwer; 2023. Table 19-4.

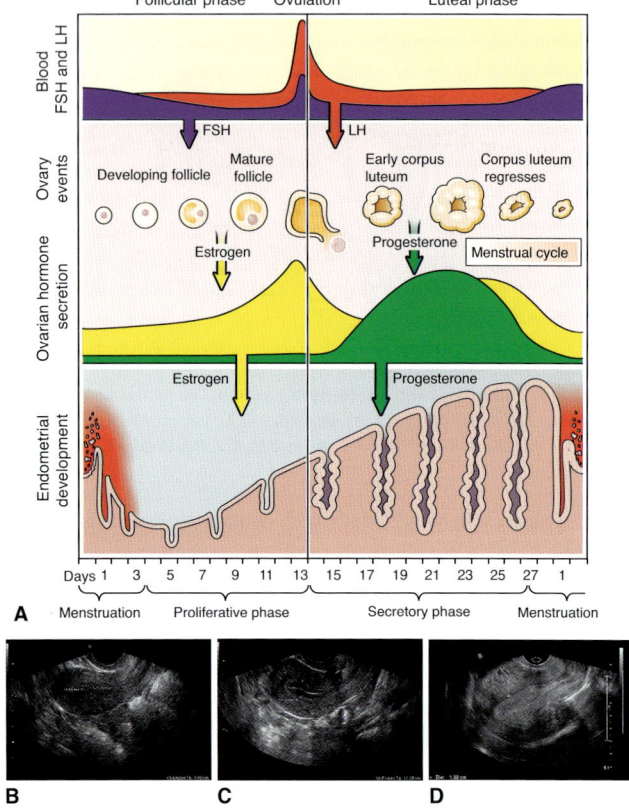

Figure 2-8. The menstrual cycle. A. Diagram of the menstrual cycle, including the hormonal changes and phases of the endometrium and ovary. B. The sonographic appearance of the thin endometrium during the early secretory phase. C. The sonographic appearance of the endometrium at midcycle is demonstrated in this image, which is also the time of ovulation. Note the three-line sign. D. The endometrium during the secretory phase appears thick and hyperechoic. (Reprinted with permission from Ismail C, Dayal M. Assisted reproductive technologies, contraception, and elective abortion. In: Stephenson SR, Dmitrieva J, eds. *Diagnostic Medical Sonography: Obstetrics & Gynecology*. 4th ed. Wolters Kluwer; 2018. Figure 12-3.)

- The ovary is stimulated by follicle-stimulating hormone produced by the anterior pituitary gland to develop follicles.
  - One follicle becomes the dominant or Graffian follicle, which contains the developing egg.
- Ovulation (day 14)
  - Ovulation is the rupture of the Graffian follicle and release of the ovum into the peritoneum.
  - Typically occurs on day 14 of the menstrual cycle.
  - A small amount of simple anechoic fluid may be noted within the posterior cul-de-sac.
- Luteal phase (days 15 to 28)
  - The ovary is stimulated by luteinizing hormone produced by the anterior pituitary gland to develop the corpus luteum.
  - The corpus luteum develops on the ovary and may be seen as a complex, solid, or cystic structure.
- Endometrial cycle
  - Proliferative phase (days 1 to 14)
    - The proliferative phase includes an early and late (periovulatory) phase.
      - The endometrium appears thin in the early proliferative phase.
      - The endometrium thickens gradually and near ovulation will have a hypoechoic functional layer and hyperechoic basal layer, which describes the three-line sign.
  - Secretory phase (days 15 to 28)
    - The secretory phase includes an early and a late phase.
    - Following ovulation, the endometrium becomes thick and echogenic.
- If pregnancy does not occur, the cycle begins anew on day 1 of menstruation.

SUGGESTED EQUIPMENT

- A sonographic examination of the female pelvis should be conducted using a sector, curved linear, and/or transvaginal transducer as needed.
- Typically, the transabdominal transducer has a range of between 3 and 5 MHz, while the transvaginal transducer ranges between 5 and 10 MHz, though this is dependent upon the available equipment.

- Though the transducer frequency and capabilities may vary, the transducer should be adjusted to operate at the highest frequency appropriate for the clinical circumstance, realizing that there is a trade-off between resolution and beam penetration.

CLINICAL INVESTIGATION FOR SONOGRAPHY OF THE FEMALE PELVIS

- Laboratory findings can be helpful in many situations (see Table 1-3 in Chapter 1).
- Evaluate prior imaging reports and images including CT, MRI, radiographs, and any other appropriate test.
- Clinical history questions can be found in Chapter 1.

NORMAL SONOGRAPHIC DESCRIPTION OF THE ADULT UTERUS AND OVARIES

- Uterus
  - The normal adult uterus is a pear-shaped organ, with smooth, uninterrupted borders.
  - The uterine myometrium should appear homogeneous, though often, especially in women who have had children, prominent arcuate vasculature may be readily recognizable along the periphery of the myometrium.
  - Nabothian cysts are commonly noted within the cervix.
  - The endometrium will have the greatest sonographic variance in appearance during reproductive years (see Endometrial Cycle for the sonographic findings during the menstrual cycle).
  - The endometrium should always be thin in postmenopausal patients, especially those who are not on hormone replacement therapy.
- Ovaries
  - Ovaries are oval or egg-shaped.
  - During reproductive years, the ovarian cortex and medulla should be homogeneous, only being interrupted with various anechoic follicles of different sizes.
    - It is normal to see a dominant, anechoic follicle around the middle of the cycle.
  - Postmenopausal ovaries are best seen with transvaginal imaging because after menopause they typically become atrophic, lack follicular development, and blend in with the surrounding anatomy.

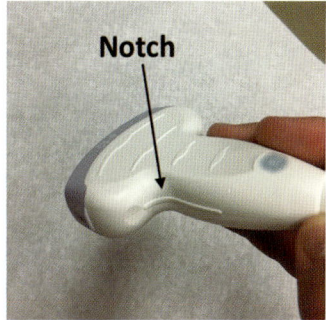

Figure 2-9. Example of a transducer used for transabdominal pelvic imaging. The notch or index on this transducer provides the reference point for image orientation. (Reprinted with permission from Huntley BJF, Goldshmid FM, Huntley ESL. Does the patient have a viable intrauterine pregnancy? In: Bornemann PH, ed. *Ultrasound for Primary Care*. Wolters Kluwer; 2021. Figure 27-4.)

IMAGE ORIENTATION

- Transabdominal imaging
  - Identify the notch or index on the transducer to orient the transducer appropriately (**Figs. 2-9** and **2-10**).
  - The patient's functional midline anatomy must be obtained (**Fig. 2-11**).
    - To obtain the functional midline, you should find the uterine cavity and orient the transducer so that the endometrium and cervical canal are aligned.
    - This may require that the transducer be placed in an oblique position, and thus away from the patient's true midline.
  - Transabdominal longitudinal imaging is performed while angling or sliding the transducer from side to side in sagittal.
    - Using a slight left lateral midline approach, angle through the bladder, to visualize the right adnexa, and vice versa to image the left adnexa.
  - Transabdominal transverse (short-axis or coronal) imaging is performed while angling or sliding the transducer from inferior to superior.
    - Angling superiorly will help you visualize the uterine fundus (normal anteverted uterine position).
    - Angling inferiorly will help you visualize the cervix and vagina (normal anteverted uterine position).

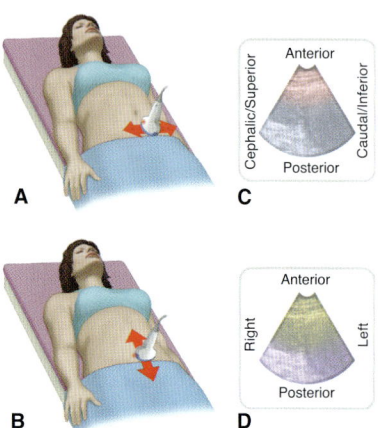

Figure 2-10. Transabdominal pelvic orientation. A. The patient in the supine position with the index (red dot on transducer) pointing toward the head, will produce a sagittal image. The transducer is angled from right to left (red arrows) B. Sagittal orientation. C. The patient in the supine position with the index (red dot on transducer) turned to the right side of the patient, creates a transverse image. The transducer is angled from superior to inferior (red arrows). D. Transverse orientation. (A and C reprinted with permission from Bornemann P. *Ultrasound for Primary Care*. Wolters Kluwer, 2020. Fig 34-2. B and D Reprinted with permission from Nolan T, Kawamura D. *Abdomen and Superficial Structures*, 5th Ed. Wolters Kluwer, 2022. Figure 2-5.)

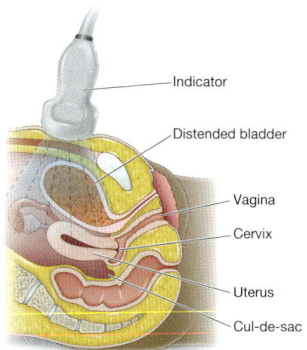

Figure 2-11. Normal sagittal transabdominal midline image. Drawing of the transabdominal midline orientation of the transducer in the sagittal plane to the uterus.

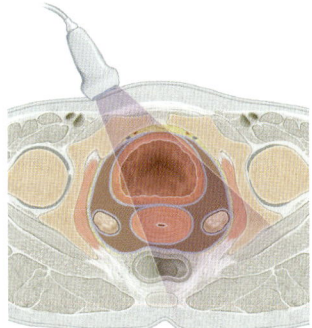

Figure 2-12. Transabdominal transverse visualization of the ovaries. Angle the transducer from the opposite side of the pelvis to image the contralateral ovary, using the distended urinary bladder as an acoustic window. (Reprinted with permission from Kupesic S. Normal anatomy of the female pelvis. In: Stephenson SR, Dmitrieva J, eds. *Diagnostic Medical Sonography: Obstetrics & Gynecology*. 4th ed. Wolters Kluwer; 2018. Figure 5-51.)

- Transabdominal transverse imaging of the ovary is best performed using the distended bladder as a sonographic window.
  - Angle the transducer from the opposite side of the pelvis to image the contralateral ovary **(Fig. 2-12)**.
- Transvaginal imaging
  - Identify the notch or index on the transducer to orient the transducer appropriately **(Fig. 2-13)**.

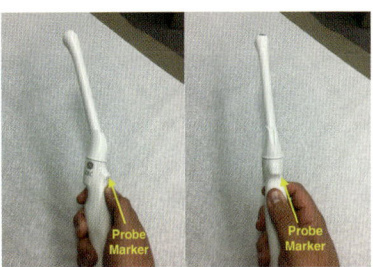

Figure 2-13. Example of a transvaginal transducer. A, B. The probe marker, notch, or index on this transducer is identified and utilized to obtain proper image orientation. (Reprinted with permission from Huntley BJF, Goldshmid FM, Huntley ESL. Does the patient have a viable intrauterine pregnancy? In: Bornemann PH, ed. *Ultrasound for Primary Care*. Wolters Kluwer; 2021. Figure 27-7.)

- Use your thumb as the notch while scanning to maintain proper orientation.
- The patient's functional midline anatomy must be obtained **(Fig. 2-14)**.
- Transvaginal longitudinal uterine images
  - To obtain the functional midline, you should find the uterine cavity and orient the transducer so that the endometrium and cervical canal are aligned.
  - This may take significant angling of the transducer away from the patient's midline.
  - Lateral imaging requires that the face of the transducer be pointed toward the patient's anatomic right for right lateral images, and pointed toward the patient's anatomic left for left lateral images.
- Transverse transvaginal uterine images
  - The transducer is rotated 90 degrees from longitudinal to obtain a transverse or coronal image of the uterus.
  - With a normal anteverted uterus, angling the face of the transducer anteriorly will assist in imaging the body and fundus of the uterus (superior uterine anatomy), whereas if the face of the transducer is angled posteriorly, the isthmus and cervix will be noted (inferior uterine anatomy) **(Fig. 2-15)**.
  - Lateral imaging requires that the face of the transducer be pointed toward the patient's anatomic right for right lateral images and pointed toward the patient's anatomic left for left lateral images.
  - For images of the adnexa, the transducer is pointed to the right side of the patient and angled anteriorly and posteriorly. The same images are obtained of the left adnexa.

SUGGESTED PROTOCOL FOR A SONOGRAM OF THE ADULT FEMALE PELVIS

- Note: The following protocol can be conducted utilizing the transabdominal or transvaginal approach but do keep in mind that the external architecture of the vagina will not be visualized well with transvaginal imaging.
  - If possible, the patient should have a distended urinary bladder and a survey conducted in both transverse and longitudinal of the pelvis utilizing the transabdominal

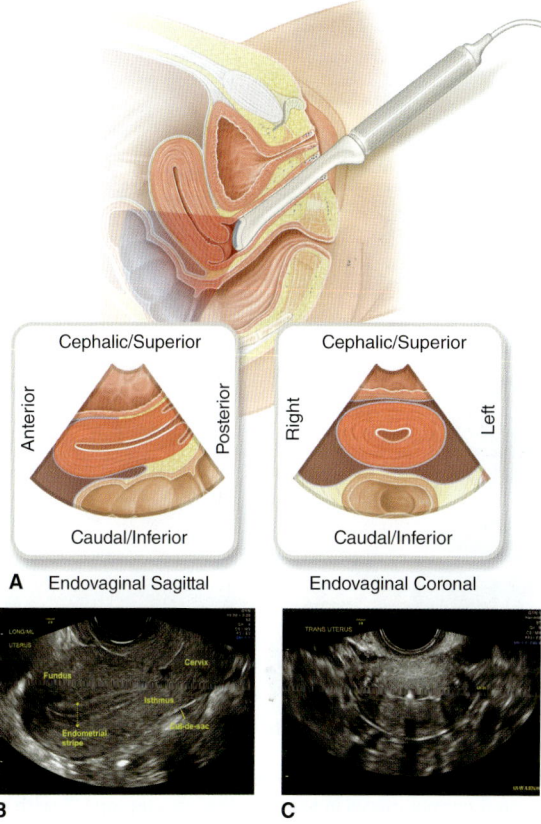

Figure 2-14. Transvaginal image orientation. A. Orientation for transvaginal scan planes. Transvaginal imaging includes sagittal and coronal scan planes. Coronal may also be labeled transverse. B. Longitudinal (Long) transvaginal representation of a normal midline of an anteverted uterus. C. Transverse uterus. This patient also has an intrauterine device within the endometrium. (A. Reprinted with permission from Hall-Terracciano B, Stephenson SR. *Workbook for Diagnostic Medical Sonography: A Guide to Clinical Practice, Obstetrics and Gynecology*. 5th ed. Wolters Kluwer; 2023:4. **B.** Reprinted with permission from Shen-Wagner J, Castleberry L. Is the patient's intrauterine device in the proper location? In: Bornemann PH, ed. *Ultrasound for Primary Care*. Wolters Kluwer; 2021. Figure 34-8. **C.** Reprinted with permission from Shen-Wagner J, Castleberry L. Is the patient's intrauterine device in the proper location? In: Bornemann PH, ed. *Ultrasound for Primary Care*. Wolters Kluwer; 2021. Figure 34-20.)

Chapter 2. Adult Female Pelvic Sonography

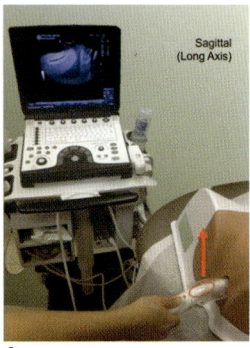

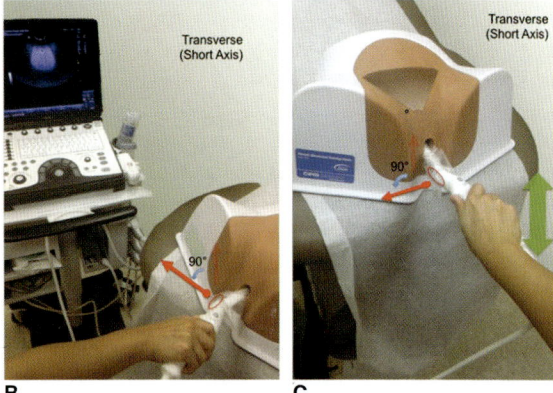

Figure 2-15. Sagittal and transverse transvaginal sonography. Simulated normal uterus in sagittal view on a laptop US with a pelvic simulator in the foreground. *Small arrow* points to probe marker. *Large arrow* indicates the orientation of the probe marker. A. Transvaginal sonography of simulated normal uterus in transverse view on a cart-based US with a pelvic simulator in the foreground. Red arrow indicates the orientation of the probe marker. B, C. With the probe marker pointed toward the patient's right, scan through the entire uterus by fanning the probe in the vertical plane. *Red arrow* indicates the orientation of the probe marker. *Green arrow* indicates the axis of fanning the probe during transverse scanning. (A. Reprinted with permission from Shen-Wagner J, Castleberry L. Is the patient's intrauterine device in the proper location? In: Bornemann PH, ed. *Ultrasound for Primary Care.* Wolters Kluwer; 2021. Figure 34-5. B. Reprinted with permission from Shen-Wagner J, Castleberry L. Is the patient's intrauterine device in the proper location? In: Bornemann PH, ed. *Ultrasound for Primary Care.* Wolters Kluwer; 2021. Figure 34-13.)

approach, given that this approach provides a global view of both the pelvis.
  - Transabdominal imaging also offers the opportunity to examine the urinary bladder and urethra.
- Empty the urinary bladder before the transvaginal examination commences and ensure that there are no foreign objects, such as tampons, within the vagina.
- Transvaginal transducer preparation and insertion
  - Explain the process of transvaginal transducer fully to the patient before commencing with the examination. Patient consent is mandatory.
  - A disinfected transvaginal transducer must be used.
  - Coupling gel is placed on the face of the transducer.
  - A sterile probe cover is placed on the transducer and air bubbles are expressed to reduce air artifacts during imaging.
  - Sterile gel is placed outside of the transducer cover over the transducer face.
  - The patient, who is in the lithotomy position or supine with legs flexed, can be asked to assist the sonographer in inserting the transducer. This may not be possible with all patients, however, when possible, this may reduce pain and anxiety.
  - The transducer should be inserted into the vagina without encountering the cervix.
  - A chaperone may be required by your institution for the transvaginal examination.
  - It is important to note that transvaginal imaging has a limited field of view.
- Longitudinal midline image of the uterus
  - This transducer should be manipulated in a direction that the patient's functional midline is obtained **(Fig. 2-16)**.
  - Measure the uterus in both longitudinal and AP dimensions **(Fig. 2-17)**.
    - Measure from the fundus to the cervix in the sagittal plane.
    - Measure the thickest AP dimension of the uterus.
    - The trace measurement tool may be utilized when there is atypical positioning of the uterus. Also, two measurements can be obtained and added together if the uterine–cervix angle produces a significant bend.
  - Examine the echogenicity and contour of the uterus for any signs of pathology.

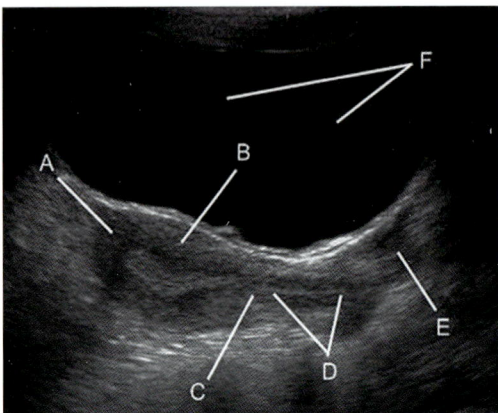

Figure 2-16. Longitudinal transabdominal image of the functional midline of the uterus. This image demonstrates the uterine fundus (*A*), uterine corpus (*B*), uterine isthmus (*C*), cervix (*D*), and vagina (*E*) posterior to the distended urinary bladder (*F*). (Reprinted with permission from Penny SM. *Examination Review for Ultrasound: Abdomen & Obstetrics and Gynecology*. 3rd ed. Wolters Kluwer; 2023. Figure 17-3.)

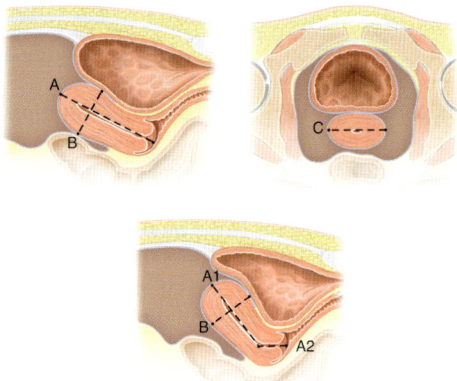

Figure 2-17. Measurement of the uterus. The uterus is measured in both longitudinal (top left) and transverse (top right). Occasionally, two measurements may be needed if there is a significant bend in the uterus (lower image). (Reprinted with permission from Kupesic S. Normal anatomy of the female pelvis. In: Stephenson SR, Dmitrieva J, eds. *Diagnostic Medical Sonography: Obstetrics & Gynecology*. 4th ed. Wolters Kluwer; 2018. Figure 5-41.)

Chapter 2. Adult Female Pelvic Sonography

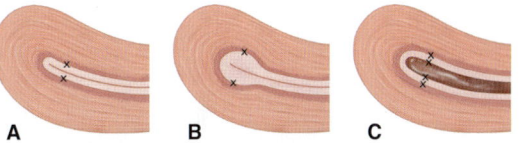

Figure 2-18. Measurement of the endometrium should be from basal layer to basal layer. It should not include the adjacent myometrium. **A.** Measurement of the thin uniform endometrium from a sagittal approach. **B.** Caliper placement for a focally thickened endometrium on a sagittal view. **C.** In the presence of intrauterine fluid, measure each endometrial layer on a sagittal plane. Those measurements can then be added together to obtain the true thickness of the endometrium.
(Reprinted with permission from Benzonelli-Blanchard S. The female cycle. In: Stephenson SR, Dmitrieva J, eds. *Diagnostic Medical Sonography: Obstetrics & Gynecology.* 4th ed. Wolters Kluwer; 2018. Figure 4-14.)

- Longitudinal image of the endometrium
  - Measure the thickness of the endometrium from basal layer to basal layer (outer-to-outer) **(Figs. 2-18** and **2-19)**.
  - Note the presence of any fluid or masses within the uterine cavity or any distortions.
  - If feasible, utilize the zoom function to better visualize the endometrium (see Fig. 2-14B).
  - Label the image with the first day of the patient's last menstrual cycle.
- Longitudinal image of the right lateral aspect of the uterus
  - Examine the echogenicity and contour of the uterus for any signs of pathology.
- Longitudinal image of the left lateral aspect of the uterus
  - Examine the echogenicity and contour of the uterus for any signs of pathology.
- Transverse uterus **(Fig. 2-20)**
  - Angle inferior to superior to image the following:
    - Vagina
    - Cervix
      - The cervix often produces edge shadowing during the transabdominal examination **(Fig. 2-21)**.
    - Corpus
      - Measure the maximum transverse dimension (see Fig. 2-20).
    - Fundus
  - Scan completely through the uterus superiorly to ensure that there is no pathology superior to the uterine fundus.

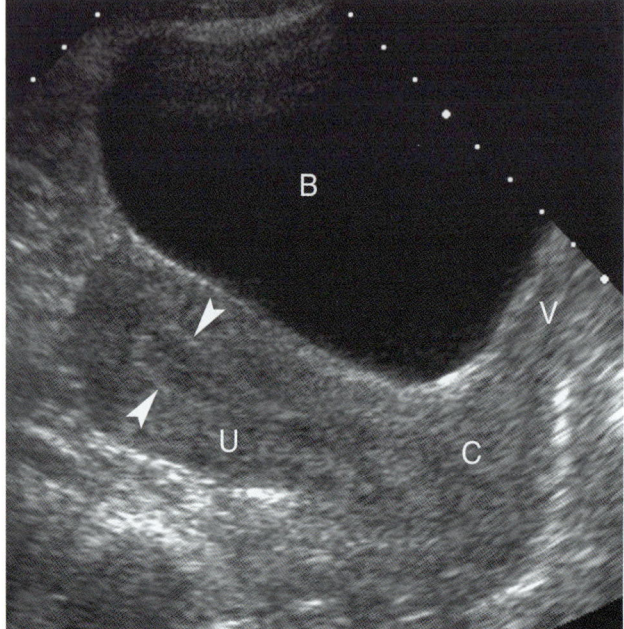

Figure 2-19. Transabdominal longitudinal measurement of the endometrium. The *arrowheads* indicate the proper placement of the electronic calipers to measure this endometrium (basal to basal). The uterus (*U*), cervix (*C*), and vagina (*V*) are all aligned. B, urinary bladder. (Reprinted with permission from Brant WE. Genital tract and bladder ultrasound. In: Brant WE, Helms CA, eds. *Fundamentals of Diagnostic Radiology*. 3rd ed. Lippincott Williams & Wilkins; 2007. Figure 37.1.)

- Obtain images and measurements in both transverse and sagittal of all uterine pathology.
- Transverse right or left ovary **(Fig. 2-22)**
  - Begin obtaining ovarian images with the ovary seen first.
  - Measure the maximum transverse dimension of the ovary.
  - Apply color Doppler to the ovary.
  - Apply pulsed-wave Doppler and attempt to obtain both arterial and venous waveforms **(Figs. 2-23 and 2-24)**.
- Longitudinal right or left ovary
  - Maintaining your focus on the previous ovary, rotate the transducer 90 degrees to obtain sagittal images of the same ovary.

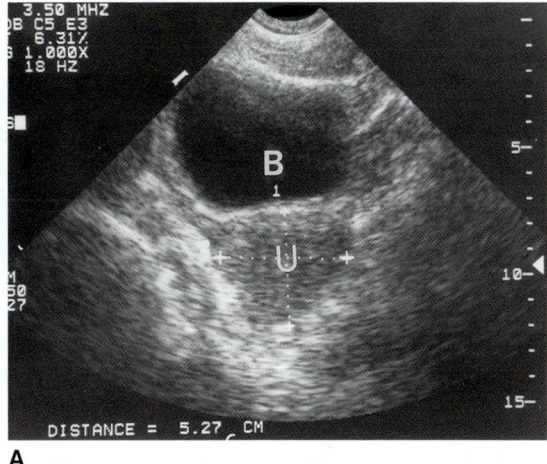

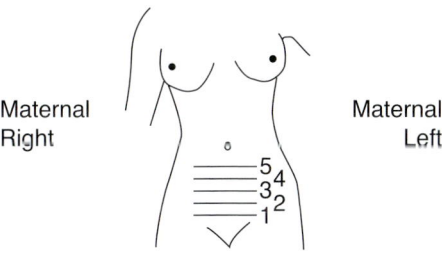

Figure 2-20. Transabdominal transverse scanning. A. The width of the uterine body and AP (which is not typically necessary if obtained in the longitudinal plane) is demonstrated. B. Image orientation is noted, as well as a schematic depicting the levels of the transverse images: *1* is the vaginal level, *2* is the cervix level, *3* is the corpus or body, *4* is the uterine fundus, and *5* is superior to the fundus. (Reprinted with permission from Menihan CA, Kopel E. *Point-of-Care Assessment in Pregnancy and Women's Health: Electronic Fetal Monitoring and Sonography.* Wolters Kluwer; 2014. Figure 9-5.)

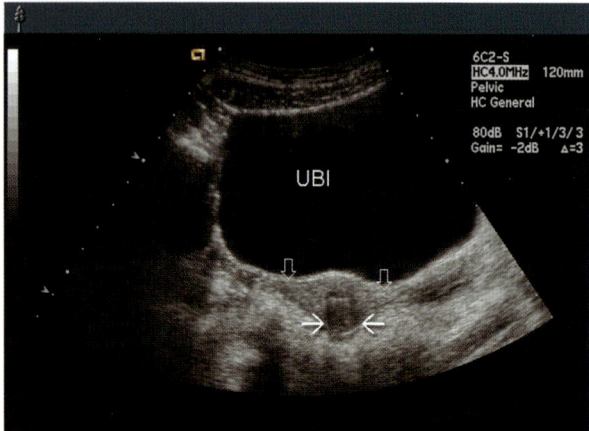

Figure 2-21. Transverse transabdominal cervix. Transverse scan at the level of the cervix often produces a shadow (*solid arrows*), which brackets a central zone of decreased echoes. This pattern is characteristic of the cervix. The *open arrows* indicate the cervical ligaments. **UBI, urinary bladder.** (Reprinted with permission from Kupesic SP, Turner T. Normal anatomy of the female pelvis. In: Stephenson SR, ed. *Diagnostic Medical Sonography: Obstetrics & Gynecology*. 3rd ed. Wolters Kluwer Health/Lippincott Williams & Wilkins; 2012. Figure 5-36.)

- Measure the maximum length and width dimensions of the ovary.
- Apply color and pulsed-wave Doppler (if not identifiable in transverse).
- Longitudinal right or left adnexa images
  - Obtain several sagittal images while scanning through each adnexa.
- Transverse right or left adnexa images
  - Obtain several transverse images while scanning through each adnexa.
- Repeat all previously listed ovarian and adnexal images of the contralateral side.

SCANNING TIPS

- Always employ the use of the distended bladder as an acoustic window while scanning transabdominally.
- Ovaries are best visualized in the transverse plane while using the transabdominal approach.

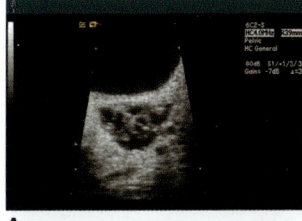
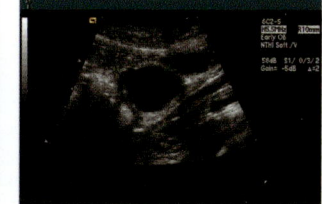

Figure 2-22. Transabdominal and transvaginal ovary images. **A.** Transabdominal transverse scan of a normal adult ovary on day 7 of the menstrual cycle. Several small follicles are seen within the ovary. **B.** Sagittal transvaginal image of a dominant follicle immediately after its rupture at ovulation. **C.** Transvaginal image of a normal ovary (*OV*). The *arrows* indicate an adjacent muscle. (**A, B.** Reprinted with permission from Kupesic S, Normal anatomy of the female pelvis. In: Stephenson SR, Dmitrieva J, eds. *Diagnostic Medical Sonography: Obstetrics & Gynecology*. 4th ed. Wolters Kluwer; 2018. Figure 5-49A-B. **C.** Reprinted with permission from Hall-Terracciano B, Stephenson SR. *Workbook for Diagnostic Medical Sonography: A Guide to Clinical Practice, Obstetrics and Gynecology*. 5th ed. Wolters Kluwer; 2023:60.)

- Remember, the ovaries can be quite high and lateral, so be sure to scan superiorly and completely lateral to the iliac vessels.
- Ovarian volume (cm^3) is obtained by calculating the length × width × height × 0.523.
- While the transvaginal transducer is inserted, watch the screen to determine proper placement and to visualize the urethra for pathology.
- Gently pressing on the patient's pelvis while performing a transvaginal exam can be helpful in determining if apparent pathology is attached to the ovary. Also, applying pressure to the patient's pelvis with your nonscanning hand can move the ovary closer to the transducer.

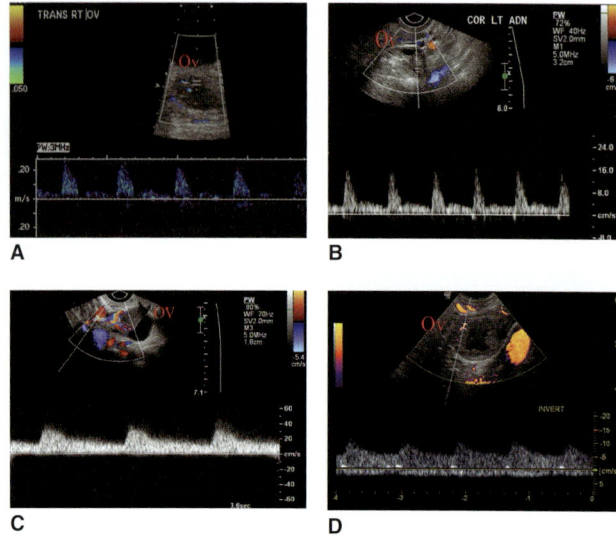

Figure 2-23. Doppler waveforms of the cyclic changes of the ovarian artery can be seen with these Doppler spectra. A. Intraovarian arterial flow during the follicular phase. **B.** Intraovarian arterial flow during the late luteal phase. **C.** Intraovarian arterial flow during the corpus luteal phase. **D.** Intraovarian flow during the corpus hemorrhagicum phase. **OV,** ovary. (Reprinted with permission from Wilson M. Doppler evaluation of the pelvis. In: Stephenson SR, ed. *Diagnostic Medical Sonography: Obstetrics & Gynecology.* 3rd ed. Wolters Kluwer Health/Lippincott Williams & Wilkins; 2012. Figure 6-15.)

- A distended urinary bladder can distort the pelvic anatomy during a transvaginal exam, and therefore the patient may need to void.
- Translabial scanning is helpful for the visualization of the cervix and vagina.
- If the patient has an overlapping abundance of abdominal tissue/fat that drapes over the pelvis, place a sheet or towel under the tissue and have the patient pull up on the fabric with both arms. Pulling the extra tissue superiorly will hopefully expose the true pubic surface superior to the pubic symphysis.
- When scanning transverse to the uterus, do not angle the transducer too much, as this will distort the anatomy. Remember, in sonographic imaging, it is best to be perpendicular to the organ or structure being scanned.

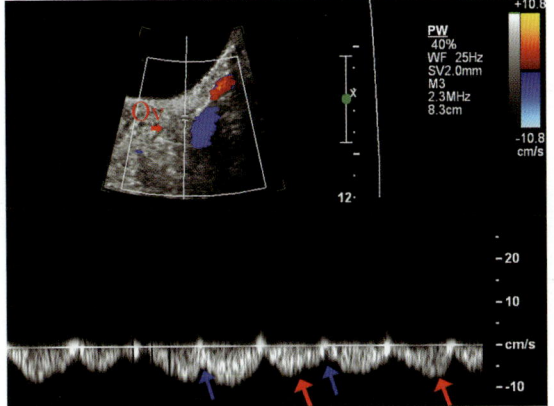

Figure 2-24. Transabdominal image of the ovarian vein. This spectral Doppler image displays the ovarian vein with continuous flow throughout the cardiac cycle. The *red arrows* depict systole, and the *blue arrows* depict diastole. OV, ovary. (Reprinted with permission from Wilson M. Doppler evaluation of the pelvis. In: Stephenson SR, ed. *Diagnostic Medical Sonography: Obstetrics & Gynecology.* 3rd ed. Wolters Kluwer Health/Lippincott Williams & Wilkins; 2012. Figure 6-18.)

- For vulvar masses, use a linear transducer, as penetration is typically not needed.
- During the transvaginal examination, the patient may have to lift her buttocks off of the examination table so that you can angle the transducer superiorly to see the fundus of the uterus and beyond.

NORMAL MEASUREMENTS

- Uterine size[3]
  - The size and shape vary with age and parity.
    - Adult nulliparous = 6 to 8.5 cm or less in length, 3 to 5 cm in width, and 2 to 4 cm in AP
    - Adult multiparous = 8 to 10.5 cm in length, 4 to 6 cm in width, and 3 to 5 cm in AP
    - Postmenopausal = 3.5 to 7.5 cm in length, 2 to 4 cm in width, and 1.7 to 3.3 cm in AP
- Endometrial thickness[2]
  - Varies with the menstrual cycle.
    - Menses = up to 4 mm
    - Early proliferative = 4 to 8 mm

- Late proliferative (periovulatory) = 6 to 10 mm
- Secretory = 7 to 14 mm
- Postmenopausal
  - No vaginal bleeding (asymptomatic)
    - Normal ≤8 mm
  - Vaginal bleeding (symptomatic)
    - Normal ≤4 to 5 mm
- Size of ovaries[4]
  - Ovarian size varies with the functional state.
    - Reproductive ovary = 2.5 to 5 cm in length, 1.5 to 3 cm in width, and 0.6 to 2.2 cm in AP
      - Ovarian volume ranges between 6 and 9 cm^3
    - Postmenopausal ovary = 1.1 cm in length (±0.6 cm), 0.7 in width, and 1.2 cm in AP (±0.3 cm)
  - Ovarian volume[2] (length × width × height × 0.523)
    - Premenopausal ovarian volume average is 9.8 cm^3.
    - Postmenopausal ovarian volume average is 5.8 cm^3.

DOPPLER OF THE FEMALE PELVIS[4]

- Venous flow
  - Spectral findings of venous flow include low resistance or a continuous recurring flow in diastole and reduced flow signal in systole.
- Arterial flow
  - Spectral findings of arterial flow include alternating quick uptake or systolic peak and a lower diastolic flow level that corresponds to the cardiac cycle.
- Normal uterine artery Doppler characteristics
  - Moderate to high velocity with a high-resistance flow in a nongravid patient
    - Resistive index in proliferative phase = 0.88 ± 0.05
    - Resistive index periovulatory = 0.84 ± 0.06
- Normal ovarian artery Doppler characteristics
  - Normal ovarian artery flow has a low velocity, with a high-resistance or impedance pattern.
    - Resistive index in follicular phase = 0.92 ± 0.08
    - Resistive index at ovulation = 0.44 ± 0.08

ESSENTIAL FEMALE PELVIC PATHOLOGY[2]

- Uterine leiomyoma (fibroid uterus)—most common benign uterine mass (Fig. 2-25)

Chapter 2. Adult Female Pelvic Sonography

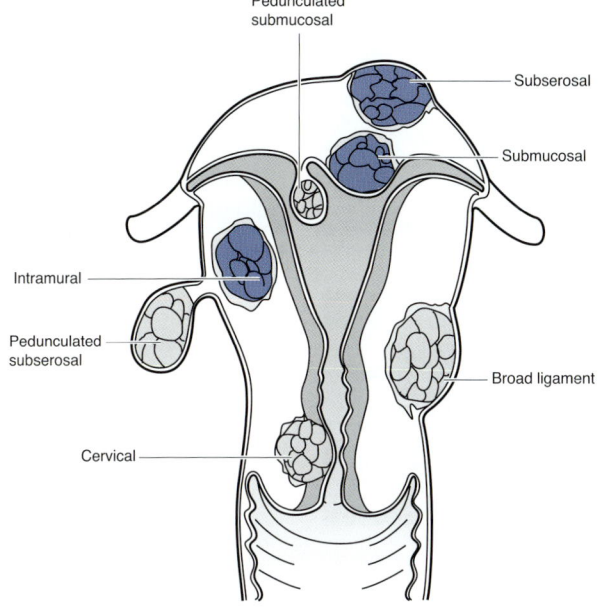

Figure 2-25. Locations of fibroids. (Reprinted with permission from Callahan TL, Caughey AB. *Blueprints Obstetrics & Gynecology*. 7th ed. Wolters Kluwer; 2018. Figure 14-5.)

- Clinical findings:
  - Menorrhagia
  - Palpable abdominal mass
  - Constipation
  - Dysuria
  - Enlarged, bulky uterus
  - Pelvic pressure and pain
  - Urinary frequency
  - Possible infertility complaints
- Sonographic findings
  - Hypoechoic mass within the uterus **(Fig. 2-26)**
    - Fibroids may be intramural, pedunculated, submucosal, subserosal, and intracavitary
  - Posterior shadowing from the mass
  - Calcifications may be present within the mass
  - Uterus may contain multiple fibroids and be enlarged

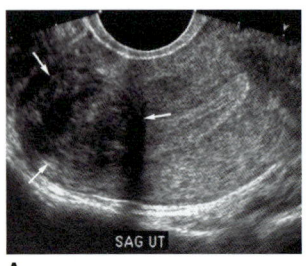
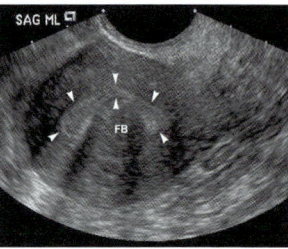
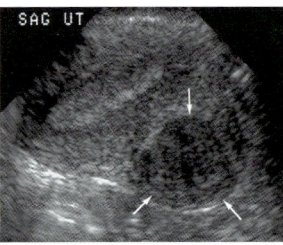

Figure 2-26. Sonograms of various fibroid locations. A. Sagittal endovaginal view of an intramural fibroid (*between arrows*). B. Sagittal endovaginal view demonstrates a submucosal fibroid (*FB*). Note the distortion of the endometrium (*arrowheads*). C. Sagittal endovaginal view of a subserosal fibroid (*long arrows*). (Reprinted with permission from Doubilet PM, Benson CB. *Atlas of Ultrasound in Obstetrics and Gynecology: A Multimedia Reference.* Lippincott Williams & Wilkins; 2003. Figure 25.1-1A-C.)

- Endometrial carcinoma—cancer of the endometrium
  - Clinical findings
    - Postmenopausal vaginal bleeding
    - Intermenstrual bleeding
    - Enlarged uterus
    - Elevation in cancer antigen-125 (CA-125)
  - Sonographic findings
    - Thickened endometrium (Fig. 2-27)
    - Heterogeneous uterus
    - Enlarged uterus with lobular contour
    - Endometrial fluid
    - Polypoid tumor within the endometrium
- Ovarian torsion—twisting of the adnexa and vasculature of the ovary which results in the interruption of either arterial or venous ovarian flow (or both)

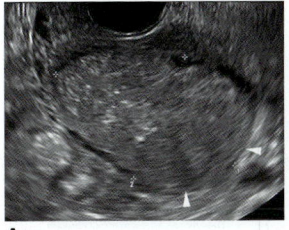 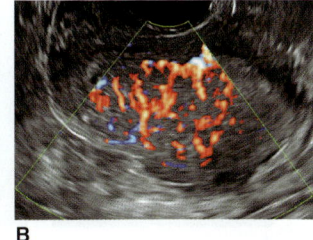

Figure 2-27. Endometrial carcinoma. A. Sagittal transvaginal view of the uterus in a patient with postmenopausal bleeding demonstrates a markedly thickened endometrium forming a mass (calipers). The endometrial–myometrial interface is obliterated at the fundus (*arrowheads*). **B.** Color Doppler reveals extensive vascularity in the endometrial mass, which proved to be invasive endometrial carcinoma. (Reprinted with permission from Doubilet PM, Benson CB, Benacerraf BR. *Atlas of Ultrasound in Obstetrics and Gynecology: A Multimedia Reference.* 3rd ed. Wolters Kluwer; 2019. Figure 30.3.3.)

- Clinical findings
  - Fever
  - Acute unilateral abdominal or pelvic pain
  - Nausea and vomiting
  - Slight leukocytosis
- Sonographic findings
  - Ovarian mass often accompanies torsion
  - Enlarged ovary **(Fig. 2-28)**
  - Multifollicular development on the ovary
  - Lack of detectable flow patterns or a significantly diminished flow
  - "Whirlpool sign"—round mass with concentric hypoechoic and hyperechoic rings that demonstrate a swirling color Doppler signature (see Fig. 3-16)
- Follicular cyst—results from the failure of the dominant follicle to ovulate; ranges in size from 3 to 8 cm; may be complex or hemorrhagic
  - Clinical findings
    - Asymptomatic
    - Pain associated with hemorrhage and enlargement
  - Sonographic findings
    - Simple ovarian cyst—anechoic, thin-walled, unilocular, round, and produces posterior enhancement **(Fig. 2-29)**

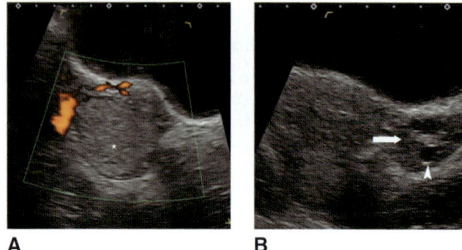

Figure 2-28. Ovarian torsion. A. Ovarian torsion. Power Doppler image of the right ovary shows the ovary to be enlarged and relatively uniformly hyperechoic, with no visible normal ovarian follicles (*asterisk*). There is no detectable blood flow in the ovary. **B.** Grayscale image of the normal left ovary for comparison shows the ovary (*arrow*) to be normal in size and echotexture, with normal-appearing ovarian follicles (*arrowhead*). (Reprinted with permission from Smith EA, Trout AT. Abdomen. In: Klein JS, Brant WE, Helms CA, Vinson EN, eds. *Brant and Helms' Fundamentals of Diagnostic Radiology*. 5th ed. Wolters Kluwer; 2019. Figure 69.49.)

- Hemorrhagic cyst—may have a complex appearance; solid appearance, fluid-debris level; web-like appearance **(Fig. 2-30)**
- Endometrioma—blood-containing mass associated with endometriosis
  - Clinical findings
    - Asymptomatic
    - Pelvic pain

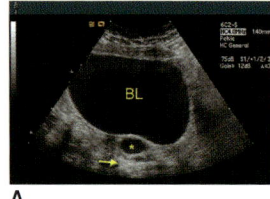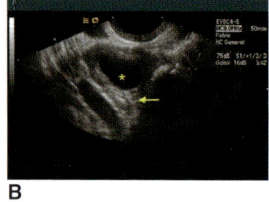

Figure 2-29. Transabdominal and transvaginal follicular cyst. A. A transabdominal sagittal image of a follicular cyst (*asterisk*) posterior to the full bladder (*BL*). Notice the posterior enhancement (*arrow*). **B.** EV image of the same patient with the follicular cyst (*asterisk*) and minimal posterior enhancement (*arrow*). (Reprinted with permission from Stephenson SR. Benign disease of the female pelvis. In: Stephenson SR, ed. *Diagnostic Medical Sonography: Obstetrics & Gynecology*. 3rd ed. Wolters Kluwer Health/Lippincott Williams & Wilkins; 2012. Figure 8-32.)

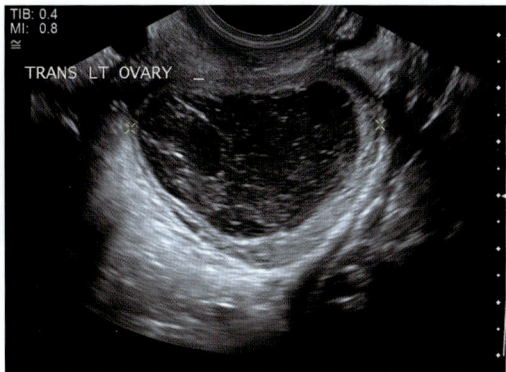

Figure 2-30. Hemorrhagic ovarian cyst. Transvaginal appearance of a hemorrhagic ovarian cyst. (Reprinted with permission from Donaldson C, Farrell TA. Pelvic imaging, including obstetric ultrasound. In: Farrell TA, ed. *Radiology 101: The Basics and Fundamentals of Imaging.* 5th ed. Wolters Kluwer; 2020. Figure 4.13.)

- Infertility
- Dysmenorrhea
- Menorrhagia
- Dyspareunia
- Painful bowel movements
- Sonographic findings
  - Mostly cystic with low-level internal echoes **(Fig. 2-31)**
  - Fluid–fluid level (see Fig. 2-31)
  - Complex
  - Homogeneous mass
- Cystic teratoma—result from the retention of an unfertilized ovum that differentiates into the three germ cell layers; may contain hair, teeth, fat, and other tissues; also referred to as a dermoid tumor
  - Clinical findings
    - Asymptomatic
    - Large teratomas can cause ovarian torsion
  - Sonographic findings
    - Complex, partially cystic mass that can contain varying amounts of solid tissues **(Fig. 2-32)**
    - Tip of the iceberg sign—only the anterior elements of the mass are seen and structures located posterior to the mass are obscured by shadowing

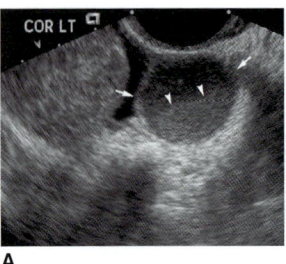 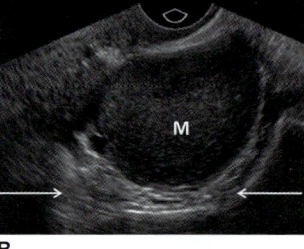

Figure 2-31. Endometrioma appearances. A. Endometrioma with fluid–fluid level. Coronal scan of the left ovary revealing a cystic adnexal mass (*arrows*) containing a fluid–fluid level (*arrowheads*). B. Transvaginal image of an ovarian hypoechoic mass (*M*) with low-level internal echoes pathologically proven to be an endometrioma. Note enhanced through transmission compatible with cystic nature, manifested as increased echogenicity (*between arrows*) behind this mass. (**A.** Reprinted with permission from Doubilet PM, Benson CB. *Atlas of Ultrasound in Obstetrics and Gynecology: A Multimedia Reference*. Lippincott Williams & Wilkins; 2003. Figure 27.6-3. **B.** Reprinted with permission from Klepchick PR, Daffner RH. Obstetric and gynecologic imaging. In: Daffner RH, Hartman MS, eds. *Clinical Radiology: The Essentials*. 4th ed. Wolters Kluwer Health/Lippincott Williams & Wilkins; 2014. Figure 10.17.)

- Dermoid plug—produces posterior shadowing
- Dermoid mesh—plug of hair
- Polycystic ovary syndrome (PCOS)—endocrinologic ovarian disorder linked with infertility
  - Clinical findings of PCOS
    - Infertility
    - Amenorrhea or oligomenorrhea
    - Hirsutism (excessive hair growth in areas where hair is usually scant)
    - Hyperandrogenism
  - Sonographic findings of PCOS
    - Many small cysts scattered around the periphery of the ovary (string of pearls sign) **(Fig. 2-33)**
    - Many small cysts noted throughout the ovary
    - Bilateral enlargement of the ovaries
      - Ovarian volume is greater than 10 mL
    - Several thresholds for diagnosis may be used including:
      - 12 or more follicle on one or both ovaries that measure between 2 and 9 mm
      - Total of 25 small follicles

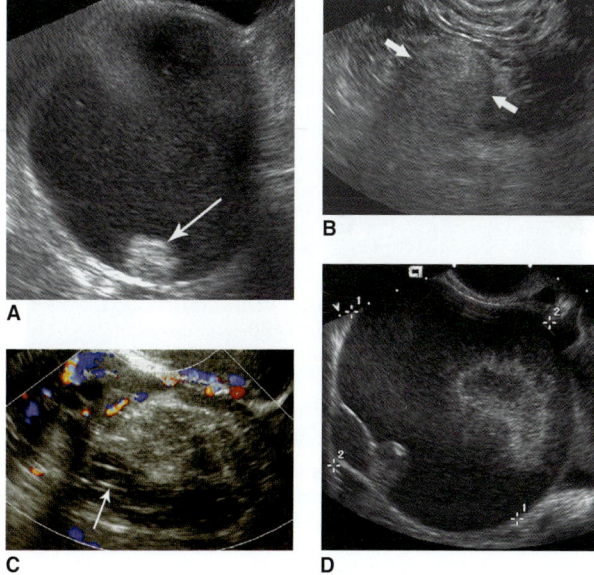

Figure 2-32. Sonographic images of the varying appearances of a cystic teratoma (dermoid). A. Predominantly cystic with floating echoes within the fluid. An echogenic nodule (*arrow*) represents a dermoid plug. B. An echogenic mass (*arrows*) with indistinct margins that fade into acoustic shadowing and reverberation. This is the typical "tip of the iceberg" appearance of a benign cystic teratoma. C. A complex ovarian mass with prominent echogenic components shows no internal blood flow. Avascular strands (*arrow*) represent hair characteristically found in benign cystic teratomas. D. This complex mass noted between calipers (+) was determined to be a dermoid. (Reprinted with permission from Brant WE. Genital tract and bladder ultrasound. In: Brant WE, Helms CA, eds. *Fundamentals of Diagnostic Radiology.* 4th ed. Wolters Kluwer Health/Lippincott Williams & Wilkins; 2012. Figure 36.20.)

- Pelvic inflammatory disease (PID)—infection of the upper genital tract most likely caused by a sexually transmitted disease (STD) like chlamydia or gonorrhea
  - Clinical findings of PID
    - Positive for an STD
    - Fever
    - Chills
    - Pelvic pain

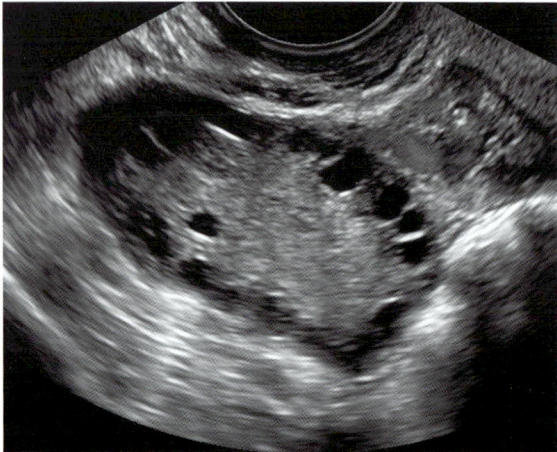

Figure 2-33. Polycystic ovary. A sonogram revealing more than 12 small peripheral follicles is a classic sonographic sign of the "string of pearls" associated with PCOS. (Reprinted with permission from Donaldson C, Farrell TA. Pelvic imaging, including obstetric ultrasound. In: Farrell TA, ed. *Radiology 101: The Basics and Fundamentals of Imaging*. 5th ed. Wolters Kluwer; 2020. Figure 4.36.)

- Purulent vaginal discharge and/or bleeding
- Dyspareunia (painful intercourse)
- Elevated white blood cell count
- Sonographic findings of PID
  - Irregular thickened endometrium
  - Irregular or unclear borders of pelvic organs
  - Dilated fallopian tubes that may contain echogenic material representing pus or blood (Fig. 2-34)
  - Multicystic and solid complex adnexal masses
- Ovarian carcinoma—cancer of the ovary
  - Clinical findings of ovarian carcinoma
    - Abdominal distension
    - Bloating
    - Weight loss
    - Elevated CA-125
  - Sonographic findings of ovarian carcinoma
    - Varying sonographic appearances
      ○ Solid wall nodules within a cystic mass (Fig. 2-35)
      ○ Thick septations greater than 3 mm within a cystic mass

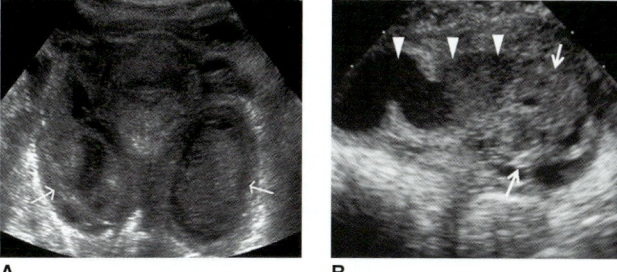

Figure 2-34. Pelvic inflammatory disease. A. Transverse transabdominal image of the female pelvis revealing bilateral complex adnexal masses (*arrows*) in the setting of an extensive pelvic infection. B. PID with pyosalpinx. Longitudinal transabdominal sonogram of the right adnexal region shows a dilated, thick-walled fallopian tube (*arrowheads*) with internal echoes and an enlarged right ovary (*arrow*). (A. Reprinted with permission from Penny SM. *Examination Review for Ultrasound: Abdomen & Obstetrics and Gynecology*. 2nd ed. Wolters Kluwer; 2018. Figure 21-1. B. Reprinted with permission from Siegel MJ. Female pelvis. In: Siegel MJ, ed. *Pediatric Sonography*. 4th ed. Wolters Kluwer Health/Lippincott Williams & Wilkins; 2011. Figure 13.31.)

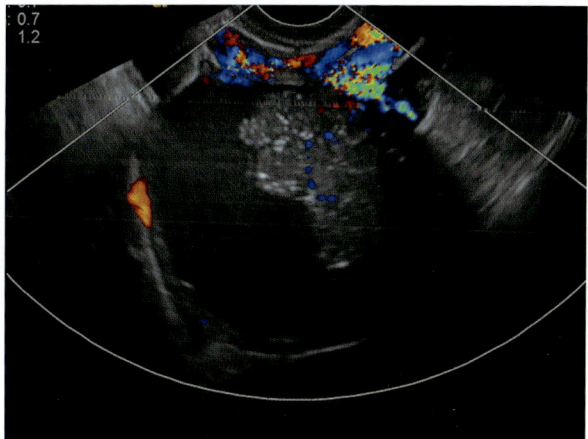

Figure 2-35. Ovarian carcinoma. Pelvic sonogram showing a partially solid ovarian mass, with a solid mural (wall) nodule containing blood flow. (Reprinted with permission from Donaldson C, Farrell TA. Pelvic imaging, including obstetric ultrasound. In: Farrell TA, ed. *Radiology 101: The Basics and Fundamentals of Imaging*. 5th ed. Wolters Kluwer; 2020. Figure 4.28.)

- Ovarian wall thickening
- Irregular walls or poorly defined margins
- Blood flow within septations, wall nodules, or other solid components
  - Doppler reveals high diastolic flow within the vessels of the mass
  - Malignant vessels tend to have resistive indices less than 0.4 and pulsatility indices less than 1.0
- Ascites is often present

WHERE ELSE TO LOOK

- Evaluate the urinary bladder carefully, scanning through completely in both sagittal and transverse.
  - The bladder wall should be thin when distended. A thickened bladder wall, especially if the bladder is distended, can be a sign of cystitis **(Fig. 2-36)**.
  - Assess the lumen of the bladder for debris and stones and the wall for focal areas of thickening which can be evidence of a bladder mass **(Fig. 2-37)**.
  - Bladder diverticulum may also be discovered **(Fig. 2-38)**.

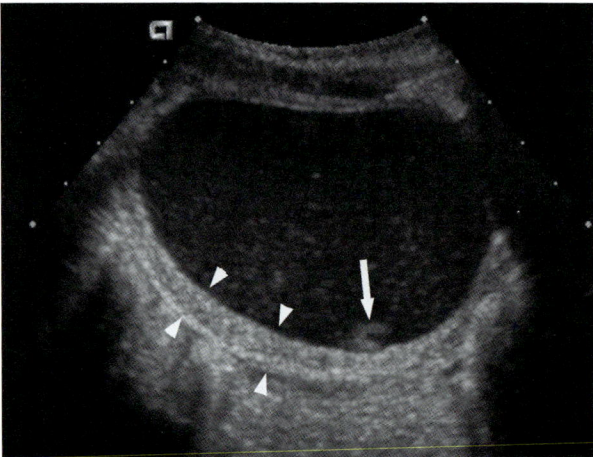

Figure 2-36. Cystitis. Sonographic image of the urinary bladder shows bladder wall thickening (*arrowheads*), echogenic intraluminal debris, and a dependent hyperechoic clot (*arrow*). (Reprinted with permission from Pizzo PA, Poplack DG. *Principles and Practice of Pediatric Oncology*. 6th ed. Wolters Kluwer Health/Lippincott Williams & Wilkins; 2011. Figure 9-67.)

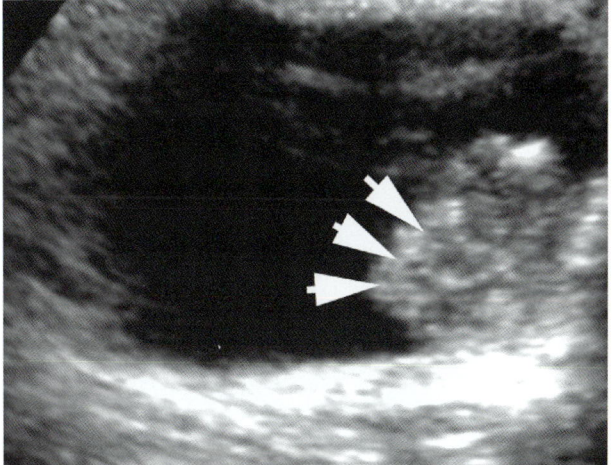

Figure 2-37. Transitional cell carcinoma of the bladder. Sonographic image of the urinary bladder in a 15-year-old girl with gross painless hematuria reveals a solid bladder mass that was proven to be transitional cell carcinoma. (Reprinted with permission from Peters CA, Traylor J, Pritzker K. Pediatric Urology. In: Emans SJH, Laufer MR, DiVasta AD, eds. *Emans, Laufer, Goldstein's Pediatric and Adolescent Gynecology.* 7th ed. Wolters Kluwer; 2020. Figure 12-1A.)

- If a large amount of free fluid is noted within the pelvis, a more thorough assessment of all four quadrants may be warranted to determine the general amount.
- Some ovarian masses are associated with pleural effusion and ascites (Meigs syndrome).
- Right lower quadrant pain can be a symptom of appendicitis. Consequently, a thorough assessment of the adnexa could reveal an enlarged appendix. A linear transducer may be most helpful to visualize the appendix, though it may be seen with transvaginal imaging occasionally **(Fig. 2-39)**.
- Congenital anomalies of the uterus often accompany congenital anomalies of the urinary tract. Therefore, the kidneys may need to be assessed as well.

OVARIAN-ADNEXAL REPORTING AND DATA SYSTEM (O-RADS)

- O-RADS Ultrasound (US) applies to the ovaries, lesions involving (or suspected to involve) the ovaries and/or

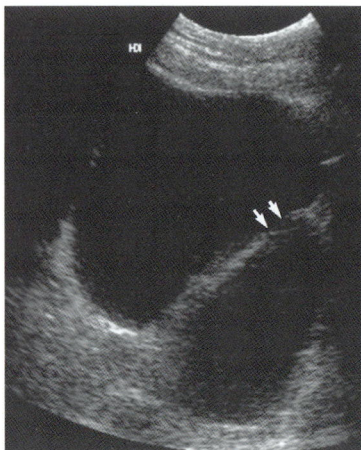

Figure 2-38. Urinary bladder diverticulum. Sagittal image of the pelvis demonstrates a fluid-filled mass posterior to the urinary bladder with a defect in the posterior wall (*arrows*) indicating the neck of a large bladder diverticulum. (Reprinted with permission from Jafri ZH, Akbar SA. The bladder, prostate, and the testis. In: Shirkhoda A, ed. *Variants and Pitfalls in Body Imaging: Thoracic, Abdominal and Women's Imaging.* 2nd ed. Wolters Kluwer Health/Lippincott Williams & Wilkins; 2011. Figure 24.16.)

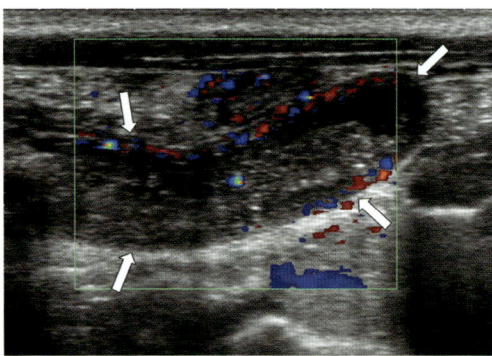

Figure 2-39. Inflamed appendix. Acute appendicitis, Doppler sonography. Longitudinal color Doppler sonogram shows a dilated, blind-ending appendix (*arrows*) with intraluminal debris and fluid. There is increased vascularity of the appendiceal walls, a sign of inflammation. (Reprinted with permission from Navarro OM, Siegel MJ. Gastrointestinal tract. In: Siegel MJ, ed. *Pediatric Sonography.* 5th ed. Wolters Kluwer; 2019. Figure 10-64.)

Chapter 2. Adult Female Pelvic Sonography

O-RADS Score	Risk Category [IOTA Model]	Lexicon Descriptors		Management	
				Pre-menopausal	Post-Menopausal
0	Incomplete Evaluation [N/A]	Lesion features relevant for risk stratification cannot be accurately characterized due to technical factors		Repeat US study or MRI	
1	Normal Ovary [N/A]	No ovarian lesion		None	
		Physiologic cyst: follicle (≤3 cm) or corpus luteum (typically ≤3 cm)		None	
2	Almost Certainly Benign [<1%]	Simple cyst	≤3 cm	N/A (see follicle)	None
			>3 cm to 5 cm	None	Follow-up US in 12 months*
			>5 cm but <10 cm	Follow-up US in 12 months*	Follow-up US in 12 months*
		Unilocular, smooth, non-simple cyst (internal echoes and/or incomplete septations)	≤3 cm	None	Follow-up US in 12 months*
		Bilocular, smooth cyst	>3 cm but <10 cm	Follow-up US in 6 months*	
		Typical benign ovarian lesion (see "Classic Benign Lesions" table)	<10 cm	See "Classic Benign Lesions" table for descriptors and management	
		Typical benign extraovarian lesion (see "Classic Benign Lesions" table)	Any size		
3	Low Risk [1 – <10%]	Typical benign ovarian lesion (see "Classic Benign Lesions" table), ≥10 cm		Imaging: • If not surgically excised, consider follow-up US within 6 months** • If solid, may consider US specialist (if available) or MRI (with O-RADS MRI score)†† Clinical: Gynecologist	
		Uni- or bilocular cyst, smooth, ≥10 cm			
		Unilocular cyst, irregular, any size			
		Multilocular cyst, smooth, <10 cm, CS ≤4			
		Solid lesion, shadowing, smooth, any size, CS = 1			
		Solid lesion, shadowing, smooth, any size, CS 2-3			
4	Intermediate Risk [10 – <50%]	Bilocular cyst without solid component(s)	Irregular, any size, any CS	Imaging: Options include: • US specialist (if available) or • MRI (with O-RADS MRI score)†† or • Per gyn-oncologist protocol Clinical: Gynecologist with gyn-oncological consultation or solely by gyn-oncologist	
		Multilocular cyst without solid component(s)	Smooth, ≥10 cm, CS <4		
			Smooth, any size, CS 4		
			Irregular, any size, any CS		
		Unilocular cyst with solid component(s)	<4 pps or solid component(s) not considered a pp, any size		
		Bi- or multilocular cyst with solid component(s)	Any size, CS 1-2		
		Solid lesion, non-shadowing	Smooth, any size, CS 2-3		
5	High Risk [≥50%]	Unilocular cyst, ≥4 pps, any size, any CS		Imaging: Per gyn-oncologist protocol Clinical: Gyn-oncologist	
		Bi- or multilocular cyst with solid component(s), any size, CS 3-4			
		Solid lesion, shadowing, smooth, any size, CS 4			
		Solid lesion, irregular, any size, any CS			
		Ascites and/or peritoneal nodules††			

GLOSSARY

Smooth and irregular: refer to inner walls/septation(s) for cystic lesions, and outer contour for solid lesions; irregular inner wall for cysts = <3 mm in height

Shadowing: must be diffuse or broad to qualify; excludes refractive artifact

CS = color score; degree of intralesional vascularity; 1 = none, 2 = minimal flow, 3 = moderate flow, 4 = very strong flow

Solid: excludes blood products and dermoid contents; solid lesion = ≥80% solid; solid component = protrudes ≥3 mm (height) into cyst lumen off wall or septation

pp = papillary projection; subtype of solid component surrounded by fluid on 3 sides

Bilocular = 2 locules; multilocular = ≥3 locules; bilocular smooth cysts have a lower risk of malignancy, regardless of size or CS

Postmenopausal = ≥1 year amenorrhea (early: <5 yrs; late: ≥5 yrs); if uncertain or uterus surgically absent, use age >50 yrs (early = >50 yrs but <55 yrs, late = ≥55 yrs)

*Shorter imaging follow-up may be considered in some scenarios (eg, clinical factors). If smaller (≥10–15% decrease in average linear dimension), no further surveillance. If stable, follow-up US at 3d months from initial exam. If enlarging (>10–15% increase in average linear dimension), consider follow-up US at 12 and 24 months from initial exam, then management per gynecology. For changing morphology, reassess using lexicon descriptors. **Clinical management with gynecology as needed.**

**There is a paucity of evidence for defining the optimal duration or interval for imaging surveillance. Shorter follow-up may be considered in some scenarios (eg, clinical factors). If stable, follow-up at 12 and 24 months from initial exam, then as clinically indicated. For changing morphology, reassess using lexicon descriptors.

† MRI with contrast has higher specificity for solid lesions, and cystic lesions with solid component(s).

Figure 2-40. O-RADS Ultrasound Risk Stratification and Management System. (Reprinted with permission from American College of Radiology Committee on O-RADS™. O-RADS™ Ultrasound Assessment Categories 2022. Accessed on June 1, 2023. https://www.acr.org/-/media/ACR/Files/RADS/O-RADS/US-v2022/O-RADS–US-v2022-Assessment-Categories.pdf)

fallopian tubes, and paraovarian cysts, when the intent is to stratify risk of malignancy.

- Some institutions may require that the sonographic participate in evaluating ovarian lesions using the O-RADS US lexicon **(Fig. 2-40)**.

IMAGE CORRELATION

- Fibroids noted on MRI **(Fig. 2-41)**
- Dermoid on CT **(Fig. 2-42)**
- Cystic mass on CT **(Fig. 2-43)**

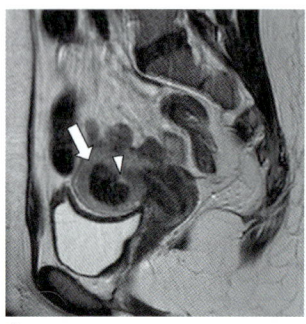 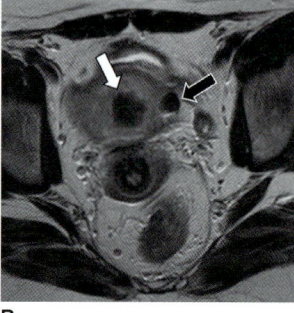

A   B

Figure 2-41. Fibroids on MRI. Fibroids in a 38-year-old woman with heavy menstrual bleeding. A. Sagittal MR image demonstrates a dominant hypointense fibroid at the uterine fundus (*arrow*). The fibroid is submucosal, projecting into the endometrium (*arrowhead*) but appears greater than 50% intramural. B. Axial MR image demonstrates a hypointense subserosal fibroid along the left lateral uterine body (*black arrow*). Dominant submucosal fibroid is also again seen (***white arrow***). (Reprinted with permission from Chung AD, Brook OR. Pelvis. In: Lee EY, Hunsaker A, Siewert B, eds. *Computed Body Tomography with MRI Correlation*. 5th ed. Wolters Kluwer; 2020. Figure 20-16A-B.)

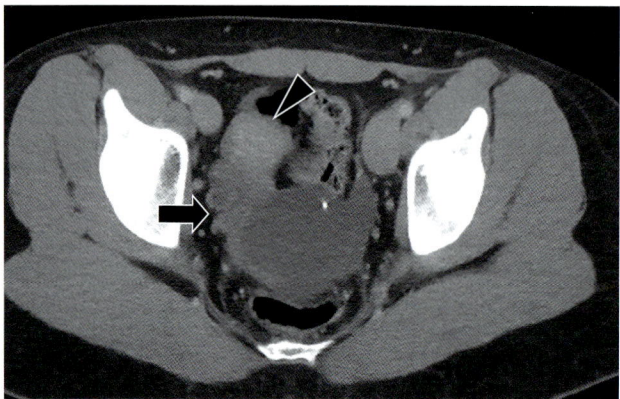

Figure 2-42. Dermoid with torsion. Axial enhanced soft tissue window setting CT image shows a partially cystic, partially calcified mass in the pelvic cul-de-sac with swirling of the right fallopian vessels (*arrow*) and displacement of the partially visualized uterus (*arrowhead*) to the **right.** (Reprinted with permission from Thacker PG, Lee EY. Pediatric Application: Abdomen and Pelvis. In: Lee EY, Hunsaker A, Siewert B, eds. Computed Body Tomography with MRI Correlation. 5th ed. Wolters Kluwer; 2020. Figure 24-108.)

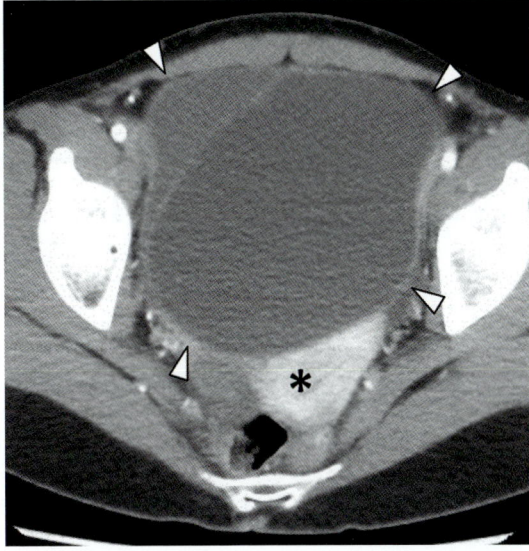

Figure 2-43. Axial CT image demonstrates a cystic mass within the midline pelvis (*arrowheads*), displacing the uterus (*asterisk*) posteriorly. Surgical pathology revealed a mucinous cystadenoma of the left ovary. (Reprinted with permission from Chung AD, Brook OR. Pelvis. In: Lee EY, Hunsaker A, Siewert B, eds. *Computed Body Tomography with MRI Correlation*. 5th ed. Wolters Kluwer; 2020. Figure 20-18C.)

REFERENCES

1. *AIUM Practice Parameter for the Performance of an Ultrasound Examination of the Female Pelvis*. Accessed on September 14, 2023. https://www.aium.org/docs/default-source/resources/guidelines/femalepelvis.pdf?sfvrsn=f5d0c38b_1
2. Penny SM. *Examination Review for Ultrasound: Abdomen & Obstetrics and Gynecology*. 3rd ed. Wolters Kluwer; 2022:11–19 & Section II.
3. Norton MN, Scoutt LM, Feldstein VA. *Callen's Ultrasonography in Obstetrics and Gynecology*. 6th ed. Elsevier; 2017:805–1075.
4. Stephenson SR, Dmitrieva J. *Diagnostic Medical Sonography: Obstetrics and Gynecology*. 5th ed. Wolters Kluwer; 2023:177–196.

CHAPTER 3

Pediatric Female Pelvic Sonography

INTRODUCTION

Transabdominal sonography provides a global view of the female patient, and it is the primary resource for imaging of the pediatric female pelvis secondary to its ease of use and lack of ionizing radiation. This brief chapter will describe the sonographic appearance of the pediatric female pelvis (infant, child, and adolescent) and provide some information regarding specific pathology that may be noted during a sonographic examination. Normal measurements will be provided as well.

RECOMMENDATIONS FOR SONOGRAPHY OF THE PEDIATRIC FEMALE PELVIS[1,2]

- Pediatric protocols and examination techniques mirror that of the adult female patient.
- The following are consistent with the practice parameters of the adult female pelvis with some pediatric information included.
- Uterus
  - The uterine size, shape, and orientation should be analyzed.
  - Measurement of the uterus should be acquired.
    - The uterine length is evaluated and obtained with electronic calipers in the sagittal view.
    - The length is measured as a straight line from the fundus to the external os of the cervix by using the outer-to-outer technique.
    - The length can also be measured by measuring from the fundal region along the endometrial lining and endocervical canal using the outer-to-outer technique.

- The uterine (depth) anteroposterior (AP) dimension is also evaluated and obtained with electronic calipers in the sagittal view.
- The calipers are placed from the anterior to posterior walls perpendicular to the length measurement.
- The maximum width is measured in the transverse or coronal view.
- A uterine volume can be obtained in the same manner as above, though the cervix should not be included.
- The various layers of the uterine wall should be evaluated, which include the myometrium and endometrium.
- The uterine appearance will vary depending on the age and functional state of the pediatric patient.
- Abnormalities of the myometrium and endometrium should be documented, including contour changes, echogenicity, masses, and cysts.
  - Myometrium
    - The anterior myometrial thickness of the uterus should also be compared for symmetry with the posterior wall.
    - The myometrium should be homogeneous, though small blood vessels may be noted. Color Doppler can be used to prove the presence of vessels.
    - There should be no heterogeneous regions, cystic spaces, or hypoechoic masses.
    - Myometrial masses are uncommon in the pediatric population.
  - Endometrium
    - The endometrium may be prominent in the perinatal period secondary to maternal hormone stimulation.
    - The endometrium in the prepubertal patient may not be seen well following the perinatal period.
    - The endometrium should be analyzed for focal abnormalities, echogenicity, and the presence of fluid or masses within the uterine cavity.
    - The endometrial thickness should be obtained.
    - The thickest part of the endometrium should be measured perpendicular to its longitudinal plane in the AP diameter from the anterior echogenic border to the posterior echogenic border (basal layer to basal layer), using the outer-to-outer technique.

- The adjacent hypoechoic myometrium is not included in this measurement.
- Intracavitary fluid is not included in this measurement. If fluid is present, the two separate endometrial layers should be measured and added together to obtain the true thickness of the endometrium.
- For postmenarchal pediatric patients and those sexually active, the patient may have an intrauterine device (IUD), and the location of the device should be documented.
- The cervix and vagina should be examined.
  - Abnormalities of the cervix and vagina, including masses, fluid, or cysts should be measured.
- The size of the uterus, which is obtained in two dimensions, and the location of clinically relevant lesions should be documented.
- Three-dimensional sonography can be helpful in many circumstances including:
  - Further analysis of the relationship of masses within the endometrial cavity
  - Uterine congenital anomalies
  - Thickened and/or heterogeneous endometrium
  - Location and orientation of an IUD
  - Integrity of the pelvic floor
- Ovaries and adnexa
  - Ovaries
    - Ovarian size may be determined by measuring the ovary in three dimensions (longitudinal, transverse, and AP diameter).
    - The views should be in two orthogonal planes (e.g., sagittal and transverse).
    - Any ovarian abnormalities should be documented.
    - If the ovaries are not visualized, this should be noted. Ovaries may not be seen if they are small or if they lack follicular development, as is often the case with prepubertal patients.
    - Perinatal ovarian cysts may be noted secondary to maternal hormonal simulation.
    - Sonograms may be requested for newborn female patients who had previously discovered cystic pelvic lesions in utero.

- Adnexa
  - The adnexa should be evaluated for abnormalities or evidence of dilated fallopian tubes.
  - The abnormality should be noted in relation to the ovaries and uterus and the sonographic appearance and size should be provided.
  - The description of the abnormality should be documented as to whether it is cystic, solid, simple, or complex.
    - Further analysis for septations (thick or thin), solid components, mural nodules, outgrowths, papillary components, and vascular characteristics should be offered.
  - Doppler sonography, including the use of spectral, color, and/or power, may be useful to evaluate the vascular characteristics of pelvic masses and to assist in the diagnosis of ovarian torsion.
- Cul-de-sac
  - An evaluation of fluid within the posterior cul-de-sac should be performed.
  - The cul-de-sac should also be evaluated for masses and those masses should be measured and their position, shape, and sonographic characteristics should be obtained.
  - The location of the mass should be compared to the relationship with the ovaries and uterus.
  - Slight probe pressure may be used to distinguish the relationship of pelvic structures and adjacent masses.
- The ALARA (As Low As Reasonably Achievable) principle should be observed for factors that affect the acoustic output by considering the transducer dwell time and total scanning time.

ESSENTIAL ANATOMY AND PHYSIOLOGY OF THE PEDIATRIC FEMALE PELVIS[2,3]

- Basic pelvic anatomy is provided in Chapter 2, along with physiology. The following section will be unique to the pediatric female pelvis.
- Uterus
  - The size and shape vary with age, especially the body-to-cervix ratio **(Fig. 3-1)**
    - Newborn uterine shape **(Fig. 3-2)**

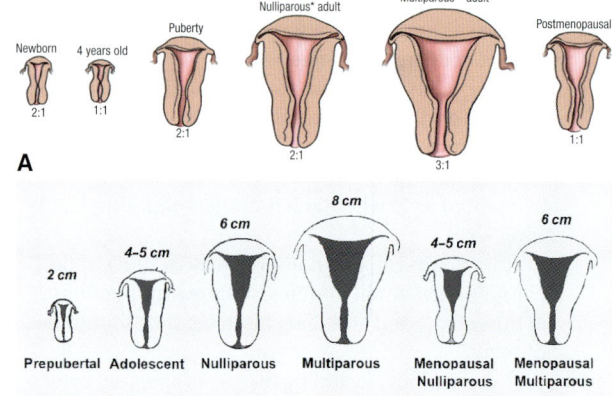

Figure 3-1. Uterine shape and size. A. Lifetime changes in the uterine body-to-cervix ratio. B. Changes in uterine size with age and parity. (**A.** Reprinted with permission from Agur AMR, Dalley AF. *Grant's Atlas of Anatomy*. 15th ed. Wolters Kluwer; 2021. Figure 5.31B. **B.** Reprinted with permission from Sanders RC. Infertility. In: Sanders RC, Hall-Terracciano B, eds. *Clinical Sonography: A Practical Guide*. 5th ed. Wolters Kluwer; 2016. Figure 14-4A.)

- The neonatal uterus will typically be prominent with a bright echogenic endometrium secondary to maternal hormonal stimulation in utero (**Figs. 3-3** and **3-4**).
- The fundus-to-cervix ratio is 1:2.

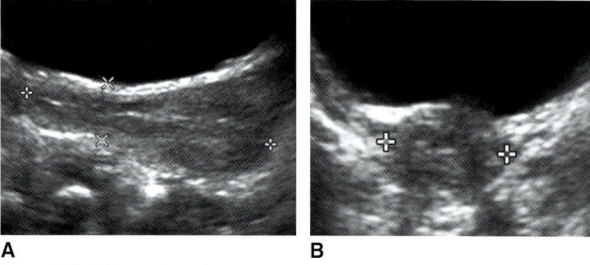

Figure 3-2. Measuring the neonatal uterus. A. Longitudinal sonogram of a normal uterus in a 2-week-old girl. Calipers have been placed to measure the superior–inferior (+) and anterior–posterior (×) dimensions. B. The transverse dimension of the uterus (+) is obtained. (Reprinted with permission from Ward VL, Estroff JA. Radiologic imaging. In: Emans SJH, Laufer MR, DiVasta AD, eds. *Emans, Laufer, Goldstein's Pediatric and Adolescent Gynecology*. 7th ed. Wolters Kluwer; 2020. Figure 37-5.)

Chapter 3. Pediatric Female Pelvic Sonography

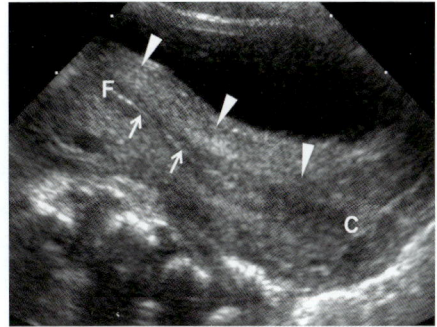

Figure 3-3. Normal neonatal uterus. Longitudinal image shows a prominent uterus (*arrowheads*) with the cervix (*C*) and fundus (*F*) having a bulbous configuration and being of similar size. Note the thin echogenic endometrial stripe (*arrows*), which is the result of in utero hormonal stimulation. (Reprinted with permission from Siegel MJ. Female pelvis. In: Siegel MJ, ed. *Pediatric Sonography*. 5th ed. Wolters Kluwer; 2019. Figure 13-43A.)

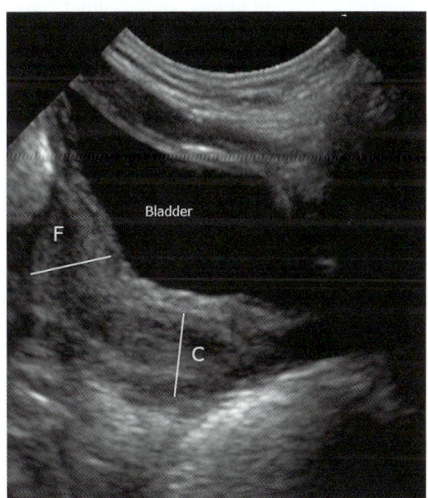

Figure 3-4. Normal 1-month-old uterus. Longitudinal view of the uterus of a 1-month-old infant shows similar anteroposterior dimensions (designated by *straight lines*) of the uterine fundus (*F*) and cervix (*C*). (Reprinted with permission from Chapman T. The female pediatric pelvis. In: Iyer RS, Chapman T, eds. *Pediatric Imaging: The Essentials*. Wolters Kluwer; 2016. Figure 22.1A.)

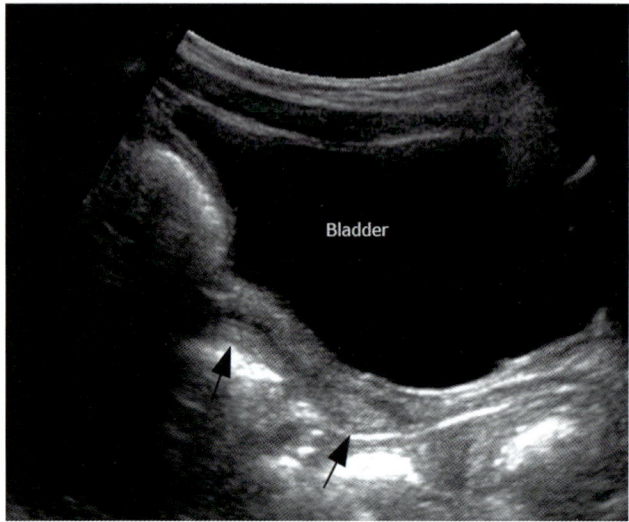

Figure 3-5. Normal 2-year-old uterus. Longitudinal view of the uterus of a 2-year-old child shows small dimensions of the uterus (*black arrows*). (Reprinted with permission from Chapman T. The female pediatric pelvis. In: Iyer RS, Chapman T, eds. *Pediatric Imaging: The Essentials*. Wolters Kluwer; 2016. Figure 22.1B.)

- Two- to 3-month-old uterine shapes up until 7 or 8 years of age (**Figs. 3-5** and **3-6**)
  - This age range will typically have a tube-shaped uterine appearance.
  - The fundus-to-cervix ratio is 1:1.
  - The endometrial stripe may not be seen well or not visualized.
- Pubertal uterus shape
  - The pubertal uterus will have more of an adult shape, which is pear-like in appearance.
  - The fundus-to-cervix ratio is 3:1.
  - The endometrial stripe will correlate with the menstrual cycle (**Figs. 3-7** and **3-8**).
- Ovaries
  - Like the testes, the ovaries develop within the upper abdomen of the fetus, and during fetal life, they descend into the pelvis.
  - Though rare, the ovaries may be located outside of the pelvis, within the abdomen.

Chapter 3. Pediatric Female Pelvic Sonography

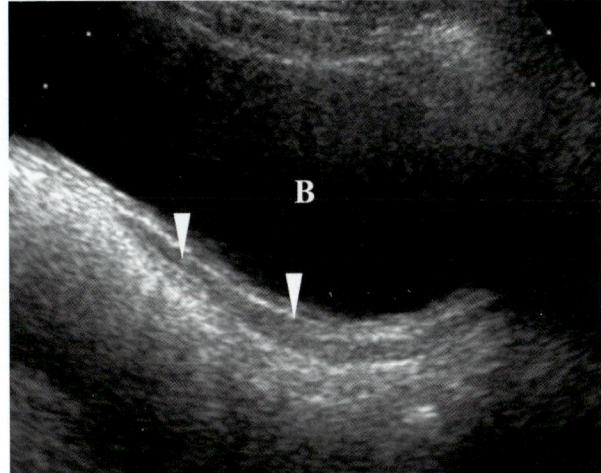

Figure 3-6. Normal 8-year-old uterus. The uterus (*arrowheads*) in an 8-year-old is smaller and tubular in configuration with no differentiation between the fundus and cervix. *B,* bladder. (Reprinted with permission from Siegel MJ. Female pelvis. In: Siegel MJ, ed. *Pediatric Sonography.* 5th ed. Wolters Kluwer; 2019. Figure 13-43B.)

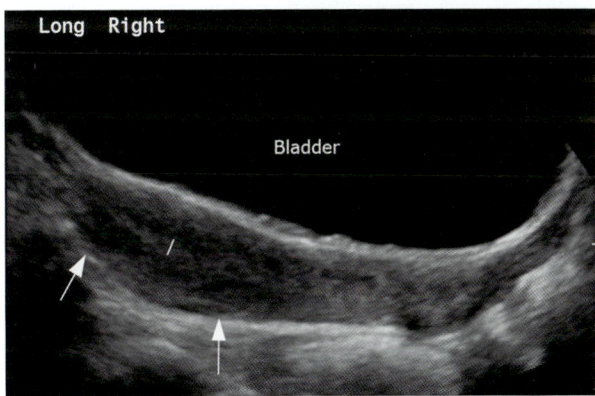

Figure 3-7. Normal 15-year-old uterus. A longitudinal image of the uterus just right of the midline in a 15-year-old shows an ellipsoid-shaped uterus (marked by *arrows*). Note the echogenic endometrial stripe (*line*). (Reprinted with permission from Chapman T. The female pediatric pelvis. In: Iyer RS, Chapman T, eds. *Pediatric Imaging: The Essentials.* Wolters Kluwer; 2016. Figure 22.3A.)

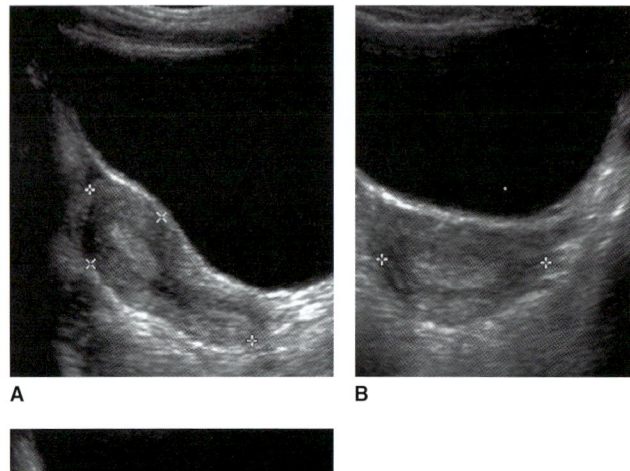

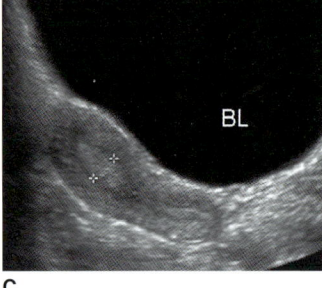

Figure 3-8. Measuring the postpurbertal uterus. A. Longitudinal image of the uterus with length (+) and AP (×) measurements. **B.** Transverse image of the uterus with width (×) measurement. **C.** Thickness (+) measurement of the endometrium in this patient was 9 mm. (Reprinted with permission from Ward VL, Estroff JA. Radiologic imaging. In: Emans SJH, Laufer MR, DiVasta AD, eds. *Emans, Laufer, Goldstein's Pediatric and Adolescent Gynecology.* 7th ed. Wolters Kluwer; 2020. Figure 37-7.)

- Ovaries are ovoid in shape.
- In the newborn, small ovarian cysts or follicles may be noted secondary to maternal hormonal stimulation. These typically resolve shortly after birth **(Fig. 3-9)**.
  - Large ovarian cysts are worrisome and may lead to ovarian torsion.
  - These ovarian cysts can exceed 9 mm.
- In infancy and before puberty, the ovaries may contain several small follicles **(Fig. 3-10)**.

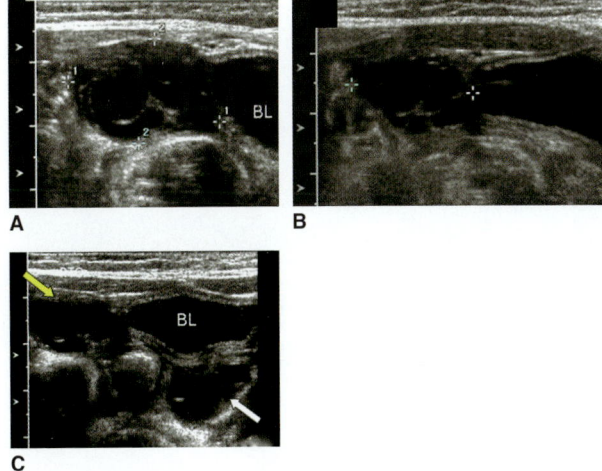

Figure 3-9. Multiple ovarian follicles in a 6-week-old girl. The multiple prominent bilateral ovarian follicles are consistent with persistent maternal hormone stimulation. A. Sagittal ultrasound (US) image of the right ovary (demarcated by *calipers*). The right ovary is located adjacent to the partially full urinary bladder (*BL*). B. Transverse US image of the right ovary (also demarcated by *calipers*). C. Transverse image of the right ovary (*yellow arrow*) and left ovary (*white arrow*) shows that both ovaries contain multiple follicles. The urinary bladder (*BL*) is seen between the ovaries. (Reprinted with permission from Ward VL, Estroff JA. Radiologic imaging. In: Emans SJH, Laufer MR, DiVasta AD, eds. *Emans, Laufer, Goldstein's Pediatric and Adolescent Gynecology.* 7th ed. Wolters Kluwer; 2020. Figure 37-9.)

- When puberty ensues, the ovaries increase in size and descend further into the pelvis.
- Multiple follicles may be present following menarche, as seen in adults.

SUGGESTED EQUIPMENT AND QUALITY CONTROL[2,3]

- Ultrasound equipment inherently varies between institutions.
- It is the institution's obligation to offer high-quality sonographic examinations, and therefore these providers should supply equipment that balances cost-effectiveness with state-of-the-art features for their sonographic practitioners to utilize.

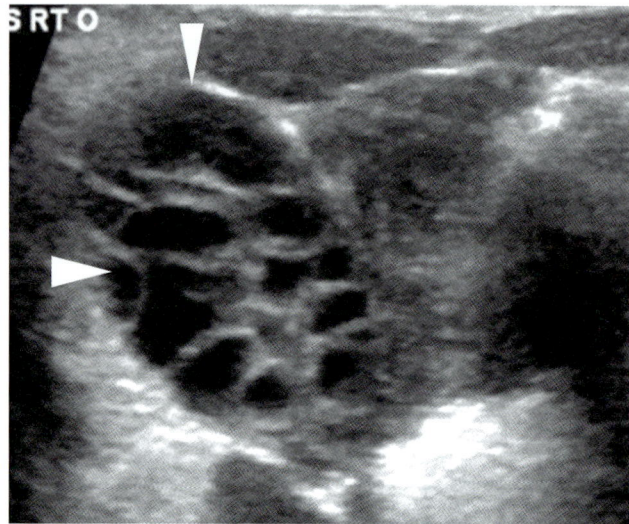

Figure 3-10. Normal prepubertal ovary. A 2-year-old girl. Longitudinal view of the right ovary (*arrowheads*) shows multiple small anechoic follicles, measuring less than 9 mm in diameter. (Reprinted with permission from Siegel MJ. Female pelvis. In: Siegel MJ, ed. *Pediatric Sonography*. 5th ed. Wolters Kluwer; 2019. Figure 13-2.)

- Both the institution and sonographic practitioner should be aware of the potential musculoskeletal injuries that can result from improper equipment or poor scanning practices and should work together to prevent such injuries.
- Ultrasound machines should be capable of standard real-time imaging, have color, power, and spectral Doppler applications, and be capable of providing adequate diagnostic imaging for interpretation by a qualified interpreting physician. These physicians should meet the specified AIUM Training Guidelines in accordance with AIUM accreditation policies.
- Sonographers performing these examinations should be appropriately credentialed in the specialty area in accordance with AIUM accreditation policies.
- Physicians not performing the examination should provide supervision as defined by Federal regulations.
- The pediatric female pelvis should be examined sonographically with a real-time scanner, preferably a 5- or

7.5-MHz sector or linear array transducer for transabdominal imaging. Lower MHz transducers may be employed for pediatric patients with larger body habitus. Some authors suggest as low as 4 MHz, with linear array transducers, often used for bowel complaints, ranging from 7 to 15 MHz.
- Transvaginal transducers, used for nonvirginal patients only, are typically 5 MHz or higher.
- Occasionally, a linear transducer may be employed as an adjunct to the examination if superficial structures need to be evaluated. For example, a linear transducer may aid the sonographer by providing higher resolution if an ovary or mass is located superficially.
- Quality control and improvement, safety, infection control, patient education, and equipment performance monitoring should be developed and implemented in accordance with the AIUM Standards and Guidelines for the Accreditation of Ultrasound Practices found at https://www.aium.org/accreditation/accreditation.aspx

CLINICAL INVESTIGATION FOR SONOGRAPHY OF THE FEMALE PELVIS

- Laboratory findings can be helpful in many situations (see Table 1-3 in Chapter 1).
- Evaluate prior imaging reports and images including CT, MRI, radiographs, and any other appropriate test.

PATIENT PREPARATION AND POSITIONING FOR PEDIATRIC GYNECOLOGIC SONOGRAPHY[2,3]

- Patient preparation
  - Transabdominal sonography
    - Transabdominal sonography is the primary imaging tool utilized to evaluate the pediatric female pelvis.
    - The patient, as with adult female pelvic sonography, is required to have a distended bladder.
    - The patient's urinary bladder can be distended to displace the bowel and to provide an acoustic window for the visualization of the uterus, ovaries, and adnexa.
    - The bladder should not be excessively distended. If this occurs, the patient may need to partially empty her bladder.
    - Proper bladder filling can be accomplished by drinking fluids, should the patient be of an age where she can

Chapter 3. Pediatric Female Pelvic Sonography

maintain a full bladder, or bladder catheterization with the instillation of sterile fluid (retrofilling of the urinary bladder) may be performed.
- ○ Patient preparation for older pediatric patients who can follow directions can prepare by drinking 24 oz of fluid 45 minutes before the examination.
- ○ Infants can be fed a bottle 30 minutes before the examination.
- ○ If the patient cannot perform preparation orally, catheterization may be required.
- Transabdominal imaging also offers the opportunity to examine the urinary bladder and urethra.
- Transvaginal sonography
  - Transvaginal sonography should not be performed in the virginal patient.
  - Empty the urinary bladder before the transvaginal examination commences and ensure that there are no foreign objects, such as tampons, within the vagina.
  - Transvaginal transducer preparation and insertion
    - ○ Preparation of transvaginal transducers between patients requires routine mandatory high-level disinfection and the use of a high-quality single-use transducer cover during each examination. (See Infection Control and Machine Maintenance in Chapter 1.)
    - ○ Explain the process of transvaginal transducer fully to the patient before commencing with the examination. Patient agreement is of course mandatory.
    - ○ A disinfected transvaginal transducer must be used.
    - ○ Coupling gel is placed on the face of the transducer.
    - ○ A sterile probe cover is placed on the transducer and air bubbles are expressed to reduce air artifacts during imaging.
    - ○ Sterile gel is placed outside of the transducer cover over the transducer face.
    - ○ The patient, who is in the lithotomy position or supine with legs flexed, can be asked to assist the sonographer in inserting the transducer. This may not be possible with all patients, however, when possible, this may reduce pain and anxiety.
    - ○ The transducer should be inserted into the vagina without encountering the cervix.

- A chaperone may be required by your institution for the transvaginal examination.
- It is important to note that transvaginal imaging has a limited field of view.
- Patient positioning
  - Transabdominal pediatric female pelvic sonogram
    - The patient is typically placed in the supine position (see Fig. 1-20).
  - Transvaginal pediatric female pelvic sonogram
    - The patient is typically placed in the lithotomy position (see Fig. 1-21).
    - The patient may be placed in the supine position with the hips elevated up from the examining table with the use of a positioning pad as well.

CLINICAL INVESTIGATION SONOGRAPHY OF THE PEDIATRIC FEMALE PELVIS

- Laboratory findings can be helpful in many situations (see Table 1-3).
- Always evaluate the results of any other imaging exams if previously conducted.
- Critical clinical history questions related to the pediatric female pelvis
  - Any vaginal bleeding or secretions? *The patient's caretaker should be able to provide this information if the patient cannot.*
  - Any palpable masses? *Enlargement of the uterus prior to puberty is uncommon; however, the ovaries may undoubtedly increase in size secondary to solid ovarian masses, cysts, and ovarian torsion. If the uterus is enlarged or the endometrium thickened in a prepubescent child, hormonal causes must be considered, and thus among other causes, an ovarian, adrenal, or possibly a brain tumor can lead to such findings. Postpubertal enlargement without vaginal bleeding may be associated with an imperforate hymen or other causes of vaginal obstruction.*
  - Any pelvic pain? *Pelvic pain may be difficult to assess in a child, though there can be many causes, including ovarian torsion, appendicitis, intussusception, and bowel obstruction. Older, sexually active pediatric females can be suffering from pelvic inflammatory disease. Though ovarian*

solid tumors are rare in children, if large enough, they can certainly lead to pain. Large ovarian masses can also result in ovarian torsion. Vaginal obstructions can lead to pain as well.
- Any disorders of puberty? *Early menarche, breast development, and other secondary sexual characteristics can lead to sonographic findings of a prominent uterus and ovaries. Malignant ovarian masses can result in an increase in hormonal circulation and thus cause the uterus to be enlarged, endometrium to thicken and hemorrhage, and lead to ovarian enlargement.*
- Ambiguous genitalia? *Occasionally, sonography may be used to analyze a patient with ambiguous genitalia. In this case, the sonographer's role is to identify the internal pelvic anatomy, including the uterus and ovaries. The abdomen may also need to be evaluated.*
- First day of the last menstrual period (postmenarchal patients)? *When relevant, this should be entered into the calculation package or documented in the exam and the sonographic findings should be correlated with the menstrual cycle.*
- Possible pregnancy (sexually active pediatric patients)? *This may not always be available if a patient provides a limited clinical history and thus a pregnancy test would be useful. If pregnancy test results are not available for a postmenarchal pediatric patient with amenorrhea, pregnancy cannot be ruled out, and thus care must be taken to evaluate the endometrium carefully for signs of an intrauterine pregnancy and the adnexa for signs of an ectopic pregnancy.*

SUGGESTED PROTOCOL FOR A SONOGRAM OF THE PEDIATRIC FEMALE PELVIS[2,3]

- Note: The following protocol can be conducted utilizing the transabdominal or transvaginal approach but do keep in mind that the external architecture of the vagina will not be visualized with transvaginal imaging.
- Longitudinal midline image of the uterus
  - The transducer should be manipulated in a direction that the patient's functional midline is viewed. This may necessitate that the transducer be angled to the right or left of the patient's actual midline.

- Measure the uterus in both longitudinal and AP dimensions.
  - Measure from the fundus to the cervix in the sagittal plane.
  - Measure the thickest AP dimension of the uterus.
  - The trace measurement tool may be utilized when there is atypical positioning of the uterus. Also, two measurements can be obtained and added together if the uterine–cervix angle produces a significant bend.
- Examine the echogenicity and contour of the uterus for any signs of pathology.
- Longitudinal image of the endometrium
  - Measure the thickness of the endometrium from basal layer to basal layer (outer-to-outer).
  - Note the presence of any fluid or masses within the uterine cavity or any distortions.
  - If feasible, utilize the zoom function to better visualize the endometrium.
  - Label the image with the first day of the patient's last menstrual cycle.
  - In prepubescent patients, the endometrium may be difficult to visualize.
- Longitudinal image of the right lateral aspect of the uterus
  - Examine the echogenicity and contour of the uterus for any signs of pathology.
- Longitudinal image of the left lateral aspect of the uterus
  - Examine the echogenicity and contour of the uterus for any signs of pathology.
- Transverse uterus
  - Image the vagina
  - Image the cervix
    - The cervix often produces edge shadowing.
  - Image the corpus
    - Measure the maximum transverse dimension.
  - Image the fundus
  - Scan completely through the uterus superiorly to ensure that there is no pathology superior to the uterine fundus.
- Obtain images and measurements in both transverse and sagittal of all uterine pathology.

- Transverse right or left ovary
  - Begin obtaining ovarian images with the ovary seen first.
  - Measure the maximum transverse dimension of the ovary.
  - Apply color Doppler to the ovary.
  - Apply pulsed-wave Doppler and attempt to obtain both arterial and venous waveforms.
- Longitudinal right or left ovary
  - Maintaining your focus on the previous ovary, rotate the transducer 90 degrees to obtain sagittal images of the same ovary.
  - Measure the maximum length and width dimensions of the ovary.
  - Apply color and pulsed-wave Doppler (if not identifiable in transverse).
- Longitudinal right or left adnexa images
  - Obtain several sagittal images while scanning through each adnexa.
- Transverse right or left adnexa images
  - Obtain several transverse images while scanning through each adnexa.
- Repeat all previously listed ovarian and adnexal images of the contralateral side.

SCANNING TIPS

- Scanning the pediatric patient may be more challenging due to a lack of cooperation.
  - Obtain assistance if needed to calm the patient.
    - Infants may be bottle-fed or provided a pacifier or toy during the examination.
  - Explain the examination using plain language for a child who can understand.
  - If they would like to, allow the patient to touch the transducer and gel prior to the examination to familiarize them with the equipment.
- Use cine loops to obtain your still images with the combative patient.
- Ovaries are best visualized in the transverse plane while using the transabdominal approach.
- Ovarian volume (cm^3) is obtained by calculating the length × width × height × 0.523.

- While the transvaginal transducer is inserted, watch the screen to determine proper placement and to visualize the urethra for pathology.
- Gently pressing on the patient's pelvis while performing a transvaginal exam can be helpful to determine if apparent pathology is attached to the ovary. Also, applying pressure to the patient's pelvis with your nonscanning hand can move the ovary closer to the transducer.
- A distended urinary bladder can distort the pelvic anatomy during a transvaginal exam, and therefore the patient may need to void.
- Translabial scanning is helpful for the visualization of the cervix and vagina.
- If the patient has an overlapping abundance of abdominal tissue/fat that drapes over the pelvis, place a sheet or towel under the tissue and have the patient pull up on the fabric. Pulling the extra tissue superiorly will hopefully expose the area superior to the pubic symphysis.
- When scanning transverse to the uterus, do not angle the transducer too much, as this will distort the anatomy. Remember, in sonographic imaging, it is best to be perpendicular to the organ or structure being scanned.
- For vulvar masses, use a linear transducer, as penetration is typically not needed.

NORMAL MEASUREMENTS[2,4]

- Uterine size
  - Uterine size changes noticeably from birth to menarche (see Fig. 3-1)
  - Neonatal uterus (possibly more prominent due to maternal hormonal stimulation)
    - Length = 2.3 to 4.6 cm
    - AP = 0.8 to 2.1 cm
  - Infantile uterus
    - Length = 2.0 to 3.3 cm in
    - AP = 0.5 to 1.0 cm in
  - Premenarchal uterus
    - Varies in size, but gradually increases with age
    - Maximum nulliparous
      - Length = 8 cm
      - Width = 5.5 cm
      - AP = 3 cm

- Size of the ovaries
  - Varies with the functional state.
  - Ovarian volume can be utilized (0.523 × width × thickness × length).
    - Ovarian volume in <1 year of age is around 1.0 cm^3.
    - Ovarian volume in >1 but <2 years of age is around 0.07 cm^3.
    - Ovarian volume in 2 to 13 years (if premenarchal) of age ranges between 0.7 and 4.2 cm^3, respectively.
    - Postmenarchal volume mean is around 9.8 cm^3.
      - Length = 2.5 to 5.0 cm
      - Width = 1.5 to 3.0 cm
      - AP = 0.6 to 1.5 cm
  - Follicle size
    - Mean follicle diameter size is around 6 to 7 mm and typically less than 9 mm.
    - Neonates may have prominent follicles greater than 9 mm due to maternal hormonal stimulation.
    - Graafian follicle (dominant follicle) prior to ovulation may measure between 15 and 30 mm.

DOPPLER OF FEMALE PELVIS[3]

- Venous flow
  - Spectral findings of venous flow include low-resistance or a continuous recurring flow in diastole and reduced flow signal in systole.
- Arterial flow
  - Spectral findings of arterial flow include alternating quick uptake or systolic peak and a lower diastolic flow level that corresponds to the cardiac cycle.
- Normal uterine artery Doppler characteristics
  - Moderate to high velocity with a high-resistance flow in a nongravid patient
    - Resistive index in proliferative phase = 0.88 ± 0.05
    - Resistive index periovulatory = 0.84 ± 0.06
- Normal ovarian artery Doppler characteristics
  - Normal ovarian artery flow has a low velocity, with a high-resistance or impedance pattern.
    - Resistive index in follicular phase = 0.92 ± 0.08
    - Resistive index at ovulation = 0.44 ± 0.08

ESSENTIAL PEDIATRIC FEMALE PELVIC PATHOLOGY

Vaginal Obstructions[3]

- Suggestive clinical signs of vaginal obstructions can be examined with sonography.
  - The patient may have a distended abdominopelvic region or palpable abdominal or pelvic mass.
  - The patient may have a bulging hymen.
- These conditions may not be noted until menarche and are often caused by an imperforate hymen, vaginal septum, duplication anomalies, or an acquired lesion that leads to obstruction of the vagina, which disallows the flow of normal secretions from the vagina.
- The vagina, cervix, and uterus may become enlarged and distended with fluids **(Table 3-1)**.
- Transperineal or translabial imaging may be helpful in evaluating patients with vaginal obstruction.

Ambiguous Genitalia[3]

- Sonography can aid in the determination of sex assignment of infants when ambiguous genitalia is present.
- True hermaphrodites are rare and have both ovarian and testicular tissue, occasionally having a combination of these tissues referred to as ovotestis.
- An enlarged clitoris (clitoromegaly) can be confused for a penis.
- A female hermaphrodite (46, XX) will have a uterus.

Table 3-1 VAGINAL OBSTRUCTION TERM WITH A DESCRIPTION

VAGINAL OBSTRUCTION TERM	DESCRIPTION
Hematocolpos **(Fig. 3-11)**	Blood in the vagina
Hematometra	Blood in the uterus
Hematometrocolpos **(Fig. 3-12)**	Blood in the uterus and vagina
Hydrocolpos **(Fig. 3-13)**	Fluid within the vagina
Hydrometra	Fluid within the uterus
Hydrometrocolpos	Fluid within the uterus and vagina

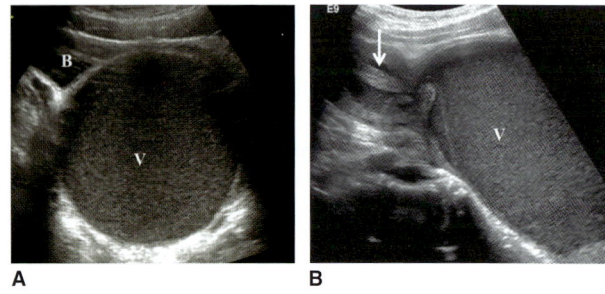

Figure 3-11. Hematocolpos in a 13-year-old girl with pelvic pain. (A) Transverse and **(B)** longitudinal images show a markedly distended vagina (*V*) and mildly dilated endometrial canal (*arrow*), both containing internal echoes representing blood. *B*, bladder. (Reprinted with permission from Siegel MJ. Female pelvis. In: Siegel MJ, ed. *Pediatric Sonography*. 5th ed. Wolters Kluwer; 2019. Figure 13-55B.)

- A chromosomal male (46, XY) with feminized external genitalia is considered a pseudohermaphrodite. It is important to identify the testes in these individuals, and they may be located anywhere, including the abdomen and within the labia.
- The sonographer's role is to identify the uterus and ovaries, thus confirming the presence of female genitalia.
- Karyotyping is most useful, though excessive hormonal distribution may result in confusing findings. These hormones may be associated with congenital adrenal hyperplasia, ovarian masses, testicular masses, and brain tumors found within the anterior pituitary gland. Clinical correlation is most useful.

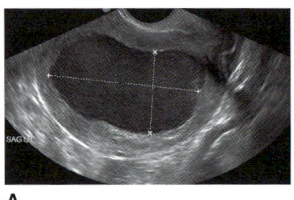
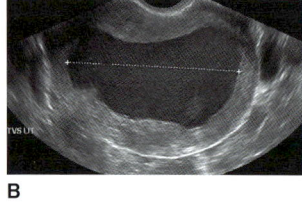

Figure 3-12. Hematometrocolpos. A. Sagittal uterus. **B.** Transverse uterus. Both images display normal myometrial texture with hypoechoic, echogenic contents. This patient was diagnosed with hematometrocolpos (*calipers*). (Reprinted from Hall-Terracciano A. Complementary imaging of the female reproductive system. In: Stephenson SR, Dmitrieva J, eds. *Diagnostic Medical Sonography: Obstetrics & Gynecology*. 4th ed. Wolters Kluwer; 2018. Figure 13-32. Images courtesy of Susan R. Stephenson.)

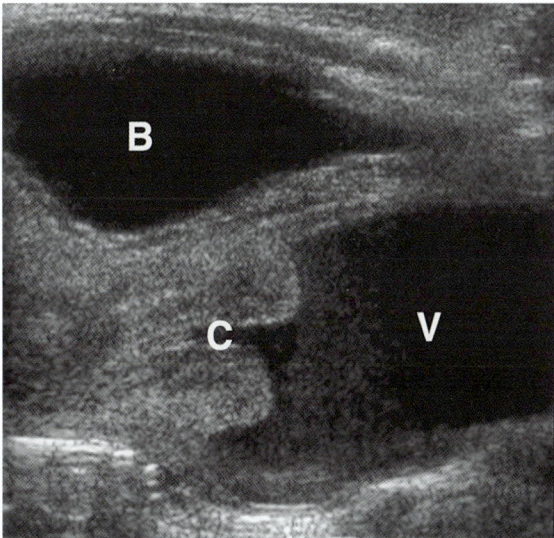

Figure 3-13. Hydrocolpos. Simple-appearing fluid is noted posterior to the urinary bladder (*B*) and inferior to the cervix (*C*) within the vagina (*V*) in this sagittal image of the neonatal pelvis. (Reprinted with permission from Siegel MJ, Coley BD. *The Core Curriculum: Pediatric Imaging.* Lippincott Williams & Wilkins; 2006. Figure 10.30.)

Precocious and Pseudoprecocious Puberty[3]

- Precocious puberty is the early onset of pubertal secondary sexual characteristics, such as menstruation, breast development, and pubic and axillary hair.
  - Precocious puberty is often associated with a brain tumor, leading to an increase in the production of hormones.
- Pseudoprecocious puberty also leads to the development of the aforementioned secondary sexual characteristics.
  - Pseudoprecocious puberty is often associated with an adrenal or ovarian mass.
  - Pseudoprecocious puberty may be associated with congenital adrenal hyperplasia.
- Sonographic findings of precocious and pseudoprecocious puberty
  - The uterus may appear enlarged with a thickened endometrium.

- The ovaries will be prominent and may contain a mass or a functional ovarian cyst.
- If allowed, analyze the adrenal glands for enlargement.

Ovarian Torsion[5]

- Ovarian torsion can occur in pediatric patients and even in utero.
- Rotation of the ovary on its vascular pedicle will lead to obstruction of the venous outflow and eventually the arterial inflow.
- Ovarian torsion most often occurs on the right side.
- Clinical findings
  - Fever
  - Loss of appetite
  - Acute unilateral abdominal or pelvic pain
  - Nausea and vomiting
  - Slight leukocytosis
- Sonographic findings
  - Ovarian mass often accompanies torsion (Fig. 3-14)
  - Enlarged ovary
  - Multifollicular development on the ovary
  - Lack of detectable flow patterns or a significantly diminished flow
  - "Whirlpool sign"—round mass with concentric hypoechoic and hyperechoic rings that demonstrate a swirling color Doppler signature (Fig. 3-15)

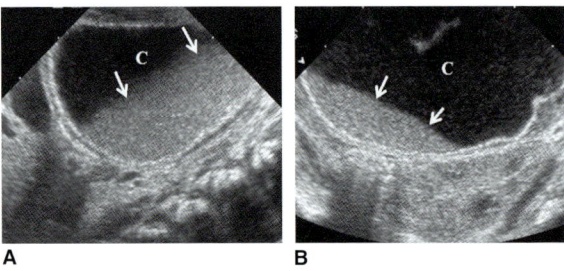

Figure 3-14. Hemorrhagic cyst and ovarian torsion. Hemorrhagic ovarian cyst complicated by torsion. Longitudinal (A) and left lateral decubitus (B) of a large hemorrhagic ovarian cyst that was associated with ovarian torsion. (Reprinted with permission from Siegel MJ. Female pelvis. In: Siegel MJ, ed. *Pediatric Sonography*. 4th ed. Wolters Kluwer Health/Lippincott Williams & Wilkins; 2011. Figure 13.9.)

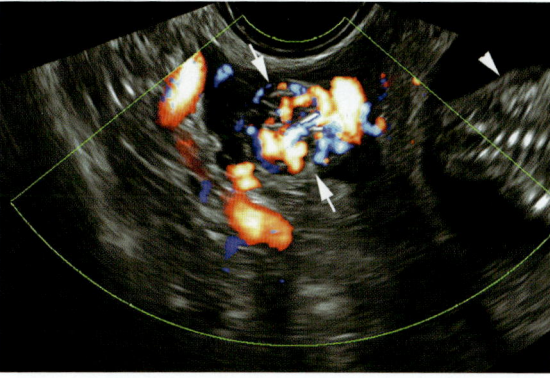

Figure 3-15. Whirlpool sign. Transvaginal view of the twisted pedicle leading to a torsed ovary, in a pregnant patient, showing the circular configuration of the adnexal vessels (*arrows*). The fetus (*arrowhead*) is visible in the uterus. (Reprinted with permission from Doubilet PM, Benson CB, Benacerraf BR. *Atlas of Ultrasound in Obstetrics and Gynecology: A Multimedia Reference.* 3rd ed. Wolters Kluwer; 2019. Figure 31.6.6.)

Pediatric Ovarian Masses

- Benign and cystic
  - Follicular cysts
    - Typically, simple appearing anechoic cysts.
    - Can grow quite large and cause clinical symptoms.
  - Corpus luteum cysts
    - May appear simple or complex and have thick rim.
  - Hemorrhagic cysts
    - Complicated cysts with internal debris and/or septations that often cause pain.
- Benign and solid
  - Cystic teratoma (dermoid)—most common solid ovarian mass seen in reproductive years.
    - Varying sonographic appearances (see Chapter 2)
  - Serous or mucinous cystadenomas
    - Varying sonographic appearances, though often are mostly cystic masses with septations
- Malignant and solid
  - Dysgerminoma—the most common pediatric malignant ovarian mass.
    - Solid hyperechoic mass **(Fig. 3-16)**

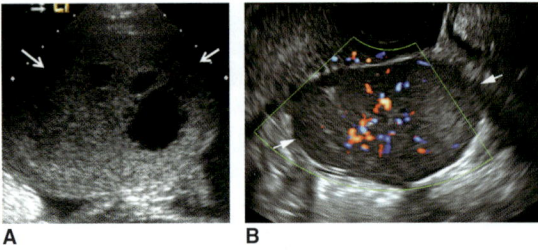

Figure 3-16. Dysgerminoma. A. This solid, hyperechoic mass containing cystic spaces was discovered in an adolescent girl and determined to be a malignant dysgerminoma (*arrows*). **B.** Transvaginal color Doppler image showing solid ovarian lesion (*arrows*) with considerable internal flow, a finding concerning for malignancy. (**A.** Reprinted with permission from Siegel MJ. Female pelvis. In: Siegel MJ, ed. *Pediatric Sonography*. 5th ed. Wolters Kluwer; 2019. Figure 13-25A. **B.** Reprinted with permission from Doubilet PM, Benson CB, Benacerraf BR. *Atlas of Ultrasound in Obstetrics and Gynecology: A Multimedia Reference*. 3rd ed. Wolters Kluwer; 2019. Figure 31.5.4.)

- May cause pseudoprecocious puberty
- Often associated with an elevated serum lactate dehydrogenase

WHERE ELSE TO LOOK[5]

- If a large amount of free fluid is noted within the pelvis, a more thorough assessment of all the quadrants may be warranted to determine the general amount.
- Some ovarian masses are associated with pleural effusion and ascites (Meigs syndrome).
- Right lower quadrant pain, especially in pediatric patients, can be a symptom of appendicitis, ovarian torsion, ovarian masses, pathology of the uterine tube, or possibly even intussusception.
- A linear transducer may be most helpful in visualizing the appendix in the pediatric patient.
  - Normal appendix ≤6 mm in diameter
  - Appendicitis ≥6 mm in diameter **(Fig. 3-17)**
- Intussusception, which is telescoping of the bowel, can cause severe intermittent abdominal pain.
  - Intussusception can appear as a solid, noncompressible cinnamon bun in the abdomen in the axial plane or have a kidney appearance in the sagittal plane **(Fig. 3-18)**.

Chapter 3. Pediatric Female Pelvic Sonography

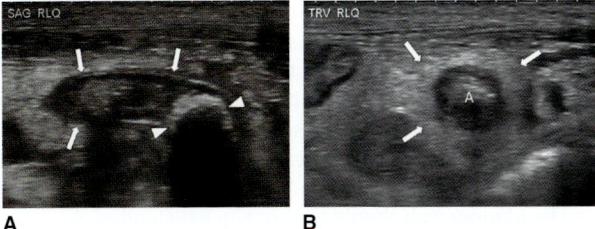

Figure 3-17. Appendicitis. A. Longitudinal sonogram shows a dilated appendix (*arrows*) with an intraluminal hyperechoic focus that causes a posterior acoustic shadow (*arrowheads*). There is increased periappendiceal echogenicity, a useful sign in the diagnosis of acute appendicitis. **B.** Transverse sonogram of the right lower quadrant shows a dilated appendix (*A*) surrounded by hyperechoic soft tissues (*arrows*), a finding that is highly suggestive of acute appendicitis. (Reprinted with permission from Navarro OM, Siegel MJ. Gastrointestinal tract. In: Siegel MJ, ed. *Pediatric Sonography*. 5th ed. Wolters Kluwer; 2019. Figures 10-62 and 10-63.)

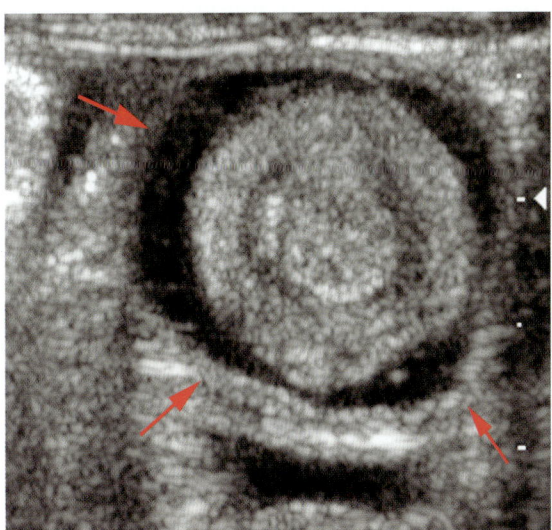

Figure 3-18. Intussusception. The bowel within the intussusception (*arrows*) is thin-walled and echogenic. (Reprinted with permission from John SD, Swischuk LE. Pediatric abdomen and pelvis. In: Brant WE, Helms CA, eds. *Fundamentals of Diagnostic Radiology*. 4th ed. Wolters Kluwer Health/Lippincott Williams & Wilkins; 2012. Figure 51.20.)

- Infants will typically have red currant jelly stool.
  - Intussuscepted bowel diameter ≥3 cm
- Congenital anomalies of the uterus often accompany congenital anomalies of the urinary tract. Therefore, the kidneys may need to be assessed as well.
- Evaluate the urinary bladder carefully, scanning through completely in both sagittal and transverse.
  - The bladder wall should be thin when distended. A thickened bladder wall, especially if the bladder is distended, can be a sign of cystitis (see Fig. 2-36).
  - Assess the lumen of the bladder for debris and stones and the wall for focal areas of thickening which can be evidence of a bladder mass (see Fig. 2-37).
  - Bladder diverticulum may also be discovered (see Fig. 2-38).

IMAGE CORRELATION

- Ovarian torsion on MRI in a pediatric patient **(Fig. 3-19)**
- Acute appendicitis on CT in a pediatric patient **(Fig. 3-20)**
- Dermoids on CT in a pediatric patient **(Fig. 3-21)**

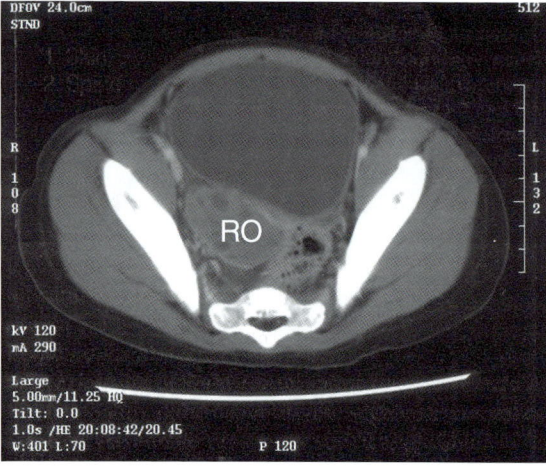

Figure 3-19. Ovarian torsion in an 8-year-old on MRI. MRI reveals an abnormally enlarged right ovary (*RO*). Subsequent laparotomy revealed a right ovarian torsion. (Reprinted with permission from Jacoby J, Heller M. Pelvic ultrasound in the nongravid patient. In: Cosby KS, Kendall JL, eds. *Practical Guide to Emergency Ultrasound*. 2nd ed. Wolters Kluwer Health/Lippincott Williams & Wilkins; 2014. Figure 14.29C.)

Chapter 3. Pediatric Female Pelvic Sonography 103

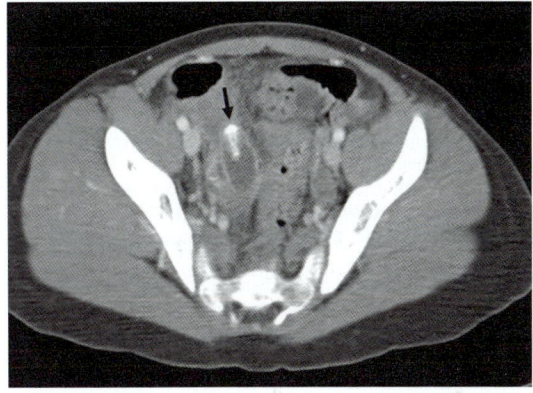

Figure 3-20. Acute appendicitis in a 6-year-old girl. CT scan with contrast demonstrates a dilated appendix (maximum dilation 15 mm) and dense appendicolith obstructing its orifice (*arrow*). Appendicitis without rupture was confirmed at laparoscopy. (Reprinted with permission from Fisher RG, Boyce TG, Correa AG. *Moffet's Pediatric Infectious Diseases: A Problem-Oriented Approach.* 5th ed. Wolters Kluwer; 2017. Figure 12-3.)

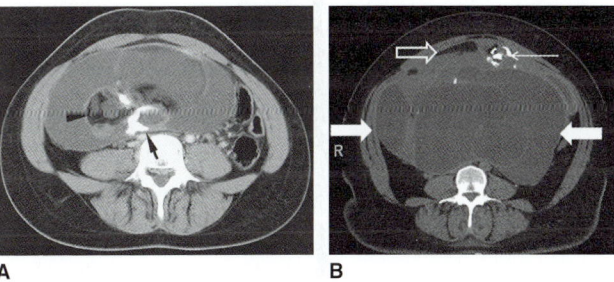

A   **B**

Figure 3-21. Dermoids on CT. A. Benign ovarian teratoma in a 15-year-old girl with pelvic pain. Contrast-enhanced CT shows a well-defined cystic pelvic mass containing calcification (*arrow*) and fat (*arrowhead*). The teratoma contained sebaceous fluid, hair, bone, and fat. B. CT scan of the abdomen shows a classic ovarian mature cystic teratoma as a large heterogeneous pelvic mass containing calcifications (*thin arrow*), fluid components (*closed arrows*), and a fat-fluid level (*open arrow*). (**A.** Reprinted with permission from Siegel MJ, Coley BD. *The Core Curriculum: Pediatric Imaging.* Lippincott Williams & Wilkins; 2006. Figure 10.24. **B.** Reprinted with permission from Klepchick PR, Daffner RH. Obstetric and gynecologic imaging. In: Daffner RH, Hartman MS, eds. *Clinical Radiology: The Essentials.* 4th ed. Wolters Kluwer Health/Lippincott Williams & Wilkins; 2014. Figure 10.21B.)

REFERENCES

1. *AIUM Practice Parameter for the Performance of an Ultrasound Examination of the Female Pelvis*. Accessed September 14, 2023. https://www.aium.org/docs/default-source/resources/guidelines/femalepelvis.pdf?sfvrsn=f5d0c38b_1
2. Siegel MJ, ed. Female pelvis. In: *Pediatric Sonography*. 5th ed. Lippincott Williams & Wilkins; 2018.
3. Stephenson SR, Dmitrieva J. *Diagnostic Medical Sonography: Obstetrics and Gynecology*. 5th ed. Wolters Kluwer; 2023:197–212.
4. Rumack CM, Levine D. *Diagnostic Ultrasound*. 5th ed. Mosby; 2017:1870–1910.
5. Penny SM. The gastrointestinal tract and abdominal wall. In: *Examination Review for Ultrasound: Abdomen & Obstetrics and Gynecology*, 3rd ed. Lippincott Williams & Wilkins; 2022.

CHAPTER 4

Sonohysterography and Three-Dimensional Gynecologic Sonography

INTRODUCTION

This short chapter will provide a brief overview of the use of sonohysterography (SIS), hysterosalpingo-contrast sonography, and three-dimensional sonography as adjuncts to the routine two-dimensional sonogram. It will demonstrate that these techniques can be exceedingly beneficial and provide further useful diagnostic information for the interpreting physician.

AIUM RECOMMENDATIONS FOR THE PERFORMANCE OF A SONOHYSTEROGRAM AND HYSTEROSALPINGO-CONTRAST SONOGRAPHY[1]

- Properly performed SIS and hysterosalpingo-contrast sonography (HyCoSy) can aid in diagnosing uterine abnormalities, including endometrial cavity pathology and fallopian tube pathology.
- SIS may also be referred to as hysterosonography **(Fig. 4-1)**.
  - The primary focus of SIS is to examine the endometrial cavity with more detail by using sterile saline as a contrast agent.
- HyCoSy may also be referred to as sonosalpingography **(Fig. 4-2)**.
  - The primary focus of HyCoSy is to examine the uterine tubes for patency by using sterile saline as a contrast agent.

CONTRAINDICATIONS OF SONOHYSTEROGRAPHY AND HYSTEROSALPINGO-CONTRAST SONOGRAPHY[1]

- These procedures are not to be performed on pregnant patients.
- SIS should not be performed on patients with pelvic infections or unexplained pelvic tenderness.

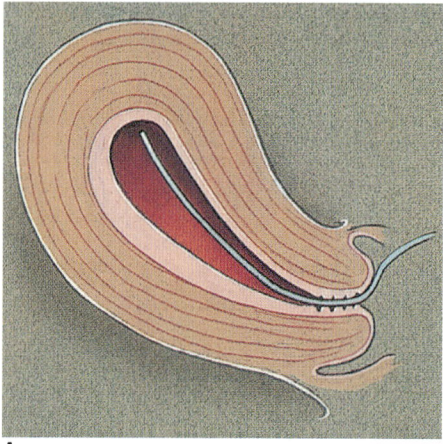

A

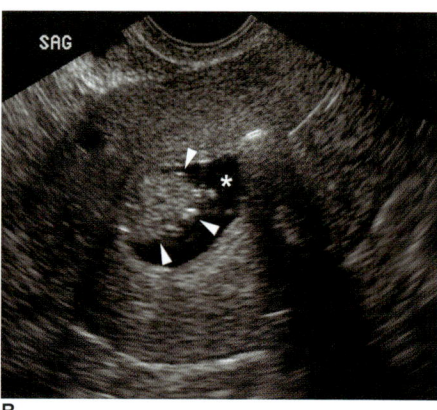

B

Figure 4-1. SIS. **A.** Saline infusion sonography (SIS) utilizes saline that is instilled into the endometrial cavity by a catheter to better visualize masses that are located within or adjacent to the uterine cavity. **B.** This woman with postmenopausal bleeding had a thickened endometrium on conventional sonography. After instillation of saline into the uterine cavity (*asterisk*), a focal polypoid mass (*arrowheads*) is seen, outlined by the fluid. (**A.** Reprinted with permission from Penny SM. *Introduction to Sonography and Patient Care.* 2nd ed. Wolters Kluwer; 2021. Figure 3-32A. **B.** Reprinted with permission from Doubilet PM, Benson CB. *Atlas of Ultrasound in Obstetrics and Gynecology: A Multimedia Reference.* 2nd ed. Wolters Kluwer Health/Lippincott Williams & Wilkins; 2012. Figure 30.1.3.)

Chapter 4. Sonohysterography and Three-Dimensional Gynecologic 107

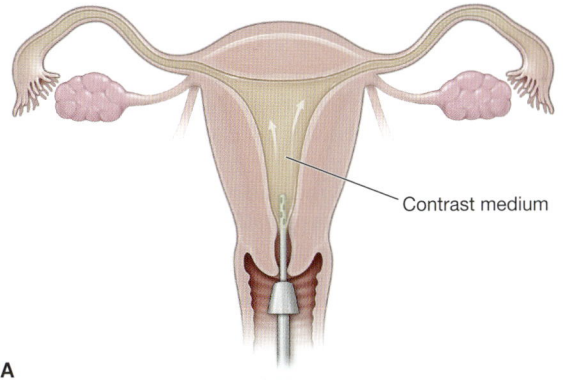

A

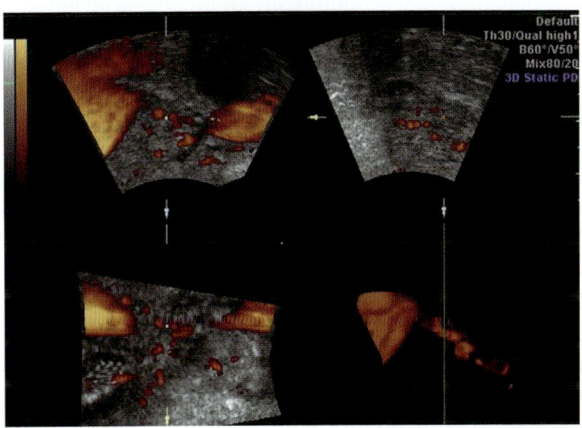

B

Figure 4-2. Hysterosalpingo-contrast sonography. A. Insertion of a contrast medium for a sonohysterosalpingogram. The contrast medium outlines the uterus and fallopian tubes on the sonogram to demonstrate patency. **B.** Fallopian tube color Doppler saline infusion sonohysterosalpingography to assess tubal patency. Three-dimensional (3D) power Doppler scan of uterine cavity after injection of isotonic saline. 3D power Doppler rendering allows simultaneous assessment of the triangular shape of uterine cavity and proximal part of tube (lower right). (**A.** Reprinted with permission from Penny SM. *Examination Review for Ultrasound: Abdomen & Obstetrics and Gynecology.* 3rd ed. Wolters Kluwer; 2023. Figure 20-10A. **B.** Reprinted from Kupesic S, Plavsic BM. 2D and 3D hysterosalpingo-contrast-sonography in the assessment of uterine cavity and tubal patency. *Eur J Obstet Gynecol Reprod Biol.* 2007;133(1):64–69. Copyright © 2006 Elsevier Ireland Ltd. With permission.)

PATIENT PREPARATION FOR SONOHYSTEROGRAPHY AND HYSTEROSALPINGO-CONTRAST SONOGRAPHY[1]

- A pregnancy test may be required if the patient is unsure about her pregnancy state or if otherwise clinically indicated.
- Patients with suspected pelvic infections may require further testing.
- The exam should be performed during the early follicular phase, just after menstrual flow has ended.
- An initial transvaginal sonogram should be performed prior to the SIS.

AIUM PROCEDURE RECOMMENDATIONS FOR SONOHYSTEROGRAPHY[1]

- The patient should be thoroughly informed and an inquiry concerning latex allergy should be conducted.
- The catheter should be flushed with sterile fluid to avoid air instillation within the uterine cavity which can lead to the creation of artifacts.
- The external os should be cleansed and the cervical canal and/or uterine cavity should be catheterized using an aseptic technique.
- Saline is most often utilized as the contrast agent.
- Real-time imaging should be performed while the contrast agent is manually injected slowly into the uterine cavity.

AIUM PROCEDURE RECOMMENDATIONS FOR HYSTEROSALPINGO-CONTRAST SONOGRAPHY[1]

- The setup and procedure for HyCoSy are exactly as noted above for a SIS.
- Typically, a balloon catheter is often used to avoid backflow (Fig. 4-3).
- Commercial devices have been created that can be used for HyCoSy that creates air-infused saline which is instilled into the uterine cavity.

AIUM PROTOCOL IMAGES FOR SONOHYSTEROGRAPHY[1]

- Under real-time imaging, the saline is instilled into the uterine cavity.
- A thorough assessment for asymmetry, irregularities, and focal lesions of the uterine cavity is performed in both sagittal and transverse.

Chapter 4. Sonohysterography and Three-Dimensional Gynecologic 109

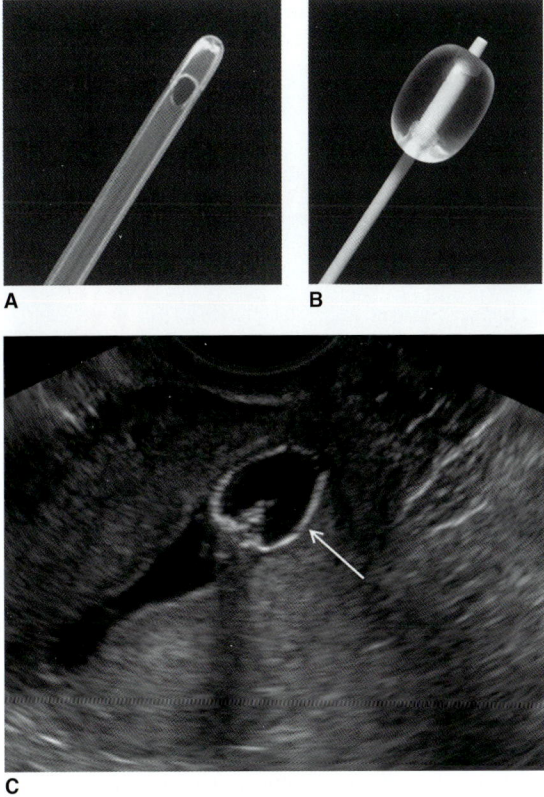

Figure 4-3. Saline infusion sonography catheters. **A.** Insemination-type. **B.** Balloon-type. **C.** Fluid-filled balloon-type catheter (*arrow*) is seen sonographically within the lower uterine segment. (**A.** Reprinted with permission from Scott JR, Gibbs RS, Karlan BY, Haney AF. *Danforth's Obstetrics and Gynecology.* 9th ed. Lippincott Williams & Wilkins; 2003. Figure 27.7. **B.** Reprinted with permission from Scott JR, Gibbs RS, Karlan BY, Haney AF. *Danforth's Obstetrics and Gynecology.* 9th ed. Lippincott Williams & Wilkins; 2003. Figure 27.6. **C.** Reprinted with permission from Barakat RR, Berchuck A, Markman M, Randall ME, eds. *Principles and Practice of Gynecologic Oncology.* 6th ed. Wolters Kluwer Health/Lippincott Williams & Wilkins; 2013. Figure 11.2B.)

- Measurements of the endometrium should be obtained in the sagittal plane. In order to document the true thickness of the endometrium, each layer of the endometrium should be obtained and then added together.

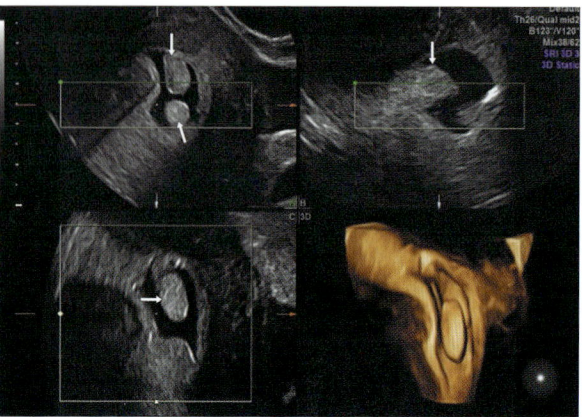

Figure 4-4. SIS and 3D sonography. 3D saline infusion study demonstrating endometrial polyps (*arrows*). (Reprinted with permission from Prince BD, Kari B. 3D Imaging. In: Sanders RC, Hall-Terracciano B, eds. *Clinical Sonography: A Practical Guide*. 5th ed. Wolters Kluwer; 2016. Figure 5-22.)

- Measurements of pathology should be obtained in three orthogonal planes.
- Three-dimensional (3D) images can be beneficial **(Fig. 4-4)**.
- Color or power Doppler can further provide vascular characteristics of identified lesions **(Fig. 4-5)**.

AIUM PROTOCOL IMAGES FOR HYSTEROSALPINGO-CONTRAST SONOGRAPHY[1]

- SIS is typically performed before a HyCoSy.
- Before instilling contrast for HyCoSy a transverse image should be obtained of the cornua of the uterus.
- Under real-time imaging, the saline should be seen to pass through both fallopian tubes.
- The accumulation of contrast in the pelvis is diagnostic for at least one patent tube. Lack of flow into and through a tube should be documented.
- Occasionally, the patient may need to be placed in an oblique position.
- 3D imaging can be helpful as well.

THREE-DIMENSIONAL GYNECOLOGIC SONOGRAPHY[2-4]

- 3D sonography is often used during the procedures discussed in this chapter.

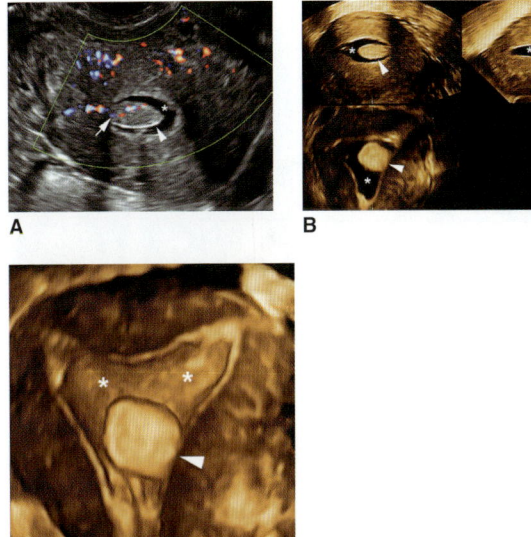

Figure 4-5. SIS, 3D imaging, and Color Doppler. Saline infusion sonohysterogram demonstrating a polyp. A. Color Doppler image from sonohysterogram in a postmenopausal woman with bleeding who had a thickened endometrium on conventional sonography. With saline distending the uterine cavity (*asterisk*), a focal polypoid mass (*arrowhead*) is seen, outlined by the fluid. A feeding vessel (*arrow*) to the polyp is visible. B. 3D rendering showing the polyp (*arrowheads*) surrounded by fluid (*asterisks*) in three orthogonal planes. C. Coronal reconstruction of a 3D volume acquired during SIS showing the uterine cavity distended with fluid (*asterisk*) outlining a large polyp (*arrowhead*).
(Reprinted with permission from Doubilet PM, Benson CB, Benacerraf BR. *Atlas of Ultrasound in Obstetrics and Gynecology: A Multimedia Reference.* 3rd ed. Wolters Kluwer; 2019. Figure 34.1.3.)

- 3D sonography can also be used as an adjunct to a routine pelvic sonogram for various reasons including, but not limited to, the following:
  - Confirmation or identification of suspected congenital uterine anomalies (also referred to as Mullerian duct anomalies) **(Fig. 4-6)**.
    - Mullerian duct anomalies are discussed in Chapter 2 as well.

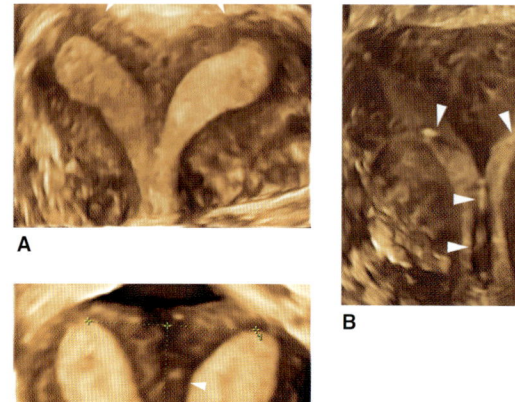

Figure 4-6. 3D uterine variants. A. A bicornuate uterus is demonstrated in this coronal reconstructed image showing indentation of the uterine fundus, splaying the uterus and endometrial cavities into two horns (*arrowheads*). **B.** IUD in a septate uterus. Coronal transvaginal view reconstructed from a 3D volume showing that an IUD (*arrowheads*) was placed in a septate uterus. The septum blocked the full insertion of the IUD, with the shaft remaining in the lower uterine segment. **C.** Subseptate uterus with 3D reconstructed coronal view showing a septum (*arrowheads*) dividing the endometrium from the fundus into the body of the uterus. The depth of the septum is measured as the distance from a line connecting the superior aspects of the endometrium on each side to the inferior part of the septum (calipers). (Reprinted with permission from Doubilet PM, Benson CB, Benacerraf BR. *Atlas of Ultrasound in Obstetrics and Gynecology: A Multimedia Reference.* 3rd ed. Wolters Kluwer; 2019. Figures 29.3.4, 30.7.6, and 29.3.7.)

- Confirmation of correct intrauterine device location or suspected perforation **(Fig. 4-7)**.
- Further analysis of intracavitary or suspected intracavitary abnormalities or pathology abutting the endometrium **(Fig. 4-8)**.

Chapter 4. Sonohysterography and Three-Dimensional Gynecologic   113

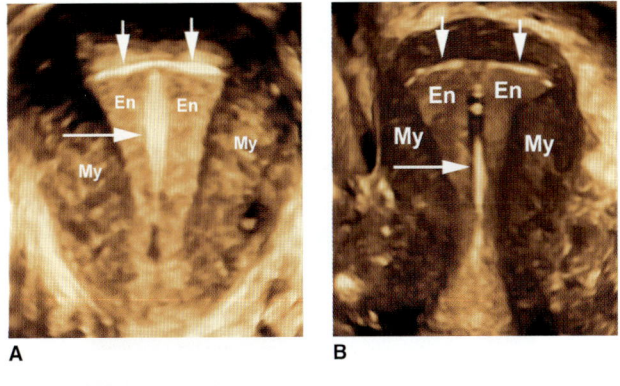

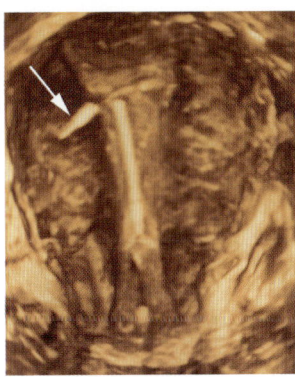

Figure 4-7. Intrauterine device (IUD) on three-dimensional (3D) ultrasound. A, B. Coronal planes of the uterus reconstructed from transvaginal 3D volumes in two patients, each displaying the shaft (*long arrow*) and arms (*short arrows*) of a normally positioned IUD. The entire IUD lies within the endometrium (En), which is brighter than the surrounding myometrium (My). The IUD appears brighter in A than B, with the difference in brightness due to different IUD types. C. Perforation of an IUD out of the endometrium (*arrow*). (Reprinted with permission from Doubilet PM, Benson CB, Benacerraf BR. *Atlas of Ultrasound in Obstetrics and Gynecology: A Multimedia Reference.* 3rd ed. Wolters Kluwer; 2019. Figures 30.7.2 and 30.7.4.)

- The ovaries may be analyzed with 3D sonography as well, especially when assessing ovarian follicles or for polycystic ovary disease (**Fig. 4-9** and **Fig. 4-10**).

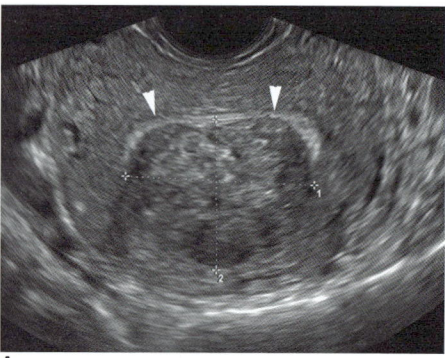

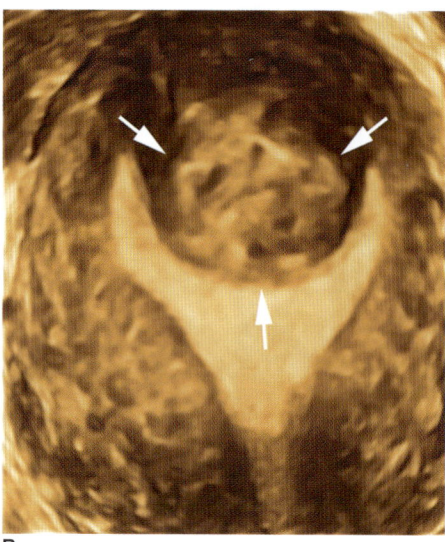

Figure 4-8. 3D ultrasound of a submucosal fibroid. A. Transverse transvaginal view of the uterus demonstrates a fibroid (calipers) indenting the endometrium (*arrowheads*). B. Coronal image of uterus reconstructed from 3D volume shows that the fibroid (*arrows*) is submucosal, projecting into the endometrium. The 3D image demonstrates the location of the fibroid with respect to the endometrium more precisely than the 2D image. (Reprinted with permission from Doubilet PM, Benson CB, Benacerraf BR. *Atlas of Ultrasound in Obstetrics and Gynecology: A Multimedia Reference.* 3rd ed. Wolters Kluwer; 2019. Figure 29.1.10.)

Chapter 4. Sonohysterography and Three-Dimensional Gynecologic 115

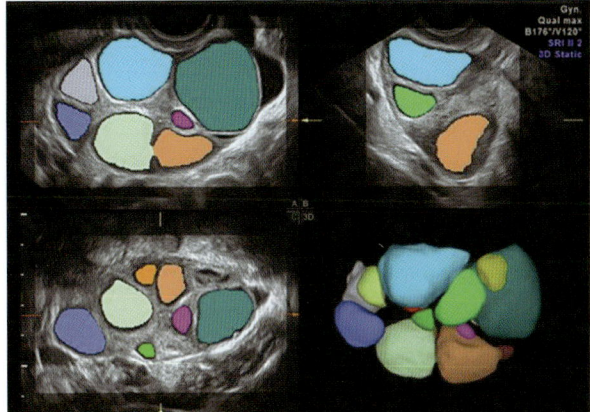

Figure 4-9. 3D ultrasound of the hyperstimulated ovary after ovulation induction. The ovary is enlarged and filled with numerous follicles that are coded in different colors. (Reprinted with permission from Kupesic SP, Turner T. Normal anatomy of the female pelvis. In: Stephenson SR, ed. *Diagnostic Medical Sonography: Obstetrics & Gynecology*. 3rd ed. Wolters Kluwer Health/Lippincott Williams & Wilkins; 2012. Figure 5-78.)

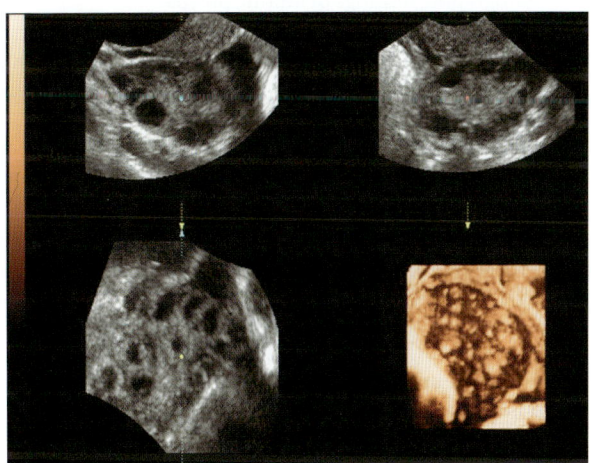

Figure 4-10. General pattern of polycystic ovary as seen by 3D ultrasound. (Reprinted with permission from Kupesic SP, Turner T. Normal anatomy of the female pelvis. In: Stephenson SR, ed. *Diagnostic Medical Sonography: Obstetrics & Gynecology*. 3rd ed. Wolters Kluwer Health/Lippincott Williams & Wilkins; 2012. Figure 5-79.)

ESSENTIAL PATHOLOGY NOTED ON SONOHYSTEROGRAPHY

- Uterine adhesions[4,5]
  - Uterine adhesions or synechiae can clearly be noted with SIS.
  - They are often associated with Asherman syndrome.
  - Asherman syndrome
    - Clinical symptoms of Asherman syndrome
      - History of dilatation and curettage, uterine trauma, or uterine surgery
      - Recurrent pregnancy loss
      - Amenorrhea or hypomenorrhea
    - Sonographic findings of Asherman syndrome
      - Echogenic bands traversing the distended endometrium with SIS (Fig. 4-11)
- Uterine polyps[4,5]
  - Uterine polyps can be clearly delineated with SIS.
  - Clinical findings of uterine polyps
    - Intermenstrual bleeding
    - Possible infertility
  - Sonographic findings of uterine polyps
    - Hyperechoic polypoid mass originating from the endometrial lining and projecting into the fluid-filled uterine cavity (Fig. 4-12)
- Uterine myoma (fibroid)[4,5]
  - Often fibroids located within the uterine cavity or those that have a submucosal location can be better delineated with SIS.
  - Clinical findings of uterine fibroid
    - Uterine enlargement
    - Dysmenorrhea
    - Menometrorrhagia
    - Pelvic pain
    - Dyspareunia
    - Boggy, tender uterus
  - Sonographic findings of uterine fibroids
    - Solid, heterogeneous, or hypoechoic mass within the myometrium
    - Distortion of the normal uterine contour
    - Ill-defined margins between the myometrium and endometrium

Chapter 4. Sonohysterography and Three-Dimensional Gynecologic 117

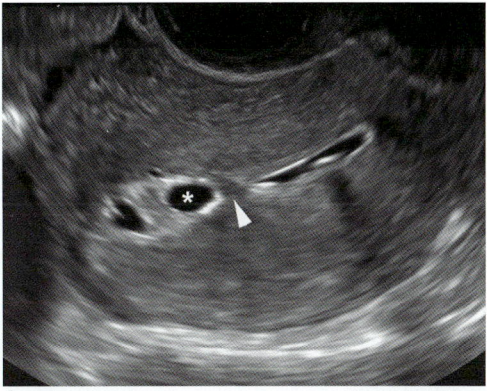

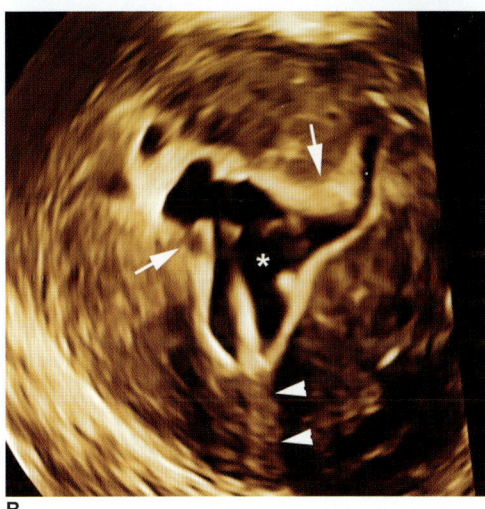

Figure 4-11. SIS of Asherman syndrome. A. Sagittal image of the uterus during a saline infusion sonohysterography (SIS) showing poor dispensability of the cavity with fluid (*asterisk*) and an adhesion (*arrowhead*) interrupting the endometrial echo. **B.** Three-dimensional reconstructed coronal view during the SIS with the catheter (*arrowheads*) in the lower uterine segment and fluid in the cavity (*asterisk*) showing marked distortion of the cavity (*arrows*) from multiple adhesions. (Reprinted with permission from Doubilet PM, Benson CB, Benacerraf BR. *Atlas of Ultrasound in Obstetrics and Gynecology: A Multimedia Reference.* 3rd ed. Wolters Kluwer; 2019. Figure 30.4.2.)

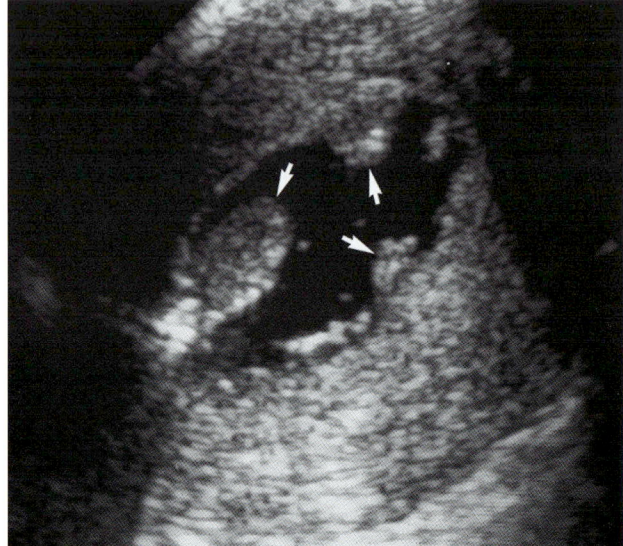

Figure 4-12. SIS and multiple endometrial polyps. After the instillation of saline, multiple polyps (*arrows*) are seen within the uterine cavity and are clearly outlined by the saline. SIS, saline infusion sonohysterography. (Reprinted with permission from Penny SM. *Examination Review for Ultrasound: Abdomen & Obstetrics and Gynecology*. 2nd ed. Wolters Kluwer; 2018. Figure 20-8.)

- Intracavitary fibroids are located within the uterine cavity and will be highlighted by the fluid during an SIS **(Fig. 4-13)**
- Submucosal fibroids will abut and distort the endometrium (see Fig. 4-13)
* Endometrial hyperplasia[4,5]
  * Clinical findings of endometrial hyperplasia
    - Abnormal uterine bleeding
    - Polycystic ovary syndrome
    - Obesity
    - Tamoxifen therapy
  * Sonographic findings of endometrial hyperplasia
    - Thickened echogenic endometrium
    - Cystic spaces within the thickened endometrium can often be better imaged with SIS **(Fig. 4-14)**

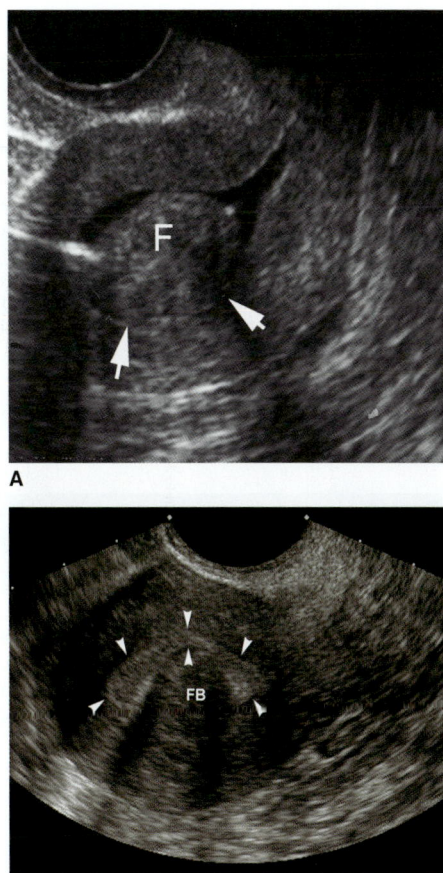

Figure 4-13. SIS and uterine myoma. **A.** Large posterior intracavitary fibroid (*F*) is outlined by saline. Note the anechoic contents with an echogenic rim typical of a myoma. The fibroid extends into the myometrium (*arrows*). **B.** Though not an SIS image, this image does demonstrate the position of a submucosal fibroid (*FB*) as it abuts the endometrium (*arrowhead*). (**A.** Reprinted with permission from Sanders RC. Vaginal bleeding with negative pregnancy test. In: Sanders RC, Hall-Terracciano B, eds. *Clinical Sonography: A Practical Guide*. 5th ed. Wolters Kluwer; 2016. Figure 19-4. **B.** Reprinted with permission from Doubilet PM, Benson CB. *Atlas of Ultrasound in Obstetrics and Gynecology: A Multimedia Reference*. 2nd ed. Wolters Kluwer Health/Lippincott Williams & Wilkins; 2012. Figure 26.1.2.)

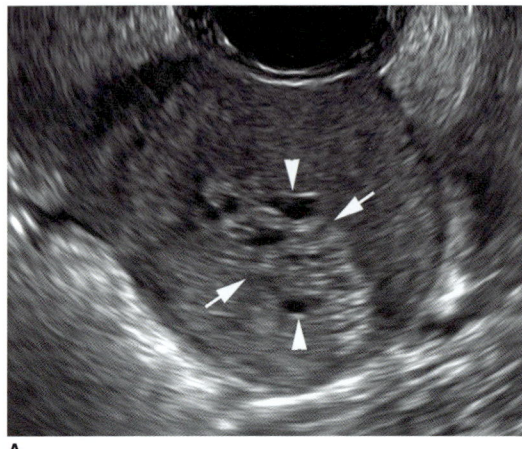

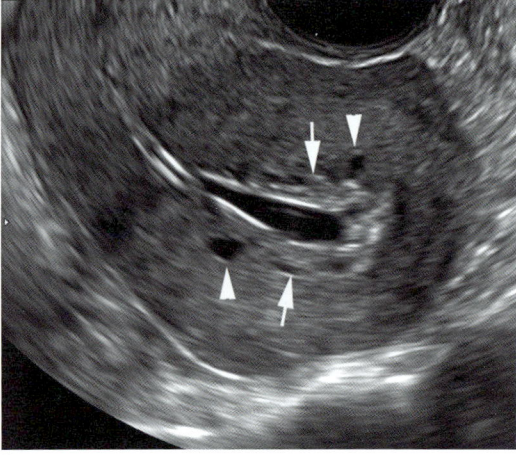

Figure 4-14. Endometrial hyperplasia caused by tamoxifen therapy. A. Transverse view of the uterus of a patient on tamoxifen showing a thickened endometrium (*arrows*) centrally containing multiple small cysts. In addition, several subendometrial cysts (*arrowheads*) are visible at the endometrial–myometrial junction. **B.** Sonohysterography shows uniform endometrial thickening (*arrows*) and several subendometrial cysts (*arrowheads*). (Reprinted with permission from Doubilet PM, Benson CB, Benacerraf BR. *Atlas of Ultrasound in Obstetrics and Gynecology: A Multimedia Reference.* 3rd ed. Wolters Kluwer; 2019. Figure 30.2.3.)

REFERENCES

1. AIUM. *Practice Parameters for the Performance of Sonohysterography and Hysterosalpingo-Contrast Sonography*. Accessed on September 14, 2023. https://www.aium.org/docs/default-source/resources/guidelines/sono-hysterography.pdf?sfvrsn=423541da_1
2. Abd elsalam SM, Abd elmegeed NE, Said AHM, Sayed MAE. Role of three-dimensional transvaginal sonography compared with magnetic resonance imaging in diagnosis of Mullerian duct anomalies. *Egypt J Radiol Nucl Med*. 2020;51(1):NA.
3. Grigore M, Popovici R, Himiniuc LM, et al. The added value of three-dimensional ultrasonography in uterine pathology. *Exp Ther Med*. 2021; 22(5):NA.
4. Douilet PM, Benson CB. *Atlas of Ultrasound in Obstetrics and Gynecology*. 2nd ed. Wolters Kluwer; 2012:412–415.
5. Penny SM. *Examination Review for Ultrasound: Abdomen & Obstetrics and Gynecology*. 3rd ed. Wolters Kluwer; 2022: Section II.

Overview of Obstetric Sonography

Obstetric Sonography — SECTION 2 — CHAPTER 5

INTRODUCTION

This chapter will provide an overview of sonography in obstetrics. American Institute of Ultrasound in Medicine indications for the standard and detailed trimester exams are also provided. General sonographic terminology, patient positioning, special considerations for the pregnant patient, and common sonographic artifacts are also offered.

AIUM INDICATIONS FOR A STANDARD FIRST-TRIMESTER ULTRASOUND EXAMINATION[1]

- First-trimester ultrasound indications include but are not limited to:
  - Confirmation of the presence of an intrauterine pregnancy
  - Confirmation of cardiac activity
  - Estimation of gestational age
  - Diagnosis or evaluation of multiple gestations, including determination of chorionicity
  - Evaluation of a suspected ectopic pregnancy
  - Evaluation of the cause of vaginal bleeding
  - Evaluation of pelvic pain
  - Evaluation of suspected gestational trophoblastic disease
  - Assessment for certain fetal anomalies, such as anencephaly
  - Measurement of the nuchal translucency when part of a screening program for fetal aneuploidy
  - Imaging as an adjunct to chorionic villus sampling, embryo transfer, and localization and removal of an intrauterine device

- Evaluation of maternal pelvic masses and/or uterine abnormalities

AIUM INDICATIONS FOR A DETAILED FIRST-TRIMESTER SONOGRAM (BETWEEN 12 WEEKS 0 DAYS AND 13 WEEKS 6 DAYS)[2]

- First-trimester detailed ultrasound indications include but are not limited to:
  - Previous fetus or child with a congenital, genetic, or chromosomal anomaly
  - Known or suspected fetal abnormality detected by ultrasound in the current pregnancy
  - Fetus at increased risk for a congenital anomaly based on the following:
    - Maternal age of 35 years or older at delivery
    - Maternal pregestational diabetes
    - Pregnancy conceived via in vitro fertilization
    - Multiple gestations
    - Teratogen exposure
    - Enlarged nuchal translucency
    - Positive screening test results for aneuploidy, including cell-free DNA screening and serum-only or combined first-trimester screening
  - Other conditions possibly affecting the pregnancy/fetus, including:
    - Maternal body mass index of 30 kg/m^2 or higher
    - Placental implantation covering the internal cervical os under a cesarean scar site or cesarean scar pregnancy diagnosed in index gestation

AIUM INDICATIONS FOR A STANDARD SECOND- AND THIRD-TRIMESTER ULTRASOUND EXAMINATION[1]

- These examinations are commonly performed to assess fetal anatomy and biometry.
- Other indications include but are not limited to:
  - Screening for fetal anomalies
  - Evaluation of fetal anatomy
  - Estimation of gestational age
  - Evaluation of suspected multiple gestation
  - Evaluation of cervical length
  - Evaluation of fetal growth

- Evaluation of a significant discrepancy between uterine size and clinical dates
- Determination of fetal presentation
- Evaluation of fetal well-being
- Suspected amniotic fluid abnormalities
- Evaluation of premature rupture of membranes and/or premature labor
- Evaluation of vaginal bleeding
- Evaluation of abdominal or pelvic pain
- Suspected placental abruption
- Suspected fetal death
- Follow-up evaluation of a fetal anomaly
- Evaluation/follow-up of placental appearance and location, including suspected placenta previa, vasa previa, and abnormally adherent placenta
- Adjunct to amniocentesis or other procedure
- Adjunct to external cephalic version
- Evaluation of suspected gestational trophoblastic disease
- Evaluation of a pelvic mass
- Suspected uterine anomalies

AIUM INDICATIONS FOR A DETAILED SECOND- AND THIRD-TRIMESTER ULTRASOUND EXAMINATION[3]

- Indications for a detailed fetal anatomic examination include, but are not limited to:
  - Previous fetus or child with a congenital, genetic, or chromosomal abnormality
  - Known or suspected fetal anomaly or known or suspected fetal growth restriction in the current pregnancy
  - Fetus at increased risk for a congenital anomaly, such as the following:
    - Maternal pregestational diabetes or gestational diabetes diagnosed before 24 weeks' gestation
    - Pregnancy conceived via assisted reproductive technology
    - Maternal body mass index of 30 kg/m^2 or higher
    - Multiple gestations
    - Abnormal maternal serum results
    - Teratogen exposure
    - First-trimester nuchal translucency measurement of 3.0 mm or greater

- Fetus at increased risk for a genetic or chromosomal abnormality, such as the following:
  - Parental carrier of a chromosomal or genetic abnormality
  - Maternal age of 35 years or older at delivery
  - Positive screening test results for aneuploidy
  - Aneuploidy marker noted on an ultrasound examination
  - First-trimester nuchal translucency measurement of 3.0 mm or greater
- Other conditions affecting the fetus, including the following:
  - Congenital infections
  - Maternal drug use
  - Alloimmunization
  - Oligohydramnios
  - Polyhydramnios
- Suspected placenta accreta spectrum or risk factors for placenta accreta spectrum such as placenta previa in the third trimester or a placenta overlying a prior cesarean scar site

EQUIPMENT SELECTION AND QUALITY CONTROL[1]

- Ultrasound equipment inherently varies between institutions.
- It is the institution's obligation to offer high-quality sonographic examinations, and therefore these providers should supply equipment that balances cost-effectiveness with state-of-the-art features for their sonographic practitioners to utilize.
- Obstetric sonograms should be conducted with real-time scanners, which confirm the presence of fetal life through observation of cardiac activity and active motion, using a transabdominal and/or transvaginal approach as the exam necessitates.
- A ≥3-MHz abdominal transducer will likely allow sufficient penetration in most patients while providing adequate resolution.
- A transvaginal transducer will likely provide superior resolution during early pregnancy and offer an optimal resolution of smaller structures that may not be seen clearly via the transabdominal

route. Transvaginal imaging is also the most accurate manner to assess the gravid cervix.
- Both the institution and sonographic practitioner should be aware of the potential musculoskeletal injuries that can result from improper equipment or poor scanning practices and should work together to prevent such injuries.

THE ALARA PRINCIPLE[4]

- The lowest possible ultrasound exposure setting should be used to obtain the necessary diagnostic information, and thus the as low as reasonably achievable (ALARA) principle should be practiced. Therefore, spectral Doppler ultrasound should not be used unless clinically indicated.
- A thermal index for soft tissue (TIs) should be used before 10 weeks gestation, and a thermal index for bone (TIb) should be used at or after 10 weeks gestation when bone ossification is evident.
- All obstetric sonograms should begin at a displayed TI of 0.7 because the total duration of a sonographic examination during pregnancy cannot be known in advance.
- The quality of a sonographic image is strongly dependent on the functionality of the ultrasound transducer used to acquire it.
- A quality control system and maintenance program should be in place.
- Regular assessment of the machine and the operation of the transducers is critical for optimal patient care.
- Quality control and improvement, safety, infection control, patient education, and equipment performance monitoring should be developed and implemented in accordance with the AIUM Standards and Guidelines for the Accreditation of Ultrasound Practices found at https://www.aium.org/accreditation/accreditation.aspx

THE TRIMESTERS AND FUNDAL HEIGHT[5]

- First trimester—conception to 12 weeks (some institutions may use up to 14 weeks) gestational age **(Fig. 5-1)**
- Second trimester—12 (to 14 weeks) up to 24 weeks (some institutions may use 28 weeks) gestational age
- Third trimester—24 weeks (to 28 weeks) up until delivery

Trimester and Fetal Development

The time from the first day of the last menstrual period to the end of a full-term pregnancy is divided into three segments called trimesters. During each trimester, a woman's body undergoes substantial changes as the fetus develops.

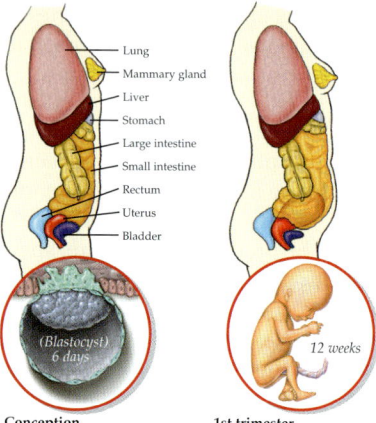

Conception

In the days immediately following conception, there is little change in the appearance of the body or position of organs.

1st trimester

(1st – 12th week)
The uterus begins to enlarge and press up into the area of the small intestine. The breasts enlarge slightly.

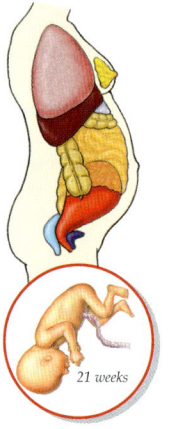

2nd trimester

(13th – 24th week)
The uterus continues to enlarge and press upward toward the small intestine, making sitting less comfortable and urination more frequent.

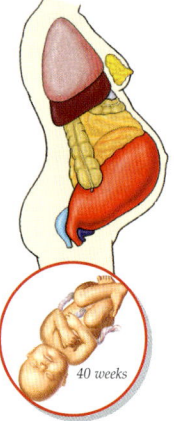

3rd trimester

(25th – 40th week)
During this stage, the uterus presses down on the bladder, and the upward expansion of the uterus on the intestines puts pressure on the stomach, liver and lungs.

Figure 5-1. Trimesters and fetal development. (Anatomical Chart Company. *Pregnancy and Birth Anatomical Chart.* Wolters Kluwer; 2008.)

- Birth weeks
  - A newborn born before 24 weeks is considered previable.
  - A newborn born between 24 weeks and 37 weeks is preterm.
  - A newborn born between 37 weeks and 42 weeks is term.
  - A newborn born after 42 weeks is post-term.
- Fundal height
  - The obstetric physician will typically measure from the pubic symphysis to the palpable, superior part of the fundus of the uterus, which yields a fundal height measurement that correlates with a given gestation **(Fig. 5-2)**.

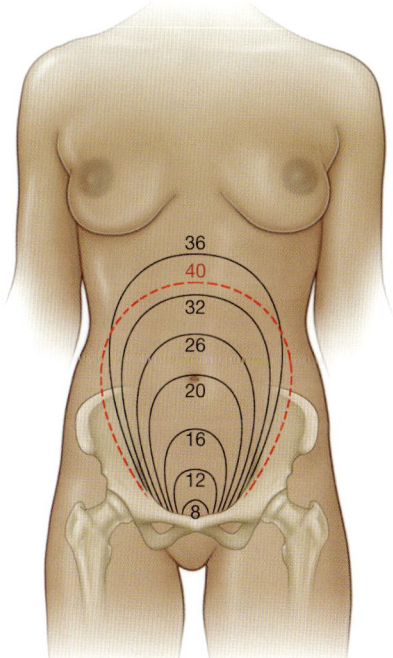

Figure 5-2. Fundal height. A common gestational measurement obtained by the obstetric physician is the fundal height, which is obtained from the superior aspect of the pubic symphysis to the fundus of the uterus. (Reprinted with permission from Casanova R, Goepfert AR, Hueppchen NA, Weiss PM, Connolly A; American College of Obstetricians and Gynecologists. *Beckmann and Ling's Obstetrics and Gynecology.* 9th ed. Wolters Kluwer; 2024. Figure 6.1.)

- A fundal height that does not match the suspected gestational age may result in an obstetric sonogram.

COMMON CLINICAL OBSTETRIC TERMS[6]

- Sonographic terms and common gynecologic artifacts can be found in Chapter 1 of this text.
- Common clinical obstetric terms are provided in Table 5-1.

Table 5-1 OBSTETRIC TERMS AND A BRIEF EXPLANATION

OBSTETRIC TERMS	EXPLANATION
Abortion (also known as a miscarriage)	Complete or partial expulsion of the conceptus • Threatened abortion—vaginal bleeding before 20 weeks gestation with a closed cervix • Complete abortion—all products of conception expelled • Incomplete abortion—part of the products of conception expelled • Missed abortion—fetal demise with a retained fetus • Inevitable abortion—vaginal bleeding with a dilated cervix
Amenorrhea	Absence of menstruation
Aneuploidy	A condition of having an abnormal number of chromosomes
Assisted reproductive therapy	Techniques used to treat infertility
Discriminatory zone	Level of human chorionic gonadotropin (hCG) beyond which an intrauterine pregnancy should be seen with sonography
Blighted ovum	When there is no evidence of a fetal pole or yolk sac within a gestational sac at the expected time; also referred to as an anembryonic gestation
Dyschezia	Painful defecation
Dysmenorrhea	Painful or difficult menses

Table 5-1	OBSTETRIC TERMS AND A BRIEF EXPLANATION (*Continued*)
OBSTETRIC TERMS	**EXPLANATION**
Dyspareunia	Painful intercourse
Embryonic (fetal) demise	Death of an embryo or fetus
Eclampsia	A condition that follows preeclampsia in which uncontrollable hypertension and proteinuria can lead to convulsion, and possible maternal and/or fetal death
Ectopic pregnancy	A pregnancy located anywhere other than the endometrium (e.g., tubal pregnancy, cervical pregnancy, abdominal pregnancy, etc.)
Estimated date of confinement	The "due date" of the pregnancy based on last menstrual period or sonographic measurements.
Fetal karyotyping	An analysis of fetal chromosomes that provides the morphology and number of chromosomes
Fetal lie	Answers the question if the fetus is in the longitudinal or transverse lie
Fetal presentation	Answers the question if the fetus is in the cephalic (head down) or breech (head up) position in relationship to the internal os
Gestational or menstrual age	Age of the pregnancy based on the first day of the last menstrual cycle
Gestational diabetes	Diabetes associated with pregnancy
Gestational trophoblastic disease (GTD)	Group of disorders associated with abnormal combination of male and female gametes • Hydatidiform molar pregnancy—can be a complete or partial mole (contains fetus) • Invasive molar pregnancy—invades into the uterus • Choriocarcinoma—malignant form of GTD
Gravida (gravidity)	Refers to the number of pregnancies

(*continued*)

Table 5-1: OBSTETRIC TERMS AND A BRIEF EXPLANATION (*Continued*)

OBSTETRIC TERMS	EXPLANATION
Hirsutism	Excessive hair growth in women in areas where hair growth is normally negligible
Hyperemesis gravidarum	Excessive vomiting during pregnancy
Infertility	The inability to conceive after 12 months of intercourse
Intrauterine device (IUD or IUCD)	Form of birth control in which a small device is placed within the endometrium to prevent pregnancy
Intrauterine growth restriction (IUGR)	A fetus that is below the 10th percentile for gestational age
Macrosomia	Estimated fetal weight greater than the 90th percentile
Menometrorrhagia	Abnormal heavy and prolonged menstruation
Metrorrhagia	Intermenstrual bleeding
Multigravida	Having had more than one pregnancy
Neural tube defects	A group of developmental abnormalities that involve the brain and spine
Nulligravida	Never been pregnancy
Para (parity)	Refers to the number of pregnancies that led to birth at or beyond 20 weeks gestational age or of an infant weighing more than 500 grams
Preeclampsia	Pregnancy-induced hypertension and proteinuria after 20 weeks
Premature rupture of membranes (PROM)	The rupture of the amniotic sac prior to the onset of labor
Primigravida	First pregnancy
Subchorionic hemorrhage	A bleed between the endometrium and gestational sac
TORCH infections	An acronym that stands for toxoplasmosis, other infections, rubella, cytomegalovirus, and herpes simplex virus

Table 5-1: OBSTETRIC TERMS AND A BRIEF EXPLANATION (*Continued*)

OBSTETRIC TERMS	EXPLANATION
TPAL	Refers to *T*erm, *P*reterm, *A*bortions, and *L*iving children
Trisomy	Having three of a single chromosome (e.g. Trisomy 21, 18, 13, etc.)

COMMON ARTIFACTS IN OBSTETRIC SONOGRAPHY[6]

- Ultrasound artifacts abound during sonographic imaging, with several of them providing useful diagnostic information **(Table 5-2)**.

BASICS OF DOPPLER IN OBSTETRIC SONOGRAPHY[7]

- Color Doppler (CD) and power Doppler (PD)
  - CD allocates varying colors to traveling red blood cells depending upon their velocity and the direction of their flow relative to the location of the transducer.

Table 5-2: COMMON ULTRASOUND ARTIFACTS

ARTIFACT	DESCRIPTION
Acoustic shadowing **(Fig. 5-3)**	Occurs when sound encounters a high attenuator
Comet tail **(Fig. 5-4)**	Type of reverberation artifact caused by small structures
Posterior acoustic enhancement (through transmission) **(Fig. 5-5)**	Occurs when sound encounters a weak attenuator
Refraction	Causes the duplication of anatomy because of the sound beam striking an interface at nonperpendicular angles
Reverberation	Bouncing of the sound beam between two or more interfaces
Ring-down	Caused by sound interacting with small air bubbles causing the bubbles to vibrate

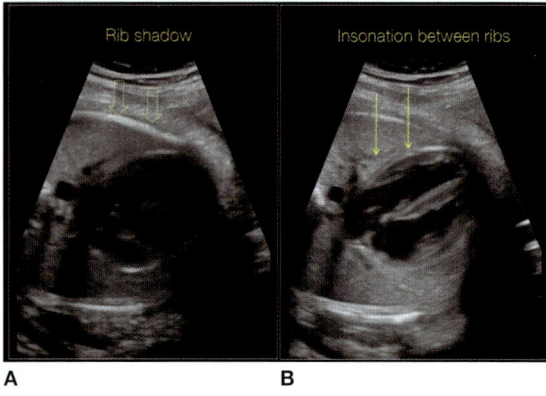

Figure 5-3. Rib shadows. Fetal bones will often produce a distinct acoustic shadow. Four-chamber views of the fetal heart in the same fetus, imaged in A through the ribs (*open arrows*) and in B with slight angulation allowing for the ultrasound beam to scan the heart through the intercostal space (*long arrows*) and between the ribs. Note the degraded image in A, resulting from the effect of rib shadowing on the fetal heart. When imaging the fetal heart, care should be taken to avoid rib shadowing during the late second and third trimesters of pregnancy. (Reprinted with permission from Abuhamad A, Chaoui R. *A Practical Guide to Fetal Echocardiography: Normal and Abnormal Hearts*. 3rd ed. Wolters Kluwer; 2016. Figure 11.8.)

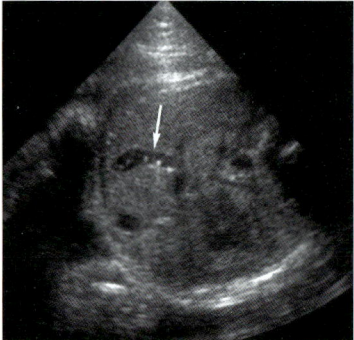

Figure 5-4. Comet tail artifact. Comet tail artifact (*arrow*) is noted emanating from debris and small stones within the fetal gallbladder. (Reprinted with permission from Layton GA. Ultrasound of the abnormal fetal chest, abdomen, and pelvis. In: Stephenson SR, ed. *Diagnostic Medical Sonography: Obstetrics & Gynecology*. 3rd ed. Wolters Kluwer Health/Lippincott Williams & Wilkins; 2012. Figure 21-19.)

Chapter 5. Overview of Obstetric Sonography

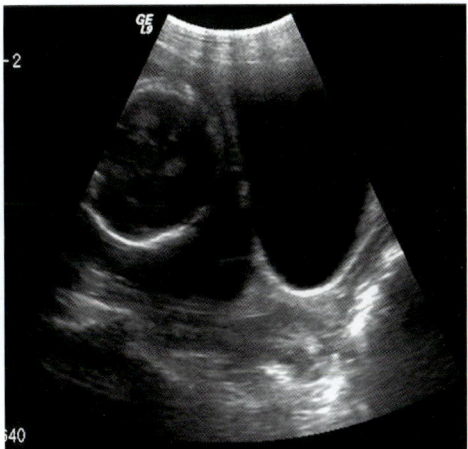

Figure 5-5. Posterior acoustic enhancement. Posterior acoustic enhancement, produced by the maternal urinary bladder, can be used to better visualize the cervix. (Reprinted with permission from Gullett J, Pigott DC. Second and third trimester pregnancy. In: Cosby KS, Kendall JL, eds. *Practical Guide to Emergency Ultrasound*. 2nd ed. Wolters Kluwer Health/Lippincott Williams & Wilkins; 2014. Figure 16.3.)

- For most ultrasound machines, flow toward the transducer is allocated red, while flow away from the transducer is allocated blue.
- Faster speeds are typically depicted with brighter colors and slower velocities are depicted with darker colors.
- Optimal CD imaging is obtained with oblique imaging, whereas a perpendicular orientation will be void of color.
- In obstetric sonographic imaging, CD is often utilized to depict flow direction within the heart, to prove abnormal openings within the heart septa, and to depict flow within the major blood vessels within the fetus. It can also be used to identify the uterine artery during pregnancy, which is useful for evaluating the pregnancy for signs of intrauterine growth restriction and fetal anemia **(Fig. 5-6)**.
- PD is a more sensitive form of CD **(Fig. 5-7)**.
  - PD exploits the amplitude of the Doppler signal.
  - PD does not typically provide flow direction.
  - PD provides evidence of flow in smaller or low-flow vessels.
  - Excessive motion can inhibit the effective use of PD.

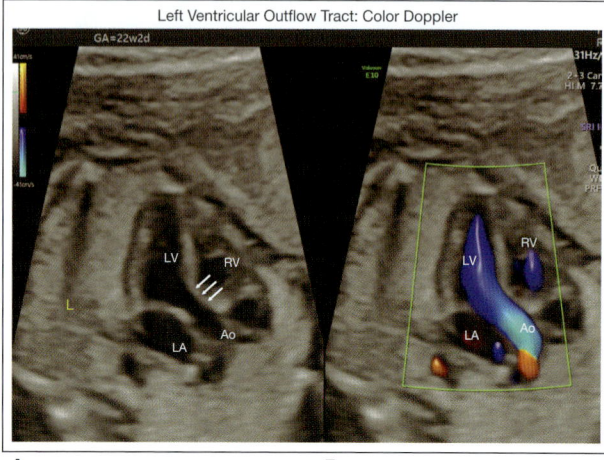

Figure 5-6. Left ventricular outflow tract view of a normal fetus imaged from an apical approach in grayscale (A) and color Doppler (B) using the dual simultaneous display mode. The septo-aortic continuity (*arrows*) is clearly recognized. The dual simultaneous display mode is a practical tool allowing simultaneous visualization of grayscale image along with their corresponding color Doppler image. L, left side of fetus; LA, left atrium; LV, left ventricle; RV, right ventricle.
(Reprinted with permission from Abuhamad A, Chaoui R. *A Practical Guide to Fetal Echocardiography: Normal and Abnormal Hearts*. 4th ed. Wolters Kluwer; 2022. Figure 8.4.)

- Pulsed-wave Doppler (PW)
  - PW is utilized to analyze the flow characteristics of specific fetal structures, with the ability to evaluate a specific area within that structure.
  - The pulsed sound is placed in a sample gate, thus providing Doppler information from the specific selected point within the chosen structure or vessel.
  - PW can provide flow direction.
  - Flow toward the transducer is often displayed above the baseline, while flow away from the transducer is often displayed below the baseline.
  - Be sure to evaluate whether the flow direction control has been inverted before making a final diagnostic conclusion.
  - Flow patterns can also be analyzed with PW. Veins typically have a continuous rhythmic flow pattern in diastole and systole.

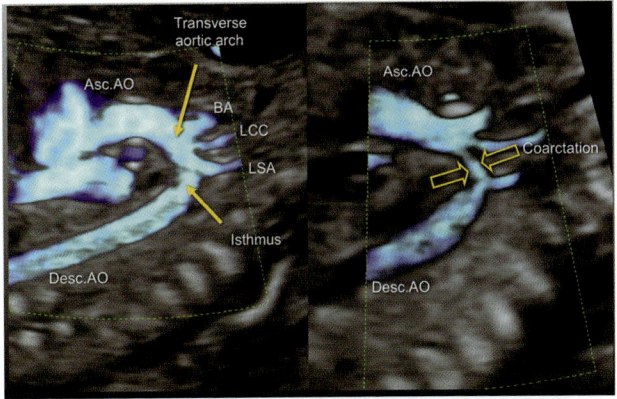

A **B**

Figure 5-7. Power Doppler (PD). PD in a sagittal view of the aortic arch in a normal fetus (A) and in a fetus with coarctation of the aorta (B). In the normal fetus (A), PD displays the ascending aorta (*Asc.AO*), the transverse aortic arch, the aortic isthmus, and the descending aorta (*Desc.AO*). In the fetus with coarctation of the aorta (B), the narrowing in the transverse aortic arch (*open arrows*) is shown between the left common carotid (*LCC*) and the left subclavian artery (*LSA*). BA, brachiocephalic artery. (Reprinted with permission from Abuhamad A, Chaoui R. *A Practical Guide to Fetal Echocardiography: Normal and Abnormal Hearts.* 3rd ed. Wolters Kluwer; 2016. Figure 23.12.)

- Resistive patterns can be depicted with PW.
  - Vessels can be described as having a low-resistant pattern or high-resistant pattern.
  - Low-resistive patterns are depicted by a biphasic systolic peak and a comparatively high level of diastolic flow.
  - High-resistive patterns are depicted by a high systolic peak and low level of diastolic flow.
- In obstetric sonography, PW is often performed on the umbilical artery and fetal heart to gather more information. It may also be used to analyze the circle of Willis within the brain and to investigate the flow within other fetal vascular structures **(Fig. 5-8)**.
- PW and CD are often used in conjunction. For example, they may be used together to depict the resistance within the uterine artery during pregnancy, which is useful for evaluating the pregnancy for signs of intrauterine growth restriction.

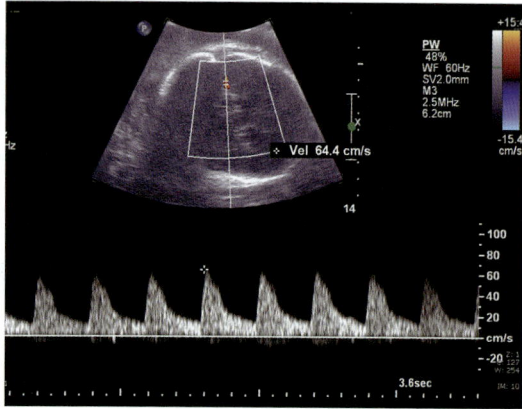

Figure 5-8. Pulsed-wave and color Doppler. Color and spectral Doppler sonography is used to obtain the peak systolic flow of the middle cerebral artery in the evaluation of fetuses at risk for anemia. (Reprinted with permission from Allen LM. Abnormalities of the placenta and umbilical cord. In: Stephenson SR, ed. *Diagnostic Medical Sonography: Obstetrics & Gynecology.* 3rd ed. Wolters Kluwer Health/Lippincott Williams & Wilkins; 2012. Figure 18-19.)

- Motion-mode (M-mode)
  - M-mode is often the preferred method for demonstrating fetal heart motion or fetal heart tones **(Fig. 5-9)**.
  - M-mode can provide beats per minute (bpm).
    - BPM varies with gestational age.
      - Normal fetal heart rate ranges from 120 to 160 bpm.
      - Tachycardia is greater than 180 bpm.
      - Bradycardia is less than 120 bpm.

SUMMARY OF MATERNAL SERUM SCREENING FOR ANEUPLOIDY[6,7]

- Blood (serum) testing of the gravid patient can be useful in the early detection of fetal abnormalities **(Table 5-3)**.
- Maternal serum labs
  - Beta-human chorionic gonadotropin (β-hCG)
    - Produced by the placenta
  - Estriol (UE3)
    - Produced by the placenta
  - Maternal serum alpha-fetoprotein (MSAFP)
    - Produced by the fetal liver

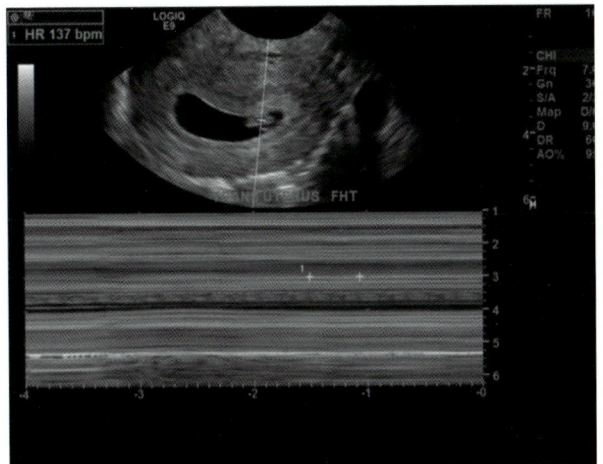

Figure 5-9. M-mode. M-mode demonstrates fetal cardiac activity at a rate of 137 beats per minute, confirming viability. (Reprinted with permission from Kanmaniraja D, Fernandez C, Murakami ME, Cernigliaro JG. Imaging in gynecologic emergencies. In: Benrubi GI, ed. *Handbook of Obstetric and Gynecologic Emergencies.* 5th ed. Wolters Kluwer; 2020. Figure 28.4B.)

Table 5-3. MATERNAL SERUM SCREENING FINDINGS IN THE MOST COMMON CHROMOSOMAL ANOMALIES AND OPEN NEURAL TUBE DEFECTS

FETAL ABNORMALITY	FIRST TRIMESTER (10–13 WEEKS 6 DAYS)	SECOND TRIMESTER (15–22 WEEKS)
Trisomy 21 (Down syndrome)	↓ PAPP-A ↑ β-hCG	↓ MSAFP ↓ UE3 ↑ β-hCG ↑ DIA
Trisomy 18 (Edwards syndrome)	↓ PAPP-A ↓ β-hCG	↓ PAPP-A ↓ β-hCG ↓ UE3
Trisomy 13 (Patau syndrome)	↓ PAPP-A ↓ β-hCG	
Open neural tube defects (Anencephaly, spina bifida, etc.)		↑ MSAFP

- Pregnancy-associated plasma protein A (PAPP-A)
  - Produced by the placenta
- Dimeric inhibin A (DIA)
  - Produced by the corpus luteum and placenta
- Triple screen
  - β-hCG, MSAFP, UE3
- Quadruple screen
  - β-hCG, MSAFP, UE3, PAPP-A
- Cell-free DNA testing (cfDNA)
  - Testing performed to analyze fetal cfDNA found within the maternal blood
  - Highly accurate for detecting Trisomies 21, 18, 13, gender, and some sex-linked disorders like Klinefelter syndrome and Turner syndrome (Monosomy X)

GENERAL CLINICAL HISTORY QUERIES

- Why did your doctor order this sonogram? *Though some patients may be poor historians, others may be capable of providing much beneficial information regarding their current and past clinical records.*
- Have you had an ultrasound for this pregnancy already? *If the patient has had a previous sonogram during the current pregnancy, the findings would be most useful, especially for dating the pregnancy if the patient had a first-trimester sonogram. The earlier measurements of a crown-rump length would be more accurate for dating than a second/third-trimester sonogram. If a report can be provided, prior sonographic findings should be analyzed so that you are completely informed.*
- When was the first day of your last menstrual period? *Obtaining this data can be useful, but do keep in mind that many patients are unsure. If the patient is sure, then the date can be entered into the calculation package of the ultrasound machine. The machine will provide an estimated gestational age.*
- Gravidity and parity score? *Gravidity refers to the number of pregnancies, parity refers to the number of pregnancies that led to birth at or beyond 20 weeks gestational age or of an infant weighing more than 500 g. Some institutions may utilize TPAL (term, preterm, abortions, and living children) to further describe the patient's history.*

- Were there any complications for live births (living children)? *This question is useful, with follow-up questions. For example, if the patient had a miscarriage, one can inquire about how early the miscarriage occurred. If the patient had full-term pregnancies, one can inquire about if there were any complications or congenital abnormalities.*
- If pain, where is your pain? *If possible, have the patient point—with one finger—to the most painful region. Assessing the area of the complaint prior to an obstetric sonogram can provide some beneficial insight. Right lower quadrant can be associated with appendicitis.*
- How long have you had pain? *This question can reveal a chronic or acute situation.*
- Are you having any vaginal bleeding? *Vaginal bleeding in early pregnancy can be a clinical indication of an ectopic pregnancy or early pregnancy failure. In the second/third trimesters, vaginal bleeding may be associated with placenta previa or early delivery.*
- Are you diabetic or have high blood pressure? *Diabetics and those suffering from high blood pressure can have related pregnancy issues. This is a good question to assess the overall health of the patient. For example, patients with pre-existing diabetes are at an increased risk for fetal anomalies. Hypertension during pregnancy can lead to a poor outcome for both the mother and fetus.*
- Are you taking any drugs or using any forms of birth control? *This would be useful to know, especially if the patient has an intrauterine device and is currently pregnant. Patients in this situation are at an increased risk for ectopic pregnancy.*
- Are you taking any fertility drugs? *Fertility drugs can lead to multiple gestations and heterotopic pregnancies. There may also be multiple ovarian follicles discovered sonographically.*
- Is there a family history of chromosomal abnormalities? *This would be useful, especially if the patient has a personal history of children with known chromosomal abnormalities.*
- Have you had any blood work performed that is related to this pregnancy/what are those findings? *Having serum screening results can be exceedingly useful for the sonographer. (See this chapter for more details.)*
- Is there a family history of multiple gestations? *A family history of multiple gestations increases the risk for multiple gestations.*

- Have you had any pelvic/obstetric surgeries, such as a Cesarean section (C-section)? *This is a general question to assess the patient for general pelvic issues and prior complaints that could affect the current pregnancy. A prior C-section increases the risk for placenta previa, placenta accreta spectrum, and vasa-previa.*

PATIENT PREPARATION AND POSITIONING FOR AN OBSTETRIC SONOGRAM

- Patient preparation for a first-trimester pelvic sonogram
  - Transabdominal first-trimester pelvic sonogram
    - The patient's urinary bladder can be distended to displace the bowel and to provide an acoustic window for the visualization of the uterus, ovaries, and adnexa (see Fig. 1-18).
    - Some authors suggest having the patient drink at least enough liquid (possibly 32 ounces of water) to distend the urinary bladder to the point where the entire fundus of the uterus is clearly visualized.
    - The bladder should not be excessively distended. If this occurs, the patient may need to partially empty her bladder.
    - If the patient has a Foley catheter in place, and the transabdominal technique has been deemed crucial for diagnostic purposes, filling the urinary bladder with sterile saline may be employed. This is termed bladder retrofilling. *Note retrofilling the urinary bladder in this manner is a protocol decision that is initiated by the institution, ordering physician, or interpreting physician. The practitioner should be instructed on how to perform this task correctly and safely.*
      - If an abnormality of the urinary bladder is noted, it should be reported as well.
  - Transvaginal first-trimester pelvic examination
    - The patient's urinary bladder should be empty for a transvaginal first-trimester pelvic sonogram.
    - Preparation of transvaginal transducers between patients requires routine mandatory high-level disinfection and the use of a high-quality single-use transducer cover during each examination. (See the heading **Infection Control and Machine Maintenance** in this chapter.)

- The patient, the sonographer, or the physician may introduce the vaginal transducer, preferably under real-time monitoring.
- Consideration of having a chaperone present should be in accordance with local policy.
- Patient positioning
  - Transabdominal obstetric sonogram
    - The patient is typically placed in the supine position (see Fig. 1-20).
  - Transvaginal obstetric sonogram
    - The patient is typically placed in the lithotomy position (see Fig. 1-21).
    - The patient may be placed in the supine position with the hips elevated up from the examining table with the use of a positioning pad as well.

LABELING OF SONOGRAPHIC EXAMINATIONS[8]

- All sonographic images, whether still-frame images or video should include the following:
  - Patient's name and other identifying information (e.g., medical record number)
  - Facility's identification information
  - Date and time of the examination
  - Output display standard (TI and mechanical index)
  - Label the anatomic location and which side of the body, when appropriate
  - Image orientation when appropriate

INFECTION CONTROL AND MACHINE MAINTENANCE[9]

- Infection control
  - Institutional guidelines should be in place for transducer disinfection to reduce the risk of iatrogenic and nosocomial infections.
  - Always follow your facility's established protocol for infection control.
  - The following is a summation of the AIUM's *Guidelines for Cleaning and Preparing External- and Internal-Use Ultrasound Transducers and Equipment Between Patients as well as Safe Handling and Use of Ultrasound Coupling Gel.*

- Transabdominal transducers
  - Preparation of transabdominal transducers between patients requires a low-level disinfection process (see Fig. 1-22).
  - Nonsterile gel is used.
  - No transducer cover is required unless there is contaminated intact skin or nonintact skin, in which case both a cover and sterile gel are recommended.
- Transvaginal transducers
  - Barriers (probe covers) used for transvaginal transducers must be single-use transducer covers that meet the sterility requirements of the procedure (see Fig. 1-23).
  - Use sterile or bacteriostatic gel.
  - Consult the manufacturer's instructions for disinfecting devices.
  - After the procedure, perform high-level disinfection. Commercially available wall or table-top disinfectant units are available for endocavity transducers (see Fig. 1-24).
  - A complete list of Food and Drug Administration (FDA)-cleared liquid sterilants and high-level disinfectants is available online.
  - Rinse to remove disinfectant.
- Equipment maintenance[10]
  - The AIUM provides the *AIUM Routine Quality Assurance of Clinical Ultrasound Equipment version 2.0* here http://aium.s3.amazonaws.com/resourceLibrary/rqa2.pdf
  - Regular interval inspection of equipment and transducers (connector, cable, housing, acoustic lens) is recommended to ensure performance. Imaging with a tissue-mimicking phantom may help reveal imaging degradation.
  - A record of quality assurance activities must be maintained and kept current. The ultrasound equipment must meet all state and federal guidelines and testing must be maintained in good operating condition and undergo routine quality assurance at least once a year or more frequently if problems arise.
  - Always report machine or equipment malfunction to facility management and remove such equipment from use.

ERGONOMICS[11]

- Ergonomics is the scientific study of creating tools and equipment that help humans adapt to the work environment.
- The use of proper ergonomics includes having the proper room design and adjustable equipment to reduce the risk of work-related musculoskeletal disorders (WRMSDs).
- Though a thorough explanation of WRMSDs is beyond the scope of this text, below are a few of the best practices:
  - Take regular breaks or micro-breaks between examinations. Relax muscles throughout the day.
  - Minimize sustained bending, twisting, reaching, lifting, pressure, and awkward positions.
  - Focus on using all your fingers and the palm, a light grip, and apply minimal or no pressure to the probe.
  - Keep your wrist in a neutral position with limited flexion and extension.
  - Use correct body mechanics when moving the patient.
  - Place the patient as close to you as possible to reduce shoulder abduction (<30 degrees). The scanning arm should be in a relaxed position, close to the body with minimal flexion.
  - Use a cable brace or support device for the cable.
  - The neck should be straight, and neck extension should be avoided.
  - Use a height-adjustable scanning table and ultrasound equipment.
  - Stand to scan occasionally and vary scanning positions to work different muscles.

SPECIAL CONSIDERATIONS FOR THE PREGNANT PATIENT DURING SONOGRAPHY[6]

- Ectopic pregnancy emergency situations
  - It is vital for the sonogram of the early pregnancy to be conducted with the patient's clinical history in mind because imaging plays a vital role in the management of ectopic pregnancy **(Fig. 5-10)**.
  - Patients who have an ectopic pregnancy often have the clinical triad of pain, vaginal bleeding, and palpable pelvic mass.
  - Patients who have a ruptured ectopic pregnancy can suffer rapidly from hemorrhagic shock.

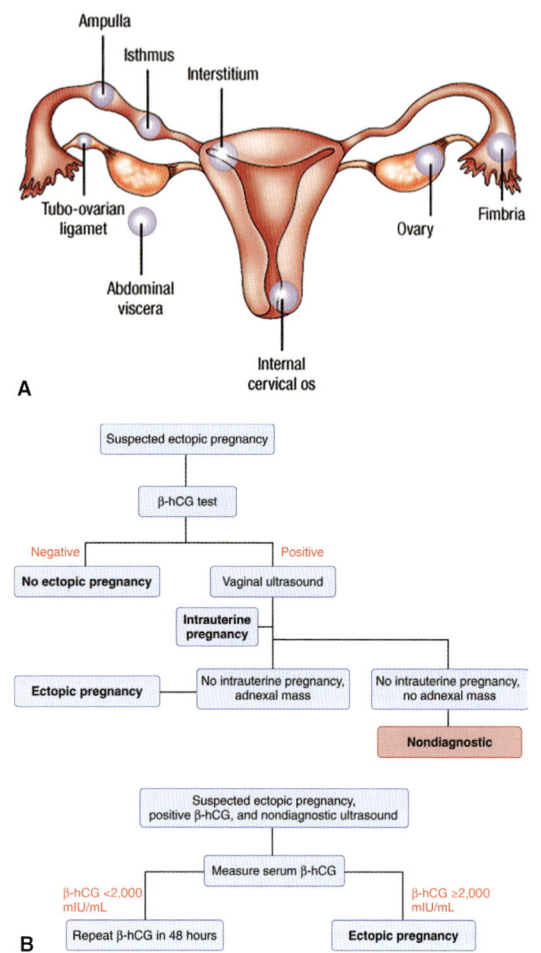

Figure 5-10. Location and the diagnostic management of ectopic pregnancy. **A.** Locations of ectopic pregnancy. The most common location is within the ampulla of the tube. **B.** Diagnostic management of ectopic pregnancy. β-hCG, β-human chorionic gonadotropin; EP, ectopic pregnancy. (**A.** Reprinted with permission from *Health Assessment Made Incredibly Visual!* 2nd ed. Wolters Kluwer Health/Lippincott Williams & Wilkins; 2011:231. **B.** Reprinted with permission from Zamstein O, Sheiner E, Wiznitzer A. Ectopic and heterotopic pregnancies. In: Reece EA, Leguizamón GF, Macones GA, Wiznitzer A, eds. *Clinical Obstetrics: The Fetus & Mother.* 4th ed. Wolters Kluwer; 2022. Algorithm 3.1.)

- Analyze the pelvis for signs of complex fluid which likely represents fluid.
- If a large amount of fluid is noted within the pelvis, a quick analysis of the right upper quadrant for signs of fluid in the right subhepatic space (Morrison pouch) is warranted.
- Supine hypotensive syndrome (aortocaval compression syndrome)
  - The pregnant patient may become uncomfortable during an extended period of scanning and may become lightheaded and have other complaints such as dizziness **(Fig. 5-11)**.
  - If this occurs, she could be suffering from supine hypotensive syndrome, which results from the compressing of the inferior vena cava and abdominal aorta by the enlarged uterus.
  - Stop the examination and place the patient in the left lateral decubitus position to decrease the pressure on the inferior vena cava and abdominal aorta.
  - Monitor the patient closely and summon an emergency response team if needed.

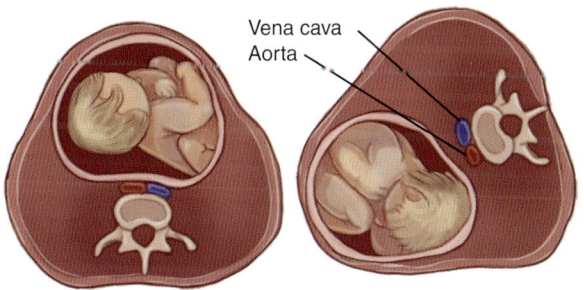

Supine position   Side-lying position

Figure 5-11. Supine hypotensive syndrome. When the pregnant woman lies flat on her back, the weight of the fetus and uterus can compress the aorta and inferior vena cava against the spine. Consequently, the amount of blood returning to the heart is compromised, pressure falls, and supine hypotensive syndrome occurs (image on the left). By placing the patient on her side (image on the right), the pressure is relieved, and the patient should feel better soon.
(Reprinted with permission from Ricci SS. *Essentials of Maternity, Newborn, and Women's Health Nursing.* 4th ed. Wolters Kluwer; 2017. Figure 11.2.)

- Maternal and gestational diabetes
  - A prior history of maternal diabetes increases the risk for fetal complications and fetal anomalies, such as congenital heart disease and other possible devastating structural fetal defects.
  - Gestational diabetes is associated with a large fetus, also referred to as macrosomia.
    - There are also complications for the mother with gestational diabetes, including preterm labor, hypertensive disorders, and an increase in a recurrence of diabetes in the future.
  - Care for women with these conditions varies **(Fig. 5-12)**.
- Preeclampsia and eclampsia
  - Preeclampia is the development of hypertension and proteinuria after 20 weeks gestation **(Fig. 5-13)**.
  - Eclampsia is the occurrence of seizure activity without other identifiable causes other than pregnancy.
- Cervical incompetence—painless dilation of the cervix in the second or early third trimester
  - The cervix should be closely examined during all stages of pregnancy.

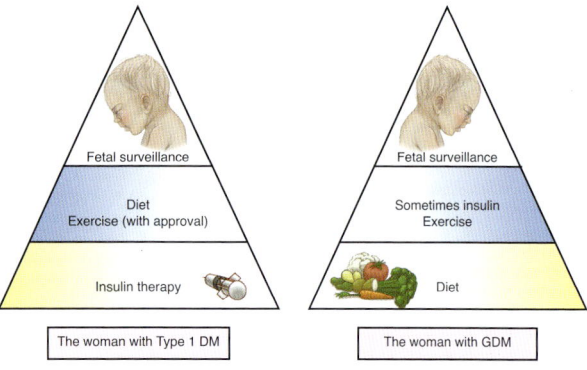

Figure 5-12. Care for patients with pregestational diabetes and gestational diabetes. Treatment overview for diabetes in pregnancy. For women with pregestational type 1 diabetes mellitus, the foundation of glycemic management is insulin therapy along with dietary management, exercise, and fetal surveillance. For the woman who develops gestational diabetes, dietary modification is generally the foundation of treatment. (Reprinted with permission from Ricci SS. *Essentials of Maternity, Newborn, and Women's Health Nursing.* 5th ed. Wolters Kluwer; 2021. Figure 20.1.)

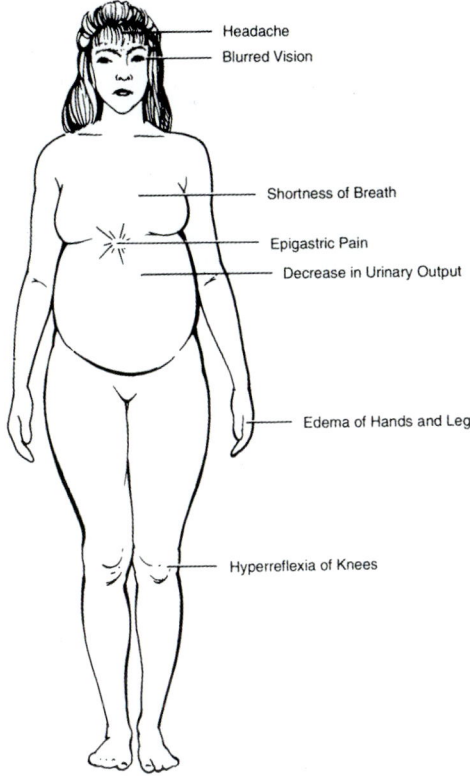

Figure 5-13. Signs and symptoms of preeclampsia. (Reprinted with permission from Sanchez-Ramos L. Hypertensive disorders of pregnancy: preeclampsia/eclampsia. In: Benrubi GI, ed. *Handbook of Obstetric and Gynecologic Emergencies*. 4th ed. Wolters Kluwer Health/Lippincott Williams & Wilkins; 2010. Figure 7.2.)

- Transvaginal is the most accurate manner to assess the cervical length.
    - Transvaginal sonography technique is performed in the typical manner as described in this chapter.
    - Care should be taken to not encounter the cervix.
    - The length of the cervix is obtained from the internal os to the external os **(Fig. 5-14)**.
    - Because the cervix is a dynamic structure, it should be watched for 5 minutes **(Fig. 5-15)**.

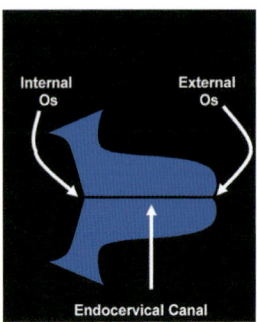 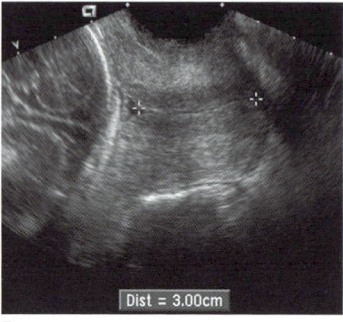

Figure 5-14. Transvaginal cervix imaging. A. Sonographic image and correlated drawing of the endocervical canal. B. Measurement of the cervix (between calipers). (**A.** Reprinted from Gomez R, Galasso M, Romero R, et al. Ultrasonographic examination of the uterine cervix is better than cervical digital examination as a predictor of the likelihood of premature delivery in patients with preterm labor and intact membranes. *Am J Obstet Gynecol.* 1994;171(4):956–964. Copyright © 1994 Elsevier. With permission. **B.** Reprinted with permission from Doubilet PM, Benson CB. *Atlas of Ultrasound in Obstetrics and Gynecology: A Multimedia Reference.* Lippincott Williams & Wilkins; 2003. Figure 3.2-1C.)

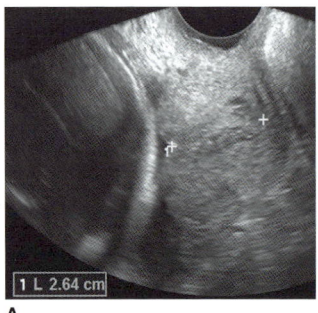 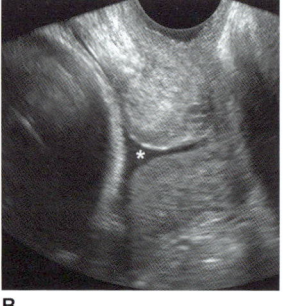

Figure 5-15. Spontaneously changing cervix. A. Sagittal transvaginal view of the cervix demonstrates a cervix measuring 2.64 cm in length (caliper). B. Approximately 20 seconds later, the cervical canal is dilated (*), mainly at the internal os. (Reprinted with permission from Doubilet PM, Benson CB, Benacerraf BR. *Atlas of Ultrasound in Obstetrics and Gynecology: A Multimedia Reference.* 3rd ed. Wolters Kluwer; 2019. Figure 20.1.3.)

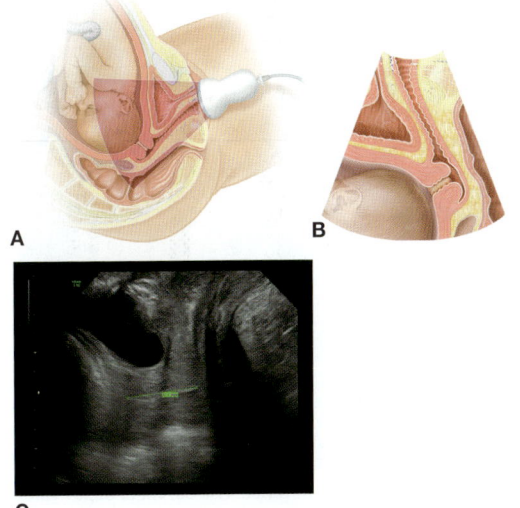

Figure 5-16. Translabial scanning. The transducer is covered and placed in a sagittal plane on the surface of labia (**A**). Schematic of the anatomy in the translabial view (**B**). **C:** The normal cervix in the translabial image measures at least 3 cm on sagittal measurements. (**A** and **B.** Reprinted with permission from Gullett J, Pigott DC. Second and third trimester pregnancy. In: Cosby KS, Kendall JL, eds. *Practical Guide to Emergency Ultrasound.* 2nd ed. Wolters Kluwer Health/Lippincott Williams & Wilkins; 2014. Figure 16.6. **C.** Reprinted with permission from Hernandez-Andrade E, Yeo L, Lo AJ, Hassan SS, Romero R. Ultrasound imaging of the uterine cervix. In: Kline-Fath BM, Bulas DI, Lee W, eds. *Fundamental and Advanced Fetal Imaging: Ultrasound and MRI.* 2nd ed. Wolters Kluwer; 2021. Figure 14.4.)

- Transperineal (translabial) imaging may be used as well to evaluate the cervix.
  - Translabial sonography technique **(Fig. 5-16)**
    - Patient permission must be granted.
    - Utilize a curved or convex transducer.
    - Place sterile lubricant on the transducer face.
    - Place a sterile drape over the transducer.
    - Place the transducer in the sagittal plane, with the index (notch) pointed anterior, against the labia.
    - Measure the internal os to the external os of the cervix.
    - The patient may have to lift her buttocks from the table due to the shadowing of the pubic symphysis.

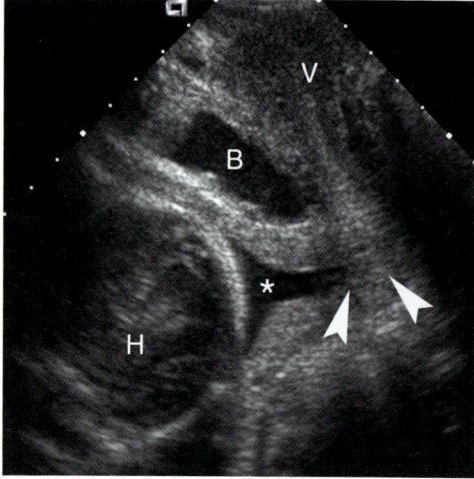

Figure 5-17. Cervical Incompetence. The cervix is best evaluated with a translabial view with the bladder (*B*) empty. The transducer is aimed down the long axis of the vagina (*V*). The cervix, measured between the internal os and the external os (*arrowheads*), is shortened to 9 mm in this patient with a history of multiple spontaneous abortions in the second trimester. The cervix is also dilated, allowing amniotic fluid (*asterisk*) to enter the endocervical canal. The fetal head (*H*) is presenting at the internal cervical os. (Reprinted with permission from Brant WE. Obstetric ultrasound. In: Brant WE, Helms CA, eds. *Fundamentals of Diagnostic Radiology*. 3rd ed. Lippincott Williams & Wilkins; 2007. Figure 38.16.)

- Funneling of the cervix is the result of the premature opening of the internal os of the cervix **(Fig. 5-17)**.
- The membranes will bulge into the cervix as the cervix dilates.
- Patients at risk for an incompetent cervix are those with uterine malformations and those who have a history of pregnancy loss in the second trimester.
- Cervical cerclage is a temporary treatment for cervical incompetence **(Fig. 5-18)**.
- Rh sensitization
  - Rh sensitization, or Rh immunization, occurs when the mother has Rh-negative blood and the fetus has Rh-positive blood.
  - During the first pregnancy, everything progresses normally, though the fetal blood cells cross into the maternal circulation where antibodies are created by the mother.

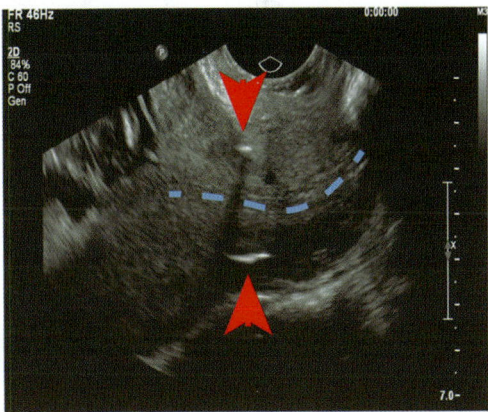

Figure 5-18. Cervical cerclage. Pelvic sonogram following postconceptional cerclage placement. Mersilene is demonstrated by *red arrows*. Resulting cervical length marked with *dotted blue line*.
(Reprinted with permission from Benabou K, Kim S, Ayhan I, Azodi M, Bahtiyar MO. Abdominal cerclage. In: Belfort MA, Shamshirsaz AA, Clark SL, Fox KA, eds. *Operative Techniques in Obstetric Surgery.* Wolters Kluwer; 2023. Tech Figure 2.4.5B.)

- During the second pregnancy, the fetal red blood cells are attacked and destroyed by the mother's white blood cells, resulting in fetal anemia, hepatosplenomegaly, and immune hydrops. This is termed erythroblastosis fetalis **(Fig. 5-19)**.
- Maternal hydronephrosis
  - Hydronephrosis is the dilation of renal collecting system and is very common during pregnancy **(Fig. 5-20)**.
  - The sonographer may be asked to investigate for signs of urolithiasis (renal stones).
  - Stones should produce a shadow, and when CD is applied, the twinkle artifact may be revealed **(Fig. 5-21)**.
- Retained products of conception (RPOC)
  - Prolonged vaginal bleeding after conception or miscarriage could be a sign of RPOC.
    - Sonographic appearance of RPOC
      - Hyperechoic material or mass may be noted within the uterine cavity.
      - Calcifications may be present.
      - CD is useful and will prove that the retained material may indeed be part of the placenta **(Fig. 5-22)**.

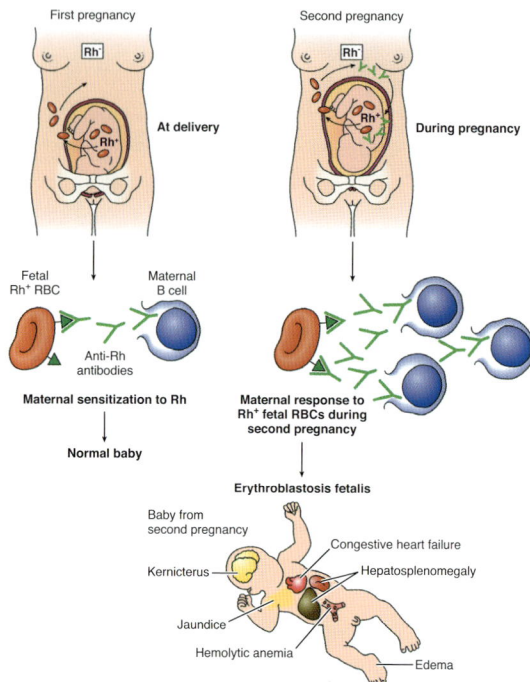

Figure 5-19. Erythroblastosis fetalis is due to maternal fetal Rh incompatibility. Sensitization of the Rh-mother with Rh+ RBCs in the first pregnancy leads to the formation of anti-Rh antibodies. These antibodies cross the placenta and damage the Rh+ fetus in subsequent pregnancies. (Reprinted with permission from Nath JL. *Using Medical Terminology*. 2nd ed. Wolters Kluwer Health/Lippincott Williams & Wilkins; 2013. Figure 10-18.)

- Pelvic masses associated with pregnancy **(Fig. 5-23)**.
  - Hemorrhagic ovarian cysts are blood-filled cysts that may represent the evolution of a corpus luteum of pregnancy.
  - Leiomyoma or fibroids are solid, benign uterine tumors.
    - Fibroids should be noted and measured, as they can grow during pregnancy, and their location can be intramural, submucosal, subserosal, intracavitary, and pedunculated (see Fig. 2-25 and Fig. 2-26).
    - Pedunculated fibroids can mimic adnexal masses, though they are attached by a stalk to the uterus.

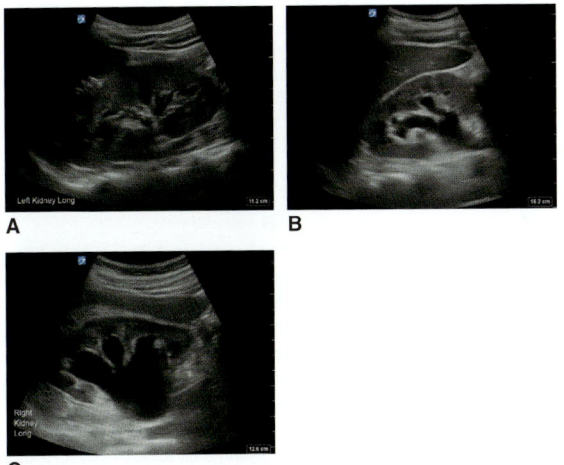

Figure 5-20. Maternal hydronephrosis. Longitudinal planes of kidneys showing different grading of hydronephrosis. **A.** Mild hydronephrosis. **B.** Moderate hydronephrosis. **C.** Marked or hydronephrosis. (Reprinted with permission from Rosario J. Point-of-care. In: Kawamura DM, Nolan TD, eds. *Diagnostic Medical Sonography: Abdomen and Superficial Structures.* 5th ed. Wolters Kluwer; 2022. Figure 25-10.)

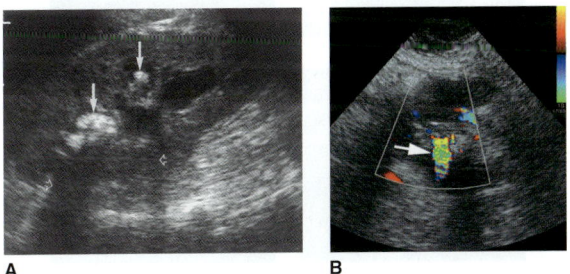

Figure 5-21. Kidney stone appearance with twinkle artifact. A. This longitudinal image of the kidney demonstrates several small hyperechoic structures (*solid arrows*) representing a kidney stone. Acoustic shadowing is seen posterior to the calculi (*arrowheads*). **B.** Color Doppler applied to small stones can reveal the twinkle sign (artifact), which is often seen posterior to kidney stones. (**A.** Reprinted with permission from Brant WE. *The Core Curriculum: Ultrasound.* Lippincott Williams & Wilkins; 2001:110. **B.** Reprinted with permission from Middleton WD, Siegel MJ, Dahiya N. Ultrasound artifacts. In: Siegel MJ, ed. *Pediatric Sonography.* 4th ed. Wolters Kluwer Health/Lippincott Williams & Wilkins; 2011. Figure 2.37.)

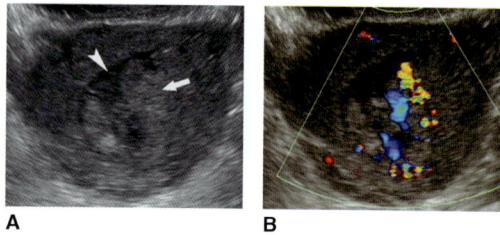

Figure 5-22. Retained products of conception. A. Transverse image of the uterus in a woman with continuing bleeding following a spontaneous abortion reveals echogenic material (*arrow*) representing retained placenta and anechoic material (*arrowhead*) representing blood and clots within the uterine cavity. **B.** Transverse color Doppler image of the uterus in the same patient documents continuing blood flow to the retained placenta. (Reprinted with permission from Brant WE. Obstetric ultrasound. In: Brant WE, Helms CA, eds. *Fundamentals of Diagnostic Radiology*. 4th ed. Wolters Kluwer Health/Lippincott Williams & Wilkins; 2012. Figure 37.12.)

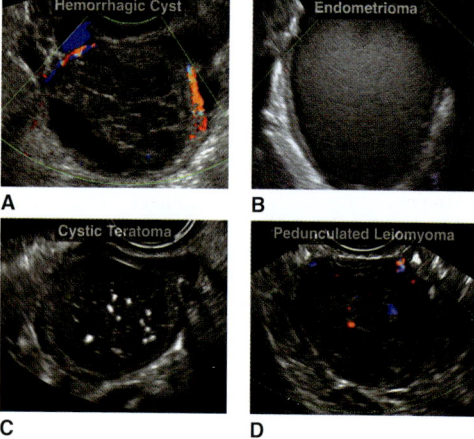

Figure 5-23. Adnexal masses are commonly seen in the first trimester of pregnancy. Hemorrhagic cyst (A) is shown with characteristic reticular pattern and fluid level, endometrioma (B) is shown with unilocular ground-glass appearance, cystic teratoma (C) with echogenic foci from the fat emulsion, and a pedunculated leiomyoma (D) with solid appearance and minimal vascularity on color Doppler. Color Doppler shows no vascular signals within the hemorrhagic cyst and endometrioma. (Reprinted with permission from Abuhamad A, Chaoui R. *First Trimester Ultrasound Diagnosis of Fetal Abnormalities*. Wolters Kluwer; 2018. Figure 5.27.)

- A cystic teratoma, also referred to as a dermoid, are complex masses that may contain teeth, hair, fat, and other tissues.
- An endometrioma is a blood-filled tumor comprised of ectopic endometrial tissue.

REFERENCES

1. AIUM–ACR–ACOG–SMFM–SRU. Practice parameter for the performance of standard diagnostic obstetric ultrasound examinations. *J Ultrasound Med*. 2018;37:E13–E24.
2. AIUM. Practice parameter for the performance of detailed diagnostic obstetric ultrasound examinations between 12 weeks 0 days and 13 weeks 6 days. *J Ultrasound Med*. 2021;40:E1–E16.
3. AIUM. Practice parameter for the performance of detailed second- and third-trimester diagnostic obstetric ultrasound examinations. *J Ultrasound Med*. 2019;38:3093–3100.
4. Prudent Use and Safety of Diagnostic Ultrasound in Pregnancy. Accessed on November 12, 2023. https://www.aium.org/resources/official-statements/view/prudent-use-and-safety-of-diagnostic-ultrasound-in-pregnancy
5. Callahan TL, Caughey AB. *Blueprints Obstetrics & Gynecology*. 6th ed. Wolters Kluwer; 2013:1–12.
6. Penny SM. *Examination Review for Ultrasound: Abdomen & Obstetrics and Gynecology*. 3rd ed. Wolters Kluwer; 2022:11–19 & Section III.
7. Kline-Fath BM, Bulas DI, Lee W. *Fundamental and Advanced Fetal Imaging: Ultrasound and MRI*. 2nd ed. Wolters Kluwer; 2020:1–156.
8. AIUM. Practice parameter for documentation of an ultrasound examination. *J Ultrasound Med*. 2020;39:E1–E4.
9. Guidelines for Cleaning and Preparing External- and Internal- Use Ultrasound Transducers and Equipment Between Patients as Well as Safe Handling and Use of Ultrasound Coupling Gel. Accessed November 12, 2023. https://www.aium.org/resources/official-statements/view/guidelines-for-cleaning-and-preparing-external-and-internal-use-ultrasound-transducers-and-equipment-between-patients-as-well-as-safe-handling-and-use-of-ultrasound-coupling-gel
10. AIUM Routine Quality Assurance of Clinical Ultrasound Equipment version 2.0. Accessed November 12, 2023. http://aium.s3.amazonaws.com/resourceLibrary/rqa2.pdf
11. Penny SM. *Introduction to Sonography and Patient Care*. 2nd ed. Wolters Kluwer; 2016:176–204.

Standard First-Trimester Sonography

INTRODUCTION

The AIUM recommends that the patient requiring a first-trimester sonogram be scanned using the transabdominal or transvaginal approach, though transvaginal is recommended when transabdominal is not definitive. This chapter will provide imaging parameters for a standard first-trimester sonogram, though some detailed components will be provided. Furthermore, it will provide both an overview of normal fetal anatomy and the essential first-trimester anatomy that should be demonstrated during a standard first-trimester sonogram. Finally, a proposed first-trimester sonogram protocol, including maternal pelvic anatomy, scanning tips, the AIUM Guidelines for Nuchal Translucency Measurements, and other normal measurements are offered.

AIUM RECOMMENDATIONS FOR THE STANDARD FIRST-TRIMESTER SONOGRAPHY (UP TO 13 6/7 WEEKS)[1]

- Perform a complete pelvic sonogram (as described in Chapter 2 of this text) to include the following:
    - Uterus and cervix
    - Adnexal structures
    - Cul-de-sacs
    - Ovaries
- The presence, location, appearance, and size of adnexal masses, including ovarian masses, should be documented.
- Uterine masses, such as fibroids, should be documented, with the measurements of the largest provided.
- Uterine anomalies should be documented.
- Assess the cul-de-sac for evidence of fluid.

Chapter 6. Standard First-Trimester Sonography

- The gravid uterus and adnexa should be evaluated for the presence of a gestational sac.
- The location and an analysis of the gestational sac should be provided, including whether a yolk sac or embryo is identified.
- If an embryo is present, a crown–rump length (CRL) measurement should be obtained. CRL is the most accurate indicator of gestational age.
- If an embryo is not identified, a mean sac diameter (MSD) should be obtained.
- Fetal cardiac activity should be documented with either a video clip or M-mode.
  - When the embryo is 2 mm or greater in length, cardiac activity can be noted.
  - If cardiac activity is not identifiable in embryo that measures less than 7 mm, then a 1-week follow-up sonogram is recommended.
- The number of fetuses should be documented.
  - If multiple gestations are noted, then chorionicity and amnionicity should be determined if possible.
- An appropriate fetal anatomic survey should be provided, including an assessment of the following:
  - Calvarium
  - Abdominal cord insertion site
  - Presence of limbs
  - Fetal nuchal region for signs of abnormalities such as a cystic hygroma
    - Measurement can be obtained (see *AIUM Guidelines for Nuchal Translucency Measurements* in this chapter.)
  - Urinary bladder and other internal structures may be identified as well.

ESSENTIAL ANATOMY AND PHYSIOLOGY OF THE FIRST TRIMESTER[2,3]

- Conception
  - Around day 14 of the menstrual cycle, the dominant follicle releases an ovum. This is called ovulation.
  - Fertilization, also referred to as conception, typically occurs within 24 hours of ovulation.
  - The structure that implants within the decidualized endometrium is referred to as the blastocyst. The

blastocyst, which implants around day 20 or 21 of the menstrual cycle, will form the gestational sac.
- Syncytiotrophoblastic cells, which produce human chorionic gonadotropin (hCG), are the cells that surround the early developing gestation.
- hCG can be detected in maternal urine or blood and thus is used as an indicator of pregnancy.
  - A urine pregnancy test can confirm pregnancy, while a blood pregnancy test can confirm the pregnancy and provide an approximate age based on the amount of hCG within the blood.
  - Normal β-hCG (beta-hCG) levels double every 48 hours.
  - The discriminatory zone, which is between 1,000 and 2,000 mIU, is the level of β-hCG at which an intrauterine pregnancy (IUP) should be seen within the uterus.
  - Using transvaginal imaging, a gestational sac can be seen as early as 1,000 mIU.
- hCG maintains the corpus luteum of pregnancy, which in turn maintains the thickness of the endometrium, readying the uterus for the implantation of early pregnancy.
  - The corpus luteum, which results from the rupture of the dominant follicle at ovulation, is the most common pelvic mass associated with pregnancy.
  - The corpus luteum is located on the ovary, and it has varying sonographic appearances, including solid, cystic, and complex, and may even present as a ring of fire (with color Doppler) on the ovary. Thus, it may be confused with an ectopic pregnancy. Clinical correlation is crucial **(Fig. 6-1)**.
- Development of early gestational structures
  - The gestational sac, also referred to as the chorionic sac, contains the amniotic cavity, which contains the embryo **(Fig. 6-2)**.
    - The amnion is the lining of the amniotic cavity.
    - The gestational sac will grow about 1 mm per week.
  - The yolk sac is located within the chorionic cavity, the space between the amnion and chorion (see Fig. 6-2).
    - The yolk sac provides nourishment for the developing embryo early in the pregnancy. By the end of the first trimester, the placenta has taken over this function and the yolk sac disappears.

Chapter 6. Standard First-Trimester Sonography

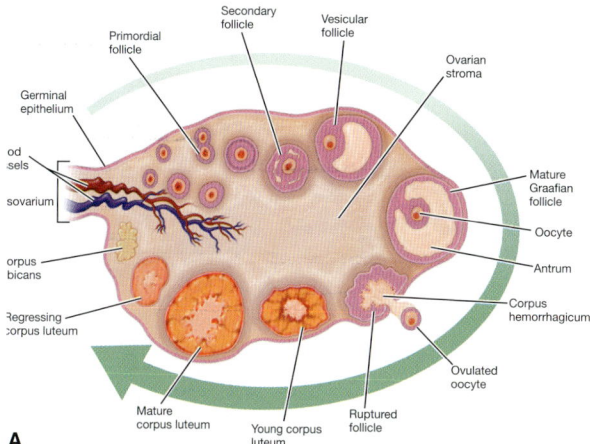

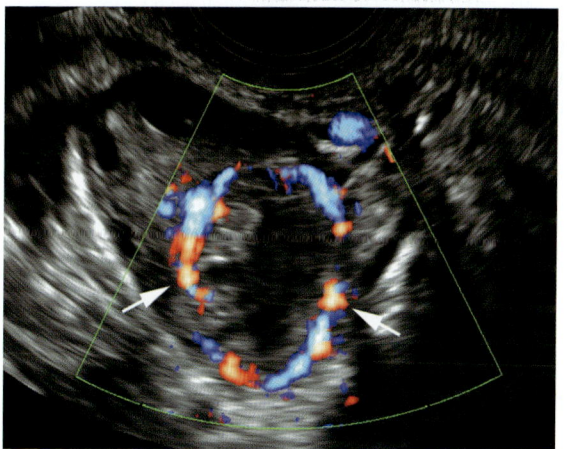

Figure 6-1. Development of the corpus luteum. A. Schematic diagram of an ovary showing the sequence of events in the origin, growth, and rupture of an ovarian follicle and the formation and retrogression of a corpus luteum. B. One sonographic appearance of the corpus luteum includes a "ring of fire," as noted in this color Doppler image. (**A.** Reprinted with permission from Penny SM. *Examination Review for Ultrasound: Abdomen & Obstetrics and Gynecology*. 3rd ed. Wolters Kluwer; 2023. Figure 18-10. **B.** Reprinted with permission from Doubilet PM, Benson CB, Benacerraf BR. *Atlas of Ultrasound in Obstetrics and Gynecology: A Multimedia Reference*. 3rd ed. Wolters Kluwer; 2019. Figure 28.1.3.)

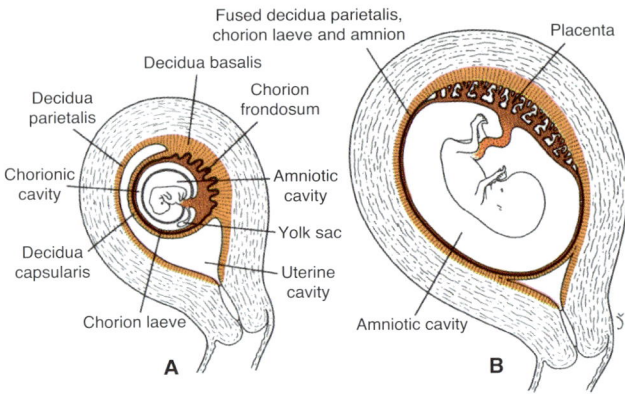

Figure 6-2. Relation of the fetal membranes to the wall of the uterus. (Reprinted with permission from Sadler TW. *Langman's Medical Embryology*. 15th ed. Wolters Kluwer; 2024. Figure 8.10.)

- The placenta will initially be recognized as a focal thickening adjacent to the gestational sac.
  - The placenta will become more well-defined as the pregnancy progresses.
  - Location of the placenta is not as important as it is in the second and third trimesters, though it can be noted, especially if it completely covers the internal os. Placenta previa can be suspected in the first trimester, but it is rarely diagnosed. Follow-up examinations are warranted.
- Development of the fetus **(Fig. 6-3)**
  - The developing embryo is located between the yolk sac and amnion at around 4 weeks gestation.
    - At 4.5 weeks, the neural plate has developed. It will give rise to the neural tube.
    - The embryo will appear initially as a solid tubular structure with a central heartbeat.
    - By 6 weeks, a tiny embryo containing a heartbeat should be identifiable adjacent to the yolk sac.
- Heart activity can be documented with M-mode or a video clip when the CRL measures 4 to 5 mm.
  - Pulsed-wave (spectral) Doppler and color Doppler are not recommended secondary to a possible increase in fetal tissues, and thus potential for bioeffects.

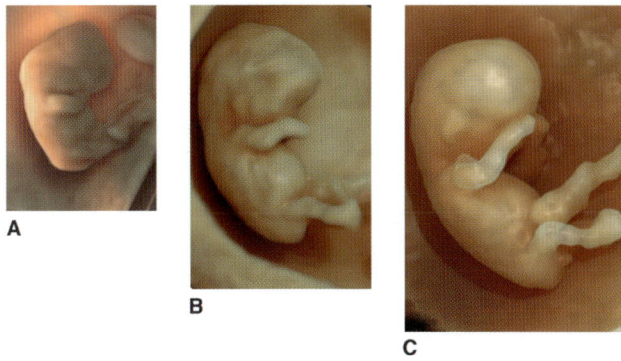

Figure 6-3. Surface mode display of 3D volumes of two normal embryos and a fetus. A, B, and C at 8, 9, and 10 weeks, respectively. Note at 8 weeks, the relatively large size of the embryo's head as compared to the body. (Reprinted with permission from Abuhamad A, Chaoui R. *First Trimester Ultrasound Diagnosis of Fetal Abnormalities*. Wolters Kluwer; 2018. Figure 3.24.)

- Most internal and external structures are in the process of forming by 6 weeks.
- The fetal lip typically closes between 7 and 8 weeks, whereas the palate closes by 12 weeks.
- Limb buds can be noted as early as 7 gestational weeks.
- The axial skeleton begins to form between 6 and 8 weeks.
- The embryo continues to grow rapidly at around 1 mm per day.
- The rhombencephalon may be seen within the fetal skull at around 7 to 8 weeks **(Fig. 6-4)**. It represents the developing fourth ventricle and other brain structures.
- The term fetus is reserved for the gestational age of ≥10 weeks and in many cases the entire fetus may be demonstrated with 3D imaging and surface mode display images **(Fig. 6-5)**.
- Beginning in the 11th week, the fetus may begin to flex and extend its body.
  - The following structures may be noted between 11 weeks 1 day and 13 weeks 6 days (especially with high-definition zoom imaging during transvaginal scanning):
- Skull (the calvarium should be ossified by 11 weeks) **(Fig. 6-6)**
  - Lateral ventricles

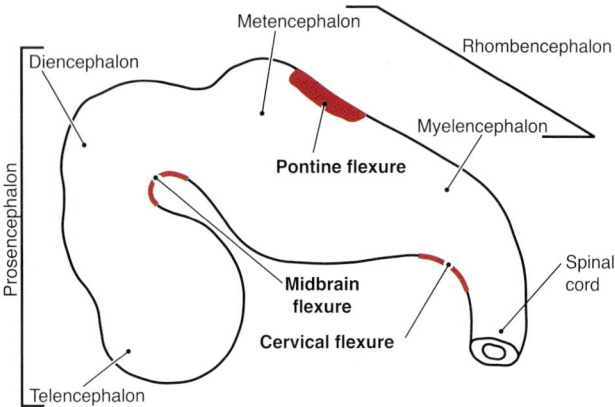

Figure 6-4. Primary vesicles. (Reprinted with permission from Bhatnagar SC. *Neuroscience for the Study of Communicative Disorders.* 4th ed. Wolters Kluwer Health/Lippincott Williams & Wilkins; 2013. Figure 2-2.)

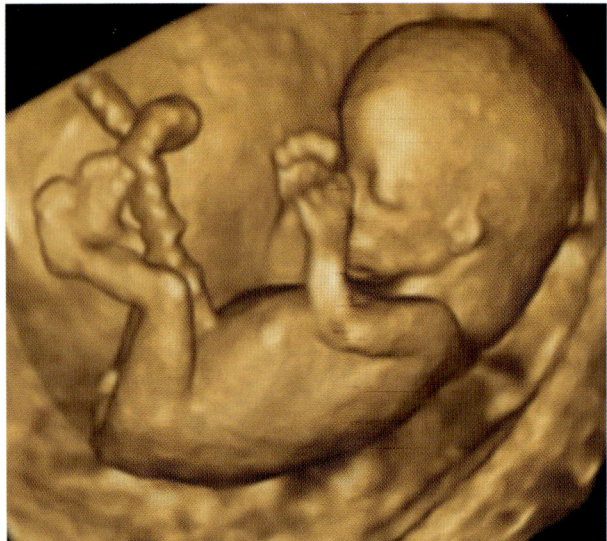

Figure 6-5. A three-dimensional image of a fetus from the lateral aspect demonstrates the head, torso, and both upper and lower extremities. (Reprinted with permission from Abuhamad A, Chaoui R. *First Trimester Ultrasound Diagnosis of Fetal Abnormalities.* Wolters Kluwer; 2018. Figure 5.24.)

Chapter 6. Standard First-Trimester Sonography

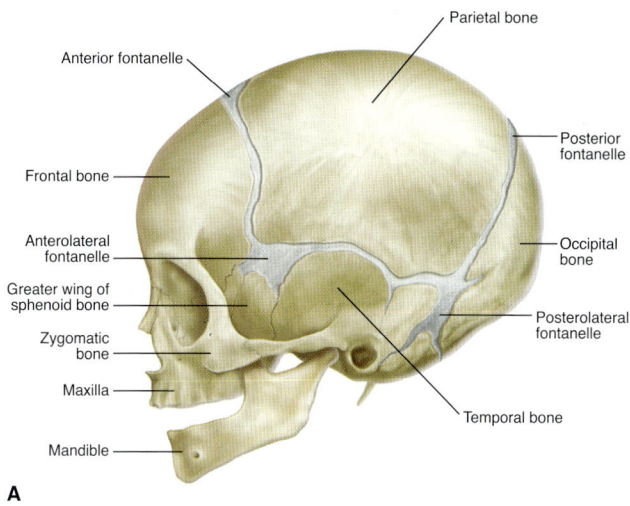

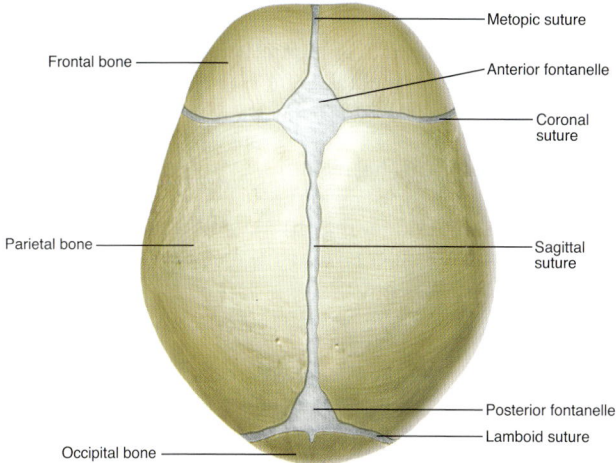

Figure 6-6. Fetal skull anatomy. Drawing A is a sagittal view and B is a superior view. (Reprinted with permission from Pansky B, Gest TR. *Lippincott's Concise Illustrated Anatomy: Head & Neck*. Vol 3. Wolters Kluwer Health/Lippincott Williams & Wilkins; 2014. Figure 2.3A-B.)

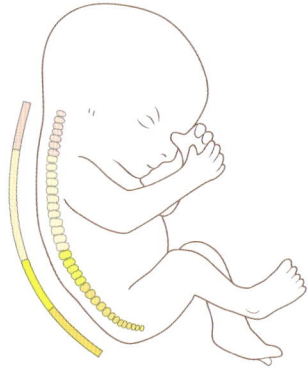

Figure 6-7. Lateral view of the curvature of the fetal vertebral column, showing cervical (*red*), thoracic (*brown*), and lumbar (*yellow*) vertebrae, and the sacrum and coccyx area (*orange*). Note the coccyx is not fully formed by term. (Reprinted with permission from Penny SM. *Examination Review for Ultrasound: Abdomen & Obstetrics and Gynecology*. 3rd ed. Wolters Kluwer; 2023. Figure 26-2C.)

- Choroid plexus within the lateral ventricles
- Small amount of cerebral tissue
- Both orbits can be visualized
- Spine (Fig. 6-7)
  - Cervical spine (nuchal region)
  - Thoracic spine (heart region)
  - Lumbar spine (kidney region)
  - Sacral spine (bladder region)
  - Coccyx (not well seen)
- Chest
  - Heart
    - The heart is fully formed by 10 weeks.
    - Though not necessary for a standard exam, a four-chamber heart can be noted with the use of zoom imaging (Fig. 6-8).
    - Having a fundamental appreciation of fetal circulation can be useful (Fig. 6-9).
    - M-mode can document fetal heart motion and beats per minute can be obtained.
- Abdomen and pelvis
  - Stomach
    - The stomach can be seen as early as 8 weeks but should be seen by 14 weeks.

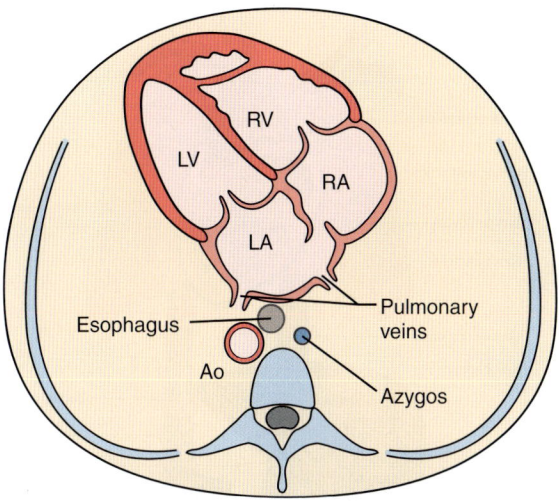

Figure 6-8. Schematic drawing of the four-chamber view showing the normal anatomic structures of the fetal chest. Note the presence of the aorta (*Ao*) to the left of the spine and the azygos vein, as a small vessel, to the right of the spine. Between the *Ao* and the left atrium (*LA*), the esophagus is found as an echogenic structure. The two inferior pulmonary veins are visualized to enter the *LA* in this plane. LV, left ventricle; RA, right atrium; RV, right ventricle. (Reprinted with permission from Abuhamad A, Chaoui R. *A Practical Guide to Fetal Echocardiography: Normal and Abnormal Hearts.* 4th ed. Wolters Kluwer; 2022. Figure 7.23.)

- The stomach should rest directly below the heart on the left side of the fetus.
- Correct situs can be determined.
- Kidneys
  - Kidneys develop in the pelvis and ascend to their normal position in the right and left upper quadrants by 9 weeks.
  - Renal function begins at 10 weeks and begins to produce most of the amniotic fluid.
  - The kidneys can be seen as early as 11 weeks with transvaginal imaging. Thus, though not required for a standard exam, kidneys may be noted with high-resolution zoom imaging.
- Umbilical cord insertion **(Fig. 6-10)**
  - Normal physiologic bowel herniation begins at 8 weeks and should resolve by 12 weeks.

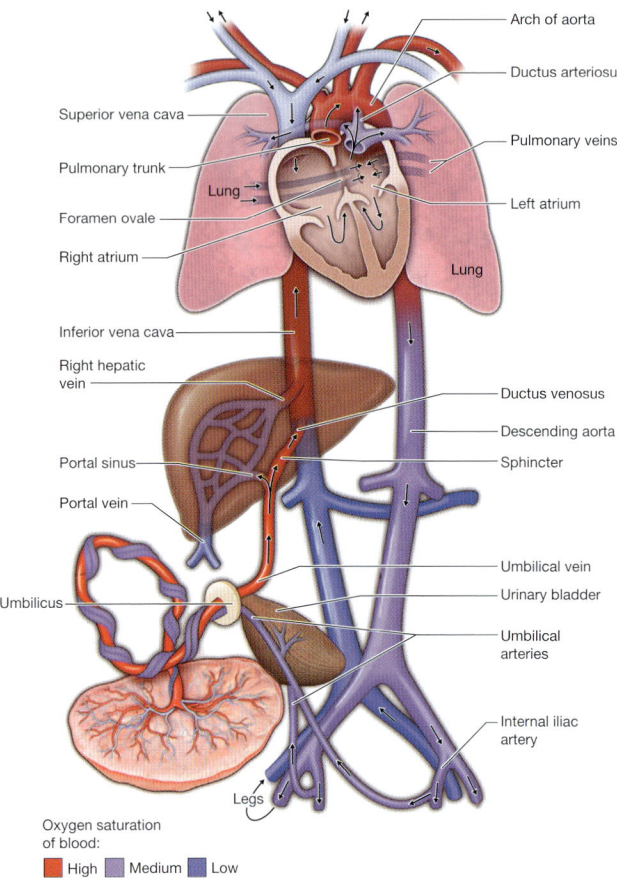

Figure 6-9. Fetal heart and circulation. Diagram of fetal circulation—*arrows* indicate the direction of blood flow; three shunts (ductus venosus, foramen ovale, ductus arteriosus) exist in utero but close shortly after birth.

- Urinary bladder
  - The bladder can be seen by 12 weeks.
- Genitalia
  - Genitalia are difficult to differentiate in the first-trimester examination and are not required for the standard examination (see Chapter 7).

Normal

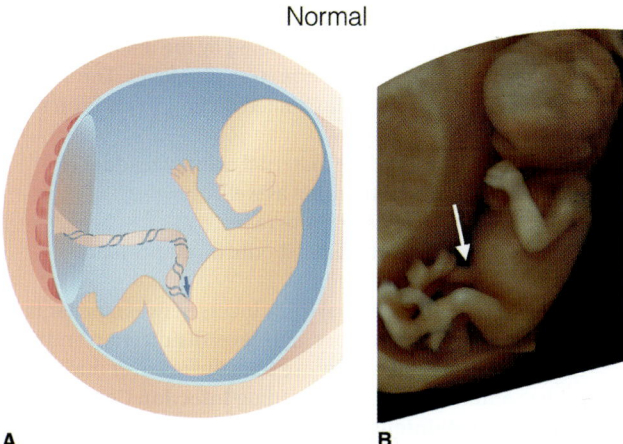

Figure 6-10. Schematic drawing (A) and corresponding 3D ultrasound image in surface mode of a fetus at 12 weeks of gestation. Note the normal insertion of the umbilical cord in the abdomen in A and B (**arrows**). (Reprinted with permission from Abuhamad A, Chaoui R. *First Trimester Ultrasound Diagnosis of Fetal Abnormalities.* Wolters Kluwer; 2018. Figure 12.9.)

- Extremities
  - Long bones can be measured as early as 12 weeks' gestation

PATIENT PREPARATION

- Transabdominal first-trimester sonogram
  - The patient's urinary bladder can be distended to displace the bowel and to provide an acoustic window for the visualization of the uterus, ovaries, and adnexa.
  - Some authors suggest having the patient drink at least enough liquid (possibly 32 ounces of water) to distend the urinary bladder to the point where the entire fundus of the uterus is clearly visualized.
  - The bladder should not be excessively distended. If this occurs, the patient may need to partially empty her bladder.
  - If the patient has a Foley catheter in place, and the transabdominal technique has been deemed crucial for diagnostic purposes, filling the urinary bladder with saline may be employed. This is termed bladder retrofilling.

- Note, retrofilling the urinary bladder in this manner is a protocol decision that is initiated by the institution, ordering physician, or interpreting physician. The practitioner should be instructed on how to perform this task correctly and safely.
  - If an abnormality of the maternal urinary bladder is noted, it should be reported as well.
- Transvaginal first-trimester sonogram
  - The patient's urinary bladder should be empty for a transvaginal pelvic sonogram.
  - Preparation of transvaginal transducers between patients requires routine mandatory high-level disinfection and the use of a high-quality single-use transducer cover during each examination. (See the heading **Infection Control and Equipment Maintenance** in this chapter.)
  - The patient, the sonographer, or the physician may introduce the vaginal transducer, preferably under real-time monitoring.
  - Consideration of having a chaperone present should follow local policy.

SUGGESTED EQUIPMENT[1]

- The female pelvis should be examined sonographically with a real-time scanner, preferably a 3.5-MHz or higher curved linear array or sector transducer for transabdominal fetal imaging.
- Transvaginal imaging offers an improved resolution of both maternal pelvic and fetal structures. The transvaginal transducer is typically 5 MHz or higher.
- As with other sonographic imaging, the frequency utilized also depends upon the approach. Furthermore, the ultrasound equipment will offer differing operating frequencies. The sonographic practitioner should ensure that the highest frequency is always utilized, appreciating that as operating frequency increases, there is a trade-off between resolution and beam penetration.
- Quality control and improvement, safety, infection control, patient education, and equipment performance monitoring should be developed and implemented following the AIUM Standards and Guidelines for the Accreditation of Ultrasound Practices found at https://www.aium.org/accreditation/accreditation.aspx

Chapter 6. Standard First-Trimester Sonography

- If the patient is actively hemorrhaging, a tissue pad should be placed under the patient's hips.

PATIENT POSITIONING

- Transabdominal female pelvic sonogram
  - The patient is typically placed in the supine position.
- Transvaginal female pelvic sonogram
  - The patient is typically placed in the lithotomy position.
  - The patient may be placed in the supine position with the hips elevated from the examining table with a positioning pad as well.

LABELING OF SONOGRAPHIC EXAMINATIONS[4]

- All sonographic images, whether still-frame images or video should include the following:
  - Patient's name and other identifying information (e.g., medical record number)
  - Facility's identification information
  - Date and time of the examination
  - Output display standard (thermal index and mechanical index)
  - Label the anatomic location and which side of the body, when appropriate
  - Image orientation when appropriate

INFECTION CONTROL AND EQUIPMENT MAINTENANCE[5]

- Infection control
  - Institutional guidelines should be in place for transducer disinfection to reduce the risk of iatrogenic and nosocomial infections.
  - Always follow your facility's established protocol for infection control.
  - The following is a summation of the AIUM's *Guidelines for Cleaning and Preparing External- and Internal-Use Ultrasound Transducers and Equipment Between Patients as well as Safe Handling and Use of Ultrasound Coupling Gel.*
    - Transabdominal transducers
      - Preparation of transabdominal transducers between patients requires a low-level disinfection process.
      - Nonsterile gel is used.

- No transducer cover is required unless there is contaminated intact skin or nonintact skin, in which case both a cover and sterile gel are recommended.
- Transvaginal transducers
  - Barriers (probe covers) used for transvaginal transducers must be single-use transducer covers that meet the sterility requirements of the procedure.
  - Use sterile or bacteriostatic gel.
  - Consult the manufacturer's instructions for disinfecting devices.
  - After the procedure, perform high-level disinfection. Commercially available wall or table-top disinfectant units are available for endocavity transducers.
  - A complete list of Food and Drug Administration (FDA)-cleared liquid sterilants and high-level disinfectants is available online.
  - Rinse to remove disinfectant.

EQUIPMENT MAINTENANCE[6]

- Regular interval inspection of equipment and transducers (connector, cable, housing, acoustic lens) is recommended to ensure performance. Imaging with a tissue-mimicking phantom may help reveal imaging degradation.
- A record of quality assurance activities must be maintained and kept current. The ultrasound equipment must meet all state and federal guidelines and testing must be maintained in good operating condition and undergo routine quality assurance at least once a year or more frequently if problems arise.
- Always report machine or equipment malfunction to facility management and remove such equipment from use.

CLINICAL INVESTIGATION

- General clinical history queries are found in Chapter 5. Some of these are the same, though more details are provided for the first trimester.
- Inquire about the first-trimester laboratory blood work obtained.
  - Patients may be under the care of a physician who has already obtained valuable laboratory findings, such as those listed in Chapter 5.
- Inquire about contraception, especially the presence of an intrauterine device.

- If possible, obtain the serum hCG level before beginning the examination. *This clinical blood test should be necessary before commencing the sonogram, though in some emergencies, this lab finding may not always be available.*
- Enter the first day of the last menstrual period within the machine's calculation package. This will provide you with an estimated due date, also referred to as an estimated date of confinement. It is important to note that some patients may be unclear about this date.
- Obtain the Gravida (number of pregnancies) Para (number of pregnancies in which the patient has given birth to a fetus at or beyond 20 weeks' gestational age or an infant weighing more than 500 g). Some institutions may utilize TPAL (term, preterm, abortions, and living children) to further describe the patient's history. *Always inquire further about any irregularities with previous pregnancies, such as ectopic pregnancy, early pregnancy loss, preterm deliveries, fetal anomalies, or chromosomal abnormalities. Always inquire about how the early pregnancy complications, such as an ectopic pregnancy were treated (e.g., medically, or surgically).*
- Have you had a previous sonogram for this pregnancy? *If so, inquire about when and if everything appeared normal. If not, more questions about the previous abnormal findings should ensue.*
- Any vaginal bleeding? *If the patient has vaginal bleeding inquire about the duration of the bleeding, color, and amount of hemorrhage. Also, inquire about the passing of clots or possible fetal tissues. Older blood will appear darker and may contain clots. Fresh blood will appear red.*
- Do your menstrual cycles occur regularly? Any menstrual abnormalities? *These are vital to note in situations where the patient is complaining of vaginal bleeding and has a positive pregnancy test.*
- Are you having any pelvic pain, and if so, where is the pain? *The classic clinical triad of an ectopic pregnancy is pain, vaginal bleeding, and palpable pelvic mass. Patients may also have shoulder or chest pain with an ectopic pregnancy secondary to the aggravation of the diaphragm by intraperitoneal hemorrhage.*
- Any previous pelvic surgery or pathology (e.g., ovarian cysts, ectopic pregnancies, uterine leiomyoma, etc.)? *It is important*

to note if the patient has had any previous pelvic surgery, such as those requiring the removal of an ovary or for ectopic pregnancies, before commencing the examination.
- Any history of multiple gestations? *This question would be best asked before the examination begins and not during the examination.*
- Are you undergoing any fertility treatment? *This is important to note, as fertility treatment can have many complications, including ectopic, multiple gestations, and heterotopic pregnancies. Inquire about what treatment the patient is undergoing.*

NORMAL SONOGRAPHIC ANATOMY OF THE FIRST TRIMESTER[1-3]

- Decidualized endometrium and intradecidual sign
  - The first sonographic sign of pregnancy, though it is nonspecific. Decidual thickening also occurs with an ectopic pregnancy, blighted ovum, and other first-trimester pathologies.
  - The intradecidual sign is the appearance of a small gestational sac in the uterine cavity surrounded by the thickened, echogenic endometrium **(Fig. 6-11)**.
- Gestational sac
  - The gestational or chorionic sac is the first definitive sign of an IUP.
  - An MSD measurement can be obtained by measuring the length, width, and height and entering those measurements in the calculation package **(Fig. 6-12)**.

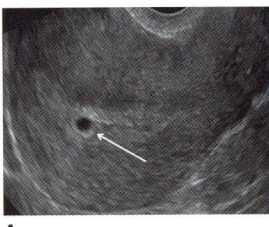 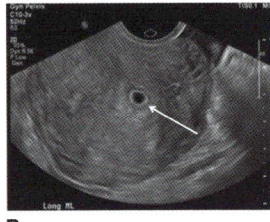

A   B

Figure 6-11. Intradecidual sign. A, B. Transvaginal longitudinal images in two different patients demonstrating an intrauterine fluid collection eccentrically placed in the endometrium with a rind of echogenic decidual reaction (*long arrows*), compatible with an early gestational sac.
(Reprinted with permission from Kanmaniraja D, Fernandez C, Murakami ME, Cernigliaro JG. Imaging in gynecologic emergencies. In: Benrubi GI, ed. *Handbook of Obstetric and Gynecologic Emergencies*. 5th ed. Wolters Kluwer; 2020. Figure 28.1.)

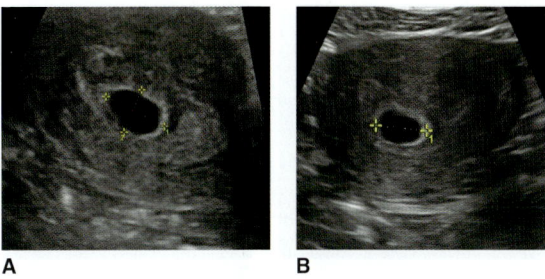

Figure 6-12. Mean sac diameter. A, B. Measurements of the mean sac diameter (MSD) of a gestational sac at 5 weeks. The MSD is calculated as the arithmetic mean diameters derived from its greatest sagittal (1), anteroposterior (2) in **A**, and coronal planes (1) in **B**. (Reprinted with permission from Abuhamad A, Chaoui R. *First Trimester Ultrasound Diagnosis of Fetal Abnormalities.* Wolters Kluwer; 2018. Figure 4.12.)

- Yolk sac
  - The secondary yolk sac will appear as a perfectly round anechoic structure with a hyperechoic rim **(Fig. 6-13)**.
  - The yolk sac is located within the chorionic cavity.
  - The yolk sac can be measured. It is measured from inside to inside **(Fig. 6-14)**.
    - An abnormal yolk sac will measure larger than 7 mm.
    - An abnormal yolk sac may also be calcified and shadow.

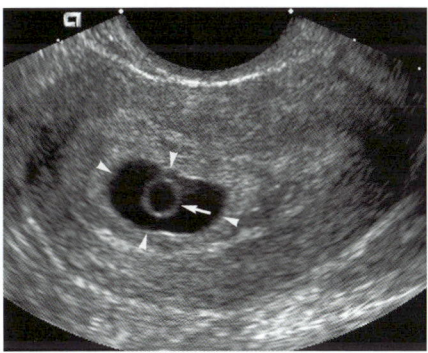

Figure 6-13. Gestational sac and secondary yolk sac at 5.5 gestational weeks. The gestational sac (*arrowheads*) contains the secondary yolk sac (*arrow*). **No embryo is seen at this time.** (Reprinted with permission from Doubilet PM, Benson CB. *Atlas of Ultrasound in Obstetrics and Gynecology: A Multimedia Reference.* Lippincott Williams & Wilkins; 2003. Figure 1.1-2.)

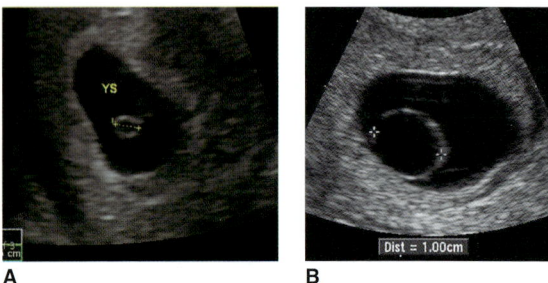

Figure 6-14. Normal and abnormal yolk sac. A. Gestational sac containing a normal-appearing yolk sac (*YS*). **B.** Probable pregnancy failure. Intrauterine gestational sac with enlarged yolk sac (calipers), measuring 10 mm in diameter, indicating probable failed pregnancy. (**A.** Reprinted with permission from Menihan CA, Kopel E. *Point-of-Care Assessment in Pregnancy and Women's Health: Electronic Fetal Monitoring and Sonography.* Wolters Kluwer; 2014. Figure 11-4. **B.** Reprinted with permission from Doubilet PM, Benson CB, Benacerraf BR. *Atlas of Ultrasound in Obstetrics and Gynecology: A Multimedia Reference.* 3rd ed. Wolters Kluwer; 2019. Figure 5.1.7.)

- Embryo/fetus <10 weeks
  - Embryo
    - The embryo will initially appear as a linear structure adjacent to the yolk sac **(Fig. 6-15)**.
    - The vitelline duct (omphalomesenteric duct) may be noted around 6 weeks. It connects the yolk sac and the embryo **(Fig. 6-16)**.
    - Limb buds may be noted as early as 7 weeks **(Fig. 6-17)**.

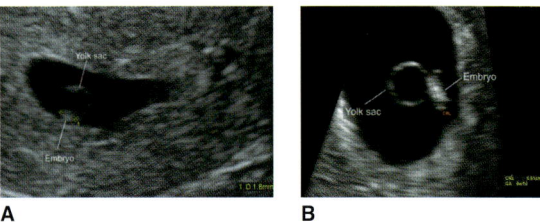

Figure 6-15. Early embryo images. A. Transvaginal sonogram of a gestational sac with an embryo measuring 1.8 mm in size. Note the proximal location of the yolk sac to the embryo. **B.** Gestational sac at 6 weeks with an embryo measuring 5.1 mm in crown–rump length (**CRL**). Reprinted with permission from Abuhamad A, Chaoui R. *First Trimester Ultrasound Diagnosis of Fetal Abnormalities.* Wolters Kluwer; 2018. Figures 4.7 and 4.8.)

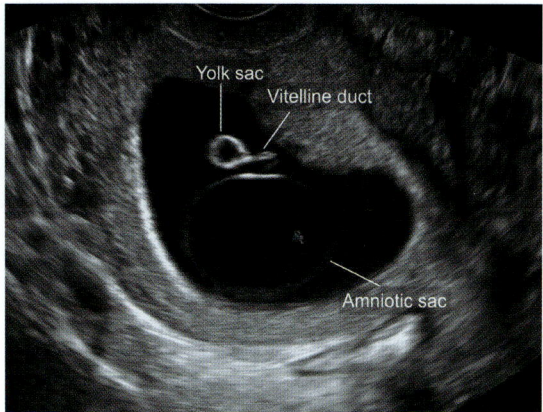

Figure 6-16. Gestational sac at 7 weeks of gestation. The amniotic sac is seen as a thin reflective circular membrane. The yolk sac and vitelline duct are seen as extra-amniotic structures. (Reprinted with permission from Abuhamad A, Chaoui R. *First Trimester Ultrasound Diagnosis of Fetal Abnormalities.* Wolters Kluwer; 2018. Figure 4.6.)

- The rhombencephalon may be noted within the skull as an anechoic structure at around 8 weeks **(Fig. 6-18)**.
- The embryo will be noted within the amniotic sac **(Fig. 6-19)**.
- Physiologic bowel herniation may be noted after 8 weeks at the base of the umbilical cord, but it will typically resolve by 12 weeks **(Fig. 6-20)**.

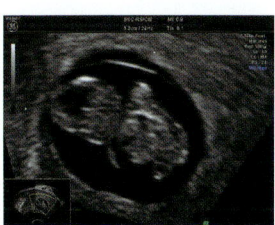
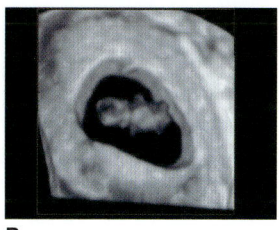

A **B**

Figure 6-17. Limb buds at 8 weeks. A. A 2D image demonstrating limb buds. Note the amnion/chorion separation. B. A 3D surface reconstruction demonstrating limb buds in an 8-week embryo. (Reprinted with permission from Woletz P. The Use of ultrasound in the first trimester. In: Stephenson SR, ed. *Diagnostic Medical Sonography: Obstetrics & Gynecology.* 3rd ed. Wolters Kluwer Health/Lippincott Williams & Wilkins; 2012. Figure 13-19.)

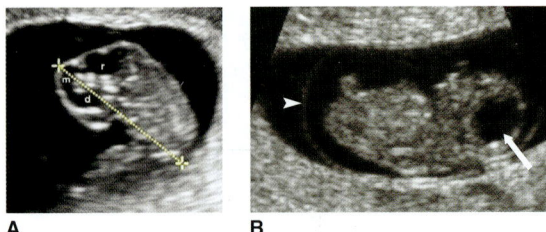

Figure 6-18. Sagittal view of an 8-week gestation. A. Sagittal view of an 8-week gestation. Calipers, CRL measurement; d, diencephalon; m, mesencephalon; r, rhombencephalon. **B.** A 7-week embryo has a prominent cystic structure (*arrow*) within the cranium. This is the normal cystic phase of development of the rhombencephalon that is seen between 6 and 8 weeks gestational age. Development of the rhombencephalon results in normal structures in the posterior fossa. The amnion (*arrowhead*) is evident. (**A.** Reprinted with permission from Sonek JD, Retzke JD, Hyett J. Normal fetal ultrasound survey. In: Kline-Fath BM, Bulas DI, Bahado-Singh R, eds. *Fundamental and Advanced Fetal Imaging: Ultrasound and MRI.* Wolters Kluwer; 2015. Figure 1.3. **B.** Reprinted with permission from Brant WE. Obstetric ultrasound. In: Klein JS, Brant WE, Helms CA, Vinson EN, eds. *Brant and Helms' Fundamentals of Diagnostic Radiology.* 5th ed. Wolters Kluwer; 2019. Figure 52.6.)

- Fetus (≥10 weeks gestational age)
  - After 10 weeks, it may be challenging to obtain an accurate CRL, but a fetus in the neutral position will yield the truest measurement **(Fig. 6-21)**.

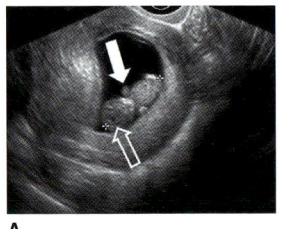
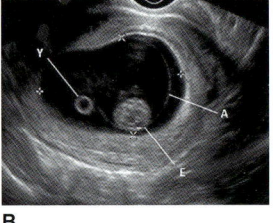

Figure 6-19. Embryo at 8 weeks 2 days. A. The head (*open arrow*) and arm bud (*closed arrow*) are clearly visible at this gestational age. The calipers (+) measure head to rump length. **B.** Transverse view through the gestational sac showing the embryo (*E*), yolk sac (*Y*), and amnion (*A*). (Reprinted with permission from Klepchick PR, Daffner RH. Obstetric and gynecologic imaging. In: Daffner RH, Hartman MS, eds. *Clinical Radiology: The Essentials.* 4th ed. Wolters Kluwer Health/Lippincott Williams & Wilkins; 2014. Figure 10.4.)

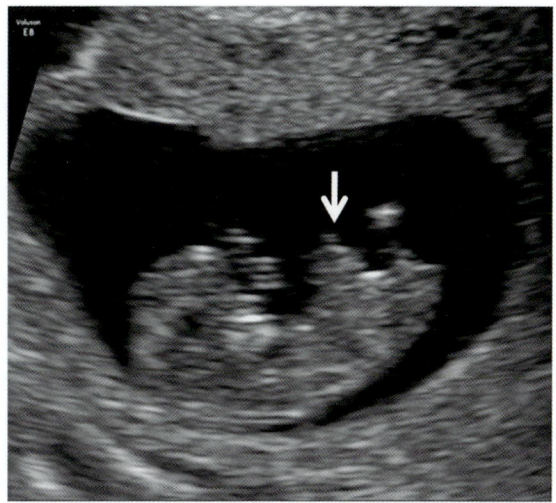

Figure 6-20. Physiologic bowel herniation. Sagittal view of a 10- to 11-week fetus demonstrating a normal physiologic bowel herniation (*arrow*). (Reprinted with permission from Sonek JD, Retzke JD, Hyett J. Normal fetal ultrasound survey. In: Kline-Fath BM, Bulas DI, Bahado-Singh R, eds. *Fundamental and Advanced Fetal Imaging: Ultrasound and MRI*. Wolters Kluwer; 2015. Figure 1.1.)

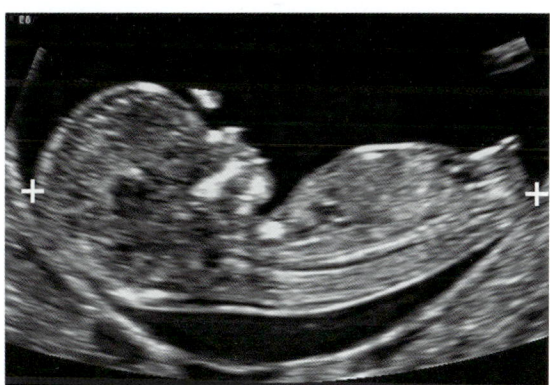

Figure 6-21. Sagittal view of an 11- to 12-week fetus. The fetus is in a neutral position. Calipers, CRL measurement. (Reprinted with permission from Sonek JD, Retzke JD, Hyett J. Normal fetal ultrasound survey. In: Kline-Fath BM, Bulas DI, Bahado-Singh R, eds. *Fundamental and Advanced Fetal Imaging: Ultrasound and MRI*. Wolters Kluwer; 2015. Figure 1.4.)

180   Chapter 6. Standard First-Trimester Sonography

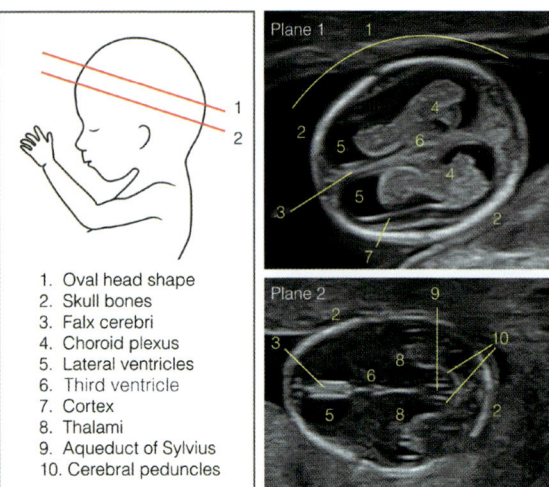

1. Oval head shape
2. Skull bones
3. Falx cerebri
4. Choroid plexus
5. Lateral ventricles
6. Third ventricle
7. Cortex
8. Thalami
9. Aqueduct of Sylvius
10. Cerebral peduncles

Figure 6-22. Fetal first-trimester brain anatomy. Planes 1 and 2 of four axial planes for the anatomic assessment of the head: Plane 1 corresponds to the transventricular plane and plane 2 corresponds to the transthalamic plane. Planes 1 and 2 are obtained from fetuses at 13 weeks of gestation. (Reprinted with permission from Abuhamad A, Chaoui R. *First Trimester Ultrasound Diagnosis of Fetal Abnormalities.* Wolters Kluwer; 2018. Figure 5.7.)

- The fetal brain and calvarium may be assessed clearly if the fetus is in an optimal position (**Figs. 6-22** to **6-24**).
  - Acrania can be diagnosed in the first trimester **(Fig. 6-25)**.
- The fetal neck can be assessed for signs of increased nuchal translucency and cystic hygroma **(Fig. 6-26)**.
  - AIUM Guidelines for Nuchal Translucency Measurements between 11 and 14 weeks **(Fig. 6-27)**
    - The margins of the NT edges must be clear with the angle of insonation perpendicular to the NT line.
    - The fetus must be in the midsagittal plane. The tip of the nose, palate, and diencephalon should be seen.
    - The image must be magnified so that it is filled by the fetal head, neck, and upper thorax.
    - The fetal neck must be in a neutral position, with the head in line with the spine, not flexed and not hyperextended.
    - The amnion must be seen as separate from the NT line.

Chapter 6. Standard First-Trimester Sonography

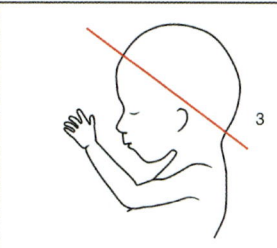
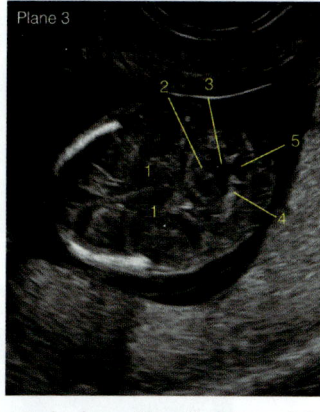

1. Thalami
2. Developing cerebellum
3. Fourth ventricle (IT)
4. Choroid plexus of Fourth ventricle
5. Future cisterna magna

Figure 6-23. Fetal first-trimester posterior fossa. Plane 3 of four axial planes for the anatomic assessment of the head: Plane 3 is a slightly oblique plane at the level of the posterior fossa, demonstrating the developing cerebellum and fourth ventricle as intracranial translucency (*IT*). (Reprinted with permission from Abuhamad A, Chaoui R. *First Trimester Ultrasound Diagnosis of Fetal Abnormalities*. Wolters Kluwer; 2018. Figure 5.8.)

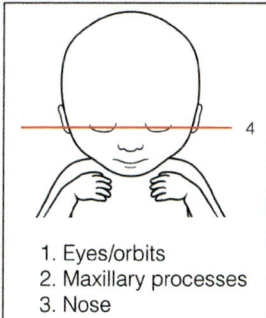
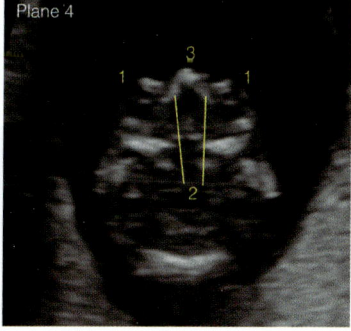

1. Eyes/orbits
2. Maxillary processes
3. Nose

Figure 6-24. Fetal first-trimester orbital assessment. Plane 4 of four axial planes for the anatomic assessment of the head: Plane 4 is an axial plane obtained at the level of the orbits demonstrating two orbits, the eyes, and the nose in between. (Reprinted with permission from Abuhamad A, Chaoui R. *First Trimester Ultrasound Diagnosis of Fetal Abnormalities*. Wolters Kluwer; 2018. Figure 5.9.)

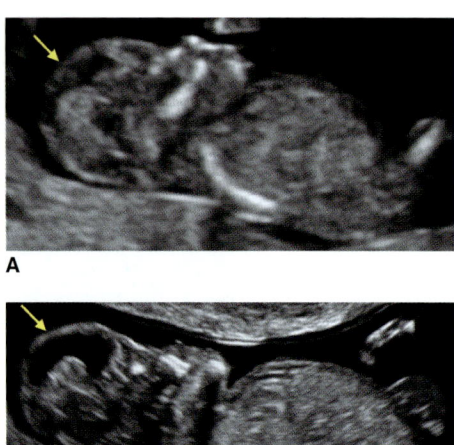

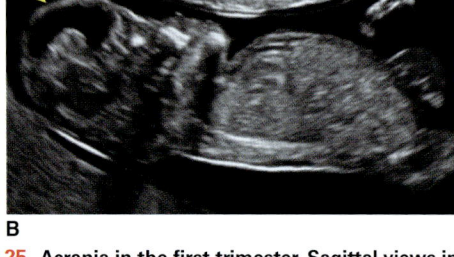

Figure 6-25. Acrania in the first trimester. Sagittal views in two fetuses (A, B) with absence of the calvarium (acrania) in early gestation. Note in A and B the presence of a membrane (pia mater) covering the brain tissue (*arrows*). The shape of the brain and head is similar in both fetuses. (Reprinted with permission from Abuhamad A, Chaoui R. *First Trimester Ultrasound Diagnosis of Fetal Abnormalities.* Wolters Kluwer; 2018. Figure 8.17.)

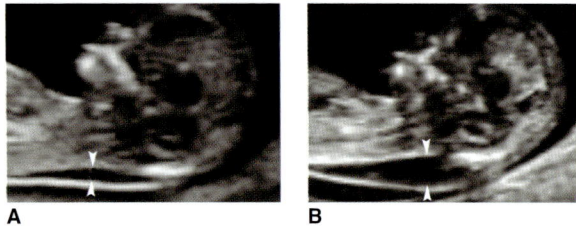

Figure 6-26. Nuchal Translucency. A. Normal nuchal translucency measurement of 2.6 mm. The measurement is precisely taken between the inner borders of the translucency (*arrowheads*). B. Abnormal nuchal translucency measurement of 3.9 mm (*between arrowheads*). Measurements greater than 3 mm are 85% predictive of the presence of Down syndrome. (Reprinted with permission from Brant WE. Obstetric ultrasound. In: Klein JS, Brant WE, Helms CA, Vinson EN, eds. *Brant and Helms' Fundamentals of Diagnostic Radiology.* 5th ed. Wolters Kluwer; 2019. Figure 52.32.)

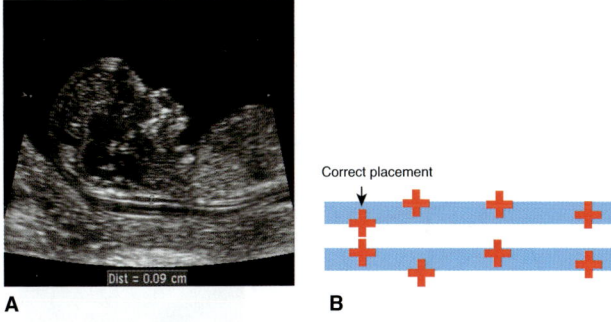

Figure 6-27. Measuring the nuchal translucency. A. Note the caliper placement on this sonographic image. **B.** The first set of calipers is the correct placement for the NT measurement according to the American Institute of Ultrasound in Medicine. (**A.** Reprinted with permission from Doubilet PM, Benson CB. *Atlas of Ultrasound in Obstetrics and Gynecology: A Multimedia Reference.* 2nd ed. Wolters Kluwer Health/Lippincott Williams & Wilkins; 2012. Figure 7.1.1.)

- The fetal abdomen and cord insertion.
  - The fetal stomach, cord insertion, and bladder can be noted **(Fig. 6-28)**.
- Normal, more well-developed fetal limbs (two upper and two lower extremities), can be demonstrated as well if possible **(Fig. 6-29)**.
- Placenta **(Fig. 6-30)**
  - The relationship of the placenta to the internal os should be noted, though placenta previa is typically not diagnosed in the first trimester.
  - The placenta and myometrial interface should be evaluated for signs of abruption.
- Corpus luteum of pregnancy, cul-de-sacs, and adnexa
  - The corpus luteum of pregnancy can have varying sonographic appearances, including having a "ring of fire" with color Doppler analysis, thus simulating an ectopic pregnancy **(Fig. 6-31)**.
    - In this situation, it is crucial that an IUP is confirmed, and if not, an ectopic pregnancy cannot be ruled out.
- The cul-de-sacs should be examined for fluid.
  - A minimal amount of simple, anechoic fluid may be seen with an IUP.

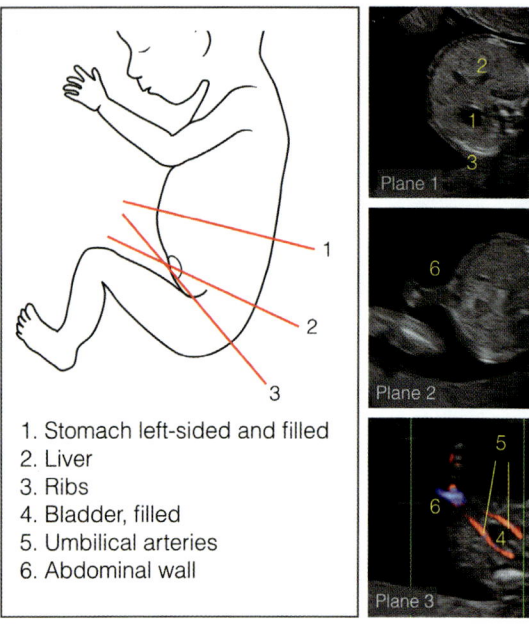

Figure 6-28. Three axial planes (planes 1 to 3) for the anatomic evaluation of the fetal abdomen. Plane 1 is at the level of the stomach and demonstrates the normal position of the stomach and liver. Plane 2 is at the level of the cord insertion in the abdomen and demonstrates an intact anterior abdominal wall and plane 3 is in color Doppler at the level of the bladder confirming its presence along with the presence of **two umbilical arteries.** (Reprinted with permission from Abuhamad A, Chaoui R. *First Trimester Ultrasound Diagnosis of Fetal Abnormalities.* Wolters Kluwer; 2018. Figure 5.14.)

- Complex fluid, which may be hemoperitoneum, is often a sign of ectopic pregnancy **(Fig. 6-32)**. The other quadrant should be assessed for fluid as well.

SUGGESTED PROTOCOL FOR A SONOGRAM OF THE STANDARD FIRST-TRIMESTER EXAMINATION

- For organizational reasons, the following protocol maintains all maternal uterus and ovary images separate from the gestational images required during a standard first-trimester sonogram. Gestation-related images can be performed at the end of the examination or at the beginning.

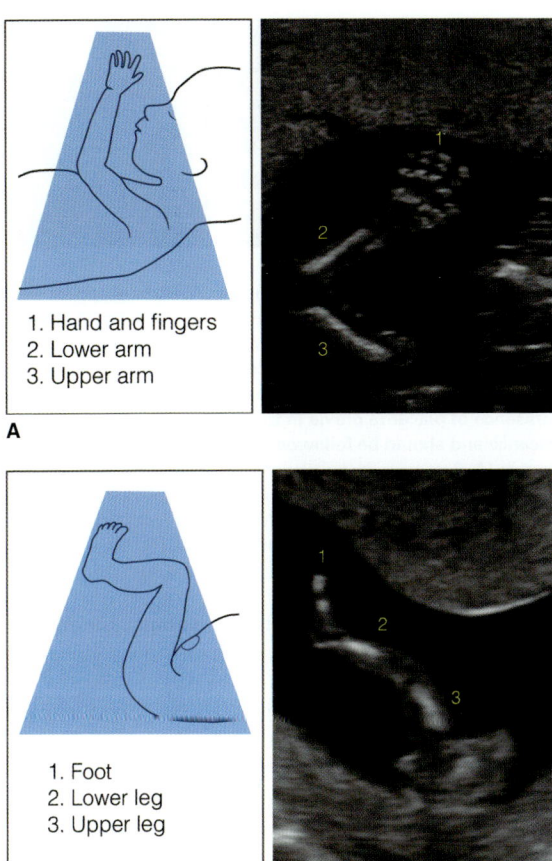

Figure 6-29. Normal upper and lower extremities in the first trimester. A. Upper extremity anatomy. B. Lower extremity anatomy. (Reprinted with permission from Abuhamad A, Chaoui R. *First Trimester Ultrasound Diagnosis of Fetal Abnormalities.* Wolters Kluwer; 2018. Figures 5.18 and 5.19.)

- The following protocol can be conducted utilizing the transabdominal or transvaginal approach but do keep in mind that the external architecture of the vagina will not be visualized with transvaginal imaging.
  - If possible, the patient should have a distended urinary bladder and a survey conducted in both transverse and

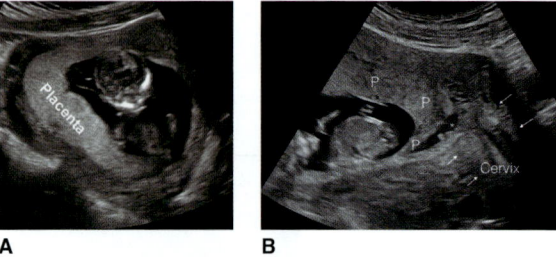

Figure 6-30. Placenta in the first trimester. **A.** Normal appearing first-trimester placenta. **B.** The position of the placenta (*P*) should be assessed in relation to the cervix (*arrows*) in the first trimester of pregnancy. Note that there is evidence of placenta (*P*) previa in this pregnancy as it is shown to cover the internal cervical os (*asterisk*). The presence of placenta previa in the first trimester is of little clinical significance and should be followed up in the second trimester of pregnancy. (**A.** Reprinted with permission from Doubilet PM, Benson CB. *Atlas of Ultrasound in Obstetrics and Gynecology: A Multimedia Reference.* 2nd ed. Wolters Kluwer Health/Lippincott Williams & Wilkins; 2012. Figure 1.3.7. **B.** Reprinted with permission from Abuhamad A, Chaoui R. *First Trimester Ultrasound Diagnosis of Fetal Abnormalities.* Wolters Kluwer; 2018. Figure 5.2.)

longitudinal of the pelvis utilizing the transabdominal approach, given that this approach provides a global view of both the pelvis.
- Transabdominal imaging also offers the opportunity to examine the urinary bladder and urethra.
- Empty the urinary bladder before the transvaginal examination commences and ensure that there are no foreign objects, such as tampons, within the vagina.
- Transvaginal transducer preparation and insertion
  - Explain the process of transvaginal transducer fully to the patient before commencing with the examination. Patient consent is mandatory.
  - A disinfected transvaginal transducer must be used.
  - Coupling gel is placed on the face of the transducer.
  - A sterile probe cover is placed on the transducer and air bubbles are expressed to reduce air artifacts during imaging.
  - Sterile gel is placed outside of the transducer cover over the transducer face.
  - The patient, who is in the lithotomy position or supine with legs flexed, can be asked to assist the sonographer in inserting the transducer. This may not be possible with

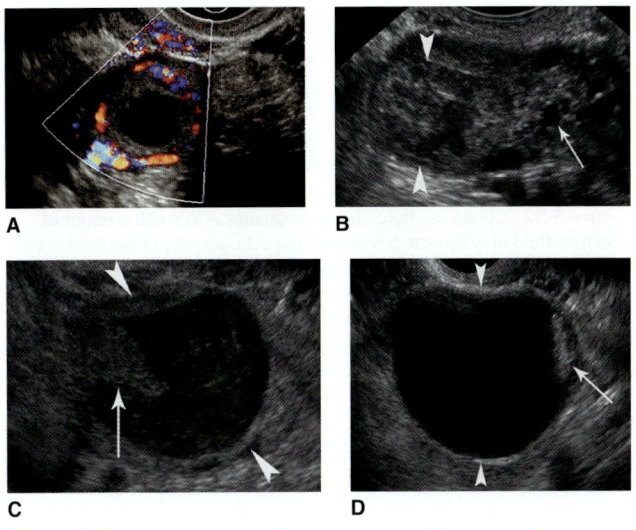

Figure 6-31. Varying sonographic appearance of the corpus luteum.
A. Transvaginal color Doppler image of the ovary reveals a 3-cm cyst surrounded by an intense ring of vascularity ("ring of fire") characteristic of the corpus luteum. This can be confused with an ectopic pregnancy. **B.** Transvaginal image of the ovary shows the collapsed cyst appearance of the corpus luteum (*between arrowheads*) that occurs just after ovulation. Note the follicles (*arrow*) that confirm the location of the structure on the ovary. **C.** The corpus luteum is prone to internal hemorrhage creating a hemorrhagic ovarian cyst (*between arrowheads*). Note the echogenic fluid and clot (*arrow*) within the cyst. **D.** A hemorrhagic corpus luteal cyst (*between arrowheads*) may enlarge to become a prominent pelvic structure and be a source of adnexal pain in early pregnancy. This corpus luteal cyst measures 5 cm in diameter. Blood clots (*arrow*) within the cyst may simulate an ectopic pregnancy containing an embryo. (Reprinted with permission from Brant WE. Obstetric ultrasound. In: Brant WE, Helms CA, eds. *Fundamentals of Diagnostic Radiology*. 4th ed. Wolters Kluwer Health/Lippincott Williams & Wilkins; 2012. Figure 37.5.)

all patients, however, when possible, this may reduce pain and anxiety.
- The transducer should be inserted into the vagina without encountering the cervix.
- A chaperone may be required by your institution for the transvaginal examination.
- It is important to note that transvaginal imaging has a limited field of view.

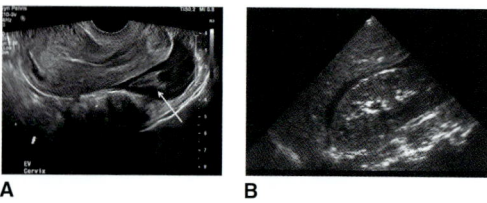

Figure 6-32. Cul-de-sac fluid during pregnancy. **A.** A small amount of anechoic fluid may be noted; however, the echogenicity of the fluid is vital to investigate. Hemorrhage (*arrow*) is noted within this fluid, which was associated with a ruptured ectopic pregnancy. **B.** The right upper quadrant should be evaluated for fluid as well. Free fluid can be seen between the liver and the right kidney in Morison pouch. (**A.** Reprinted with permission from Kanmaniraja D, Fernandez C, Murakami ME, Cernigliaro JG. Imaging in gynecologic emergencies. In: Benrubi GI, ed. *Handbook of Obstetric and Gynecologic Emergencies.* 5th ed. Wolters Kluwer; 2020. Figure 28.15. **B.** Reprinted with permission from Murakami ME, Cernigliaro JG. Imaging in gynecologic emergencies. In: Benrubi GI, ed. *Handbook of Obstetric and Gynecologic Emergencies.* 4th ed. Wolters Kluwer Health/Lippincott Williams & Wilkins; 2010. Figure 28.20C.)

- A quick sonographic survey should initially examine the pelvis for:
  - Evidence of an IUP such as:
    - Gestational sac within the endometrium
    - Yolk sac
    - Fetal pole
    - If present, an embryonic/fetal heartbeat should be noted during real-time imaging.
  - Signs of free fluid within the pelvis
    - The echogenicity and amount of the fluid should be analyzed.
    - Echogenic fluid can be a sign of hemorrhage as in the case of ruptured ectopic.
  - Evidence of an adnexal mass
- Perform the routine pelvic sonogram as noted below
  - Longitudinal midline image of the gravid uterus
    - The transducer should be manipulated in a direction that the patient's functional midline is obtained.
    - Measure the uterus in both longitudinal and anteroposterior (AP) dimensions (see Fig. 2-17).
      - Measure from the fundus to the cervix in the sagittal plane.
      - Measure the thickest AP dimension of the uterus.
      - The trace measurement tool may be utilized when there is atypical positioning of the uterus. Also, two

measurements can be obtained and added together if the uterine–cervix angle produces a significant bend.
- Examine the echogenicity and contour of the uterus for any signs of pathology.
- (If no IUP is noted) Longitudinal measurement of the endometrium.
  - If feasible, utilize the zoom function to better visualize the endometrium.
  - If evidence of a gestational sac is not seen, measure the thickness of the endometrium from basal layer to basal layer (outer-to-outer) (see Figs. 2-18 and 2-19).
    - The endometrium may need to be measured when a small gestational sac is noted.
  - Label the image with the first day of the patient's last menstrual cycle.
- Longitudinal image of the right lateral aspect of the uterus.
  - Examine the echogenicity and contour of the uterus for any signs of pathology.
- Longitudinal image of the left lateral aspect of the uterus.
  - Examine the echogenicity and contour of the uterus for any signs of pathology.
- Transverse uterus (see Fig. 2-20)
  - Angle inferior to superior to image the:
    - Vagina
    - Cervix
      - The cervix often produces edge shadowing during the transabdominal examination (see Fig. 2-21).
    - Corpus
      - Measure the maximum transverse dimension (see Fig. 2-20).
    - Fundus
  - Scan completely through the uterus superiorly to ensure that there is no pathology superior to the uterine fundus.
- Obtain images and measurements in both transverse and sagittal of all uterine pathology.
- Transverse right or left ovary (see Fig. 2-22)
  - Begin obtaining ovarian images with the ovary seen first.
  - Measure the maximum transverse dimension of the ovary.
  - Apply color Doppler to the ovary.
  - Apply pulsed-wave Doppler and attempt to obtain both arterial and venous waveforms (see Figs. 2-23 and 2-24).

- Longitudinal right or left ovary
  - Maintaining your focus on the previous ovary, rotate the transducer 90 degrees to obtain sagittal images of the same ovary.
  - Measure the maximum length and width dimensions of the ovary.
  - Apply color and pulsed-wave Doppler (if not identifiable in transverse).
- Longitudinal right or left adnexa images
  - Obtain several sagittal images while scanning through each adnexa.
- Transverse right or left adnexa images
  - Obtain several transverse images while scanning through each adnexa.
- Repeat all previously listed ovarian and adnexal images of the contralateral side.
- Gestational images
  - Initially, the intradecidual sign may be noted.
    - The intradecidual sign is evident when there is an intrauterine fluid collection eccentrically placed in the endometrium with a rind of echogenic decidual reaction (see Fig. 6-11).
  - Gestational sac measurement (sagittal and transverse)
    - Measure the length, width, and height of the gestational sac, including your measurements in the calculation package.
    - Note the shape of the gestational sac.
      - The borders should be smooth, and the size should not be too small or too large compared to the size of the embryo/fetus.
      - Irregular shaped gestational sacs can be a sign of inevitable demise and should be followed (Fig. 6-33).
      - Some institutions will not require a gestational sac measurement if a crown–rump length is obtainable.
    - Note the location of the gestational sac.
      - It should be located within the endometrium.
      - Eccentric locations can be indicative of cornual pregnancies.
      - Low gestational sac locations can be indicative of a cesarean scar pregnancy (Fig. 6-34).
      - Evaluate for other fluid collections within the endometrium.
  - Yolk sac measurement (sagittal or transverse)
    - The normal yolk sac is perfectly round.

Chapter 6. Standard First-Trimester Sonography

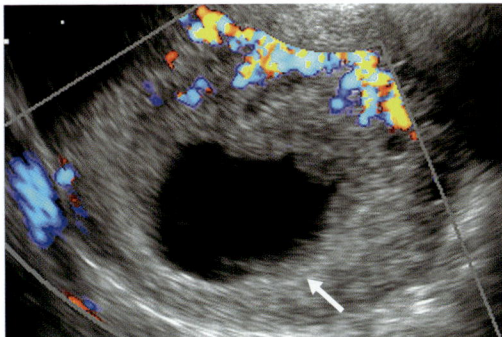

Figure 6-33. Irregular shaped gestational sac. An empty gestational sac, measuring 27 mm in MSD, is demonstrated within the uterus by transvaginal US. The margin of the sac is irregular in contour and the decidual reaction (*arrow*) is poorly defined and only weakly echogenic. Color Doppler shows blood flow only in the myometrium. An embryo should always be seen on a transvaginal sonogram when the MSD is ≥25 mm. (Reprinted with permission from Brant WE. Obstetric ultrasound. In: Klein JS, Brant WE, Helms CA, Vinson EN, eds. *Brant and Helms' Fundamentals of Diagnostic Radiology*. 5th ed. Wolters Kluwer; 2019. Figure 52.8.)

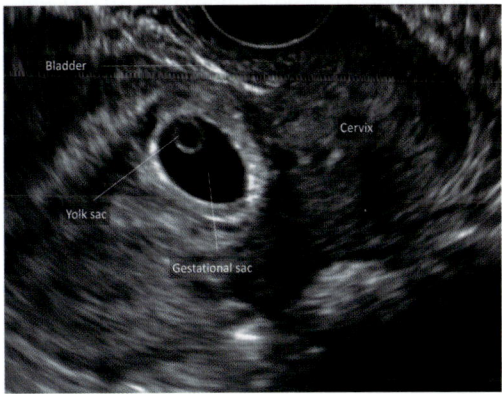

Figure 6-34. Transvaginal ultrasound of the midline sagittal plane of the uterus in a pregnancy at 7 weeks of gestation demonstrating a cesarean section scar implantation. Note that the gestational sac is imbedded into the cesarean section scar. Also note the proximity of the empty bladder to the gestational sac. (Reprinted with permission from Abuhamad A, Chaoui R. *First Trimester Ultrasound Diagnosis of Fetal Abnormalities*. Wolters Kluwer; 2018. Figure 15.20.)

- The yolk sac should not be echogenic or enlarged (see Fig. 6-14).
- A single measurement of the yolk sac should be performed, measuring inside to inside.
- Embryo/fetal pole (sagittal, transverse, or oblique)
  - Measure the CRL.
    - Measure at least three times to ensure that you have obtained the longest dimension possible.
  - Fetal cardiac activity should be documented with either a video clip or M-mode.
  - M-mode measurement is measured from the beginning of one beat to the beginning of the next (note, manufacturer guidelines must be followed as this may vary per machine).
  - Evaluate and demonstrate all anatomy that can be provided at the specific gestational age, as this can vary dramatically during the first trimester.
  - Calvarium
  - Abdominal cord insertion site
  - Presence of limbs
  - Fetal nuchal region for signs of abnormalities such as a cystic hygroma
    - Measurement can be obtained (see *AIUM Guidelines for Nuchal Translucency Measurements* in this chapter).
  - Urinary bladder and other internal structures may be identified as well.

SCANNING TIPS

- Special certifications in nasal bone, nuchal translucency, and other fetal measurements can be obtained through the Fetal Medicine Foundation.
  - Visit https://fetalmedicine.org/
- If asymmetry between the gestational sac and the size of the embryo is evident, obtain an MSD measurement for comparison (Fig. 6-35). Disagreement between these two obstetric measurements can be a sign of impending pregnancy loss.
- Overdistention of the urinary bladder should be avoided during a transvaginal sonogram because this can inhibit the possibility of obtaining valuable diagnostic images. If necessary, stop the examination and allow the patient to void.
- Implantation bleeds and subchorionic hemorrhage may mimic second gestational sacs. In these situations, no yolk sac or fetal pole will be recognized (Fig. 6-36).

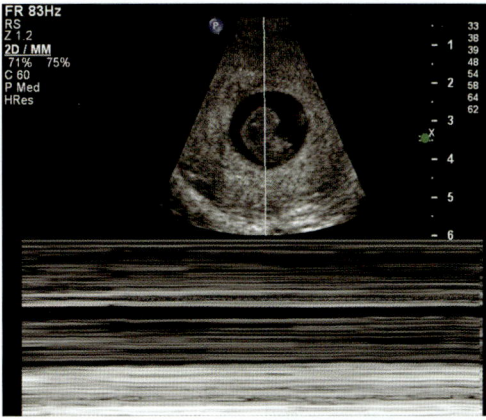

Figure 6-35. Fetal demise with gestational sac/fetal growth discrepancy. First-trimester embryonic demise proven with M-mode. Note how small the gestational sac is in relation to the size of the fetus as well. (Reprinted with permission from Gullett J, Pigott DC. Second and third trimester pregnancy. In: Cosby KS, Kendall JL, eds. *Practical Guide to Emergency Ultrasound*. 2nd ed. Wolters Kluwer Health/Lippincott Williams & Wilkins; 2014. Figure 16.25.)

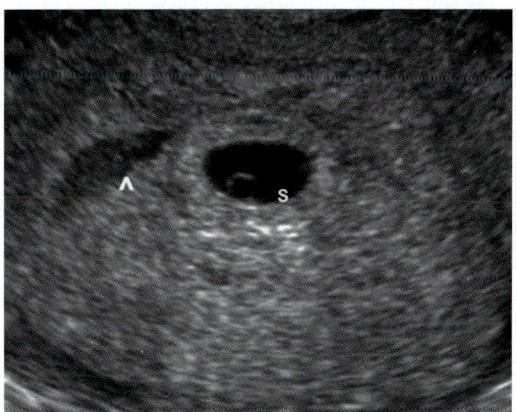

Figure 6-36. Implantation bleeding. Transverse image showing a gestational sac containing a yolk sac (*S*) and a second irregular "saclike" area (*arrowhead*) consistent with an implantation bleed. (Reprinted with permission from Drose JA. Multiple gestations. In: Stephenson SR, ed. *Diagnostic Medical Sonography: Obstetrics & Gynecology*. 3rd ed. Wolters Kluwer Health/Lippincott Williams & Wilkins; 2012. Figure 26-14.)

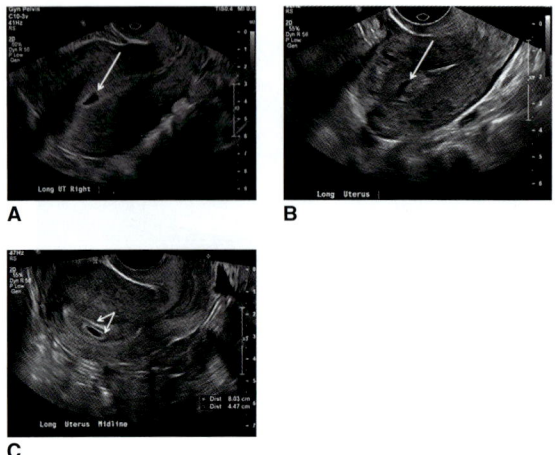

Figure 6-37. Pseudogestational sac versus intrauterine gestational sac. A, B. Small irregular appearing fluid collection (*long arrows*) in two different patients centrally located within the endometrium, compatible with a pseudogestational sac in a patient with known ectopic pregnancy. **C.** Well-circumscribed smooth, oval cystic lesion eccentrically located in the endometrium with double decidual reaction (*short arrows*), compatible with an intrauterine gestational sac of early pregnancy.
(Reprinted with permission from Kanmaniraja D, Fernandez C, Murakami ME, Cernigliaro JG. Imaging in gynecologic emergencies. In: Benrubi GI, ed. *Handbook of Obstetric and Gynecologic Emergencies*. 5th ed. Wolters Kluwer; 2020. Figure 28.14.)

- Do not confuse the amnion with the nuchal translucency. Asking the patient to cough may help to change the position of the fetus.
- Be careful not to confuse normal physiologic bowel herniation with an omphalocele. By the end of the first trimester, one should be able to differentiate the two findings.
- A pseudodecidual reaction and pseudogestational sac may be present with an ectopic pregnancy. These will both appear abnormal **(Fig. 6-37)**.

NORMAL MEASUREMENTS[7]

- hCG range according to the international reference preparation (IRP)
  - 5 weeks = 2,580 to 6,330 (IRP)
  - 6 weeks = 11,230 to 25,640 (IRP)

- 7 weeks = 36,130 to 73,280 (IRP)
- 8 weeks = 64,600 to 116,310 (IRP)
- Gestational sac
  - MSD obtained in three orthogonal planes.
  - Earliest sac will measure as small as 3 mm at around 4.6 gestational weeks.
  - Gestational sac will grow around 1 mm per day in early gestation.
  - Between 2 and 14 mm, the MSD is most accurate for dating gestation.
  - At around 14 mm, an embryo will likely be noted within the amniotic sac adjacent to the yolk sac. The MSD size and associated weeks are below.
    - 5 weeks = 5.5 mm
    - 6 weeks = 13 mm
    - 7 weeks = 19 mm
    - 8 weeks = 26 mm
    - 9 weeks = 32 mm
- CRL
  - The measurement is the longest straight line from the head of the embryo/fetus to the caudal end.
    - 5.7 weeks = 0.2 mm
    - 6 weeks = 0.4 mm
    - 7 weeks = 1.0 mm
    - 8 weeks = 1.6 mm
    - 9 weeks = 2.3 mm
    - 10 weeks = 3.1 mm
    - 11 weeks = 4.1 mm
    - 12 weeks = 5.4 mm
- Yolk sac
  - The yolk sac diameter should not exceed 7 mm.
- Fetal heart rate in beats per minute (bpm)
  - Heart rate ranges from 120 to 160 bpm
  - Bradycardia is below 120 bpm
  - Tachycardia is higher than 160 bpm

WHERE ELSE TO LOOK

- Evaluate all quadrants for free fluid if an excessive amount is noted during an obstetric sonogram.
- Evaluate the patient for urinary tract pathology such as renal stones if clinical signs and symptoms are present.

- Evaluate the appendix for signs of appendicitis if right lower quadrant pain is present.
- Evaluate the urinary bladder for pathology.
- Though rare, a heterotopic pregnancy can be present, especially if the patient is undergoing fertility treatment.

COMMON FIRST-TRIMESTER PATHOLOGY[2,3]

- Ectopic pregnancy—a pregnancy located anywhere other than the endometrial or uterine cavity
  - Clinical findings of ectopic pregnancy
    - Vaginal bleeding
    - Pelvic pain
    - Palpable pelvic mass
    - Low hematocrit
    - Shoulder pain (with intraperitoneal rupture and hemorrhage)
  - Sonographic findings of ectopic pregnancy (Fig. 6-38)
    - Extrauterine gestational sac that may contain a yolk sac and embryo
    - Adnexal ring demonstrating a ring of fire with color Doppler
    - Complex adnexal mass
    - Free fluid in the posterior cul-de-sac (may be complex fluid representing hemorrhage)
    - Pseudogestational sac
    - Poor decidual reaction
- Anembryonic gestation—a gestation lacking an embryo (also referred to as a blighted ovum)
  - Clinical findings of anembryonic gestation
    - Vaginal bleeding
    - Low hCG
    - Loss of or decreased pregnancy symptoms
  - Sonographic findings of anembryonic gestation (see Fig. 6-33)
    - Large, irregular gestational sac lacking a fetal pole and yolk sac
    - Poor decidual reaction
- Molar pregnancy—a group of disorders, also referred to as gestational trophoblastic disease, in which there is an abnormal combination of male and female gametes
  - Clinical findings of a molar pregnancy

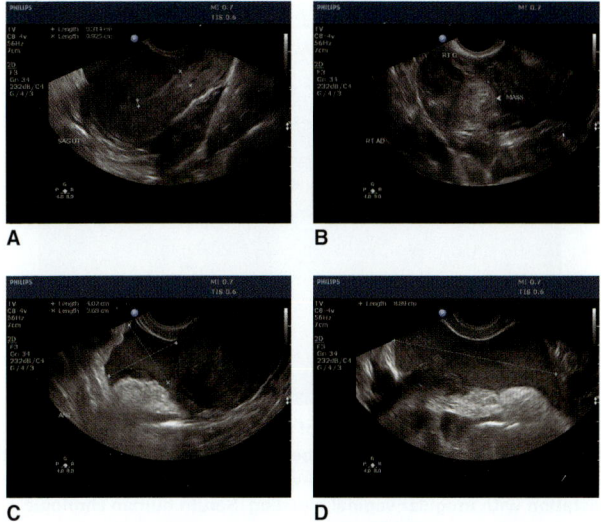

Figure 6-38. Sonographic signs of ectopic pregnancy. A. Endovaginal ultrasound in a sagittal plane demonstrates an empty uterus in a pregnant patient. **B.** Transverse endovaginal image demonstrates a mass in the right adnexal area. RT O, right ovary. **C.** Transverse image demonstrating complex free fluid in the right adnexal area. **D.** Sagittal endovaginal image of the same fluid, which was determined surgically to be blood. (Reprinted with permission from Auckland A. Sonographic assessment of the ectopic pregnancy. In: Stephenson SR, Dmitrieva J, eds. *Diagnostic Medical Sonography: Obstetrics & Gynecology.* 4th ed. Wolters Kluwer; 2018. Figure 17-23.)

- Hyperemesis gravidarum (excessive vomiting during pregnancy)
- Markedly elevated hCG level
- Heavy vaginal bleeding
- Enlarged uterus
- Hypertension
- Sonographic findings of a molar pregnancy **(Fig. 6-39)**
  - Complex mass representing an enlarged heterogeneous placenta within the uterus ("vesicular snowstorm appearance")
  - Variable-sized cysts replacing normal placental tissue with hydropic villi
  - Partial molar pregnancy will have a fetus that is likely triploid

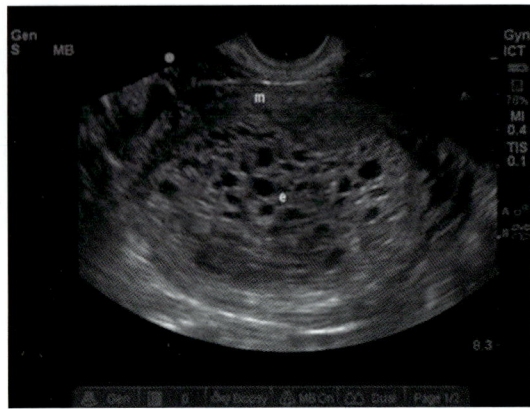

Figure 6-39. Sonographic signs of molar pregnancy. Sonogram showing multiple vesicular endometrial structures (*e*) consistent with a complete molar pregnancy. A 26-year-old presented at 10 weeks' gestation with irregular vaginal bleeding. Serum human chorionic gonadotropin was 1,20,000 mIU/mL. m, myometrium. (Reprinted with permission from Berkowitz RS, Horowitz NS, Goldstein DP. Gestational trophoblastic disease. In: Berek JS, Hacker NF, eds. *Berek & Hacker's Gynecologic Oncology*. 7th ed. Wolters Kluwer; 2021. Figure 15.1.)

- Bilateral ovarian theca-lutein cysts which will appear as enlarged cystic ovaries
- Embryonic demise—death of the embryo
  - Clinical findings of an embryonic demise
    - Vaginal bleeding
    - Small for date
    - Low hCG (based on last menstrual period)
  - Sonographic findings of an embryonic demise (see Fig. 6-35)
    - No detectable heartbeat in a 4- to 5-mm embryo (follow-up may be warranted)
    - Irregular shaped fetus
    - Irregular sized or shaped gestational sac
    - Irregular appearing yolk sac (e.g., calcified, enlarged, misshapen, etc.)
- Miscarriage—termination of a pregnancy before viability
  - Clinical findings of a miscarriage
    - Vaginal bleeding
    - Pelvic cramping
    - Passage of the products of conception

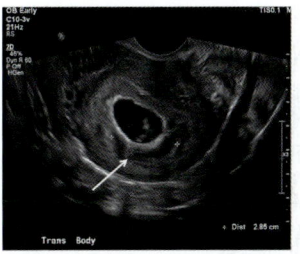 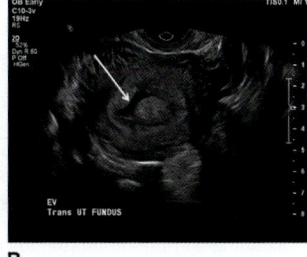

A   **B**

Figure 6-40. Subchorionic hemorrhage. Subchorionic hemorrhage. A, B. Transvaginal image in the same patient shows a large subchorionic hemorrhage (*long arrows*) adjacent to the gestational sac. (Reprinted with permission from Kanmaniraja D, Fernandez C, Murakami ME, Cernigliaro JG. Imaging in gynecologic emergencies. In: Benrubi GI, ed. *Handbook of Obstetric and Gynecologic Emergencies*. 5th ed. Wolters Kluwer; 2020. Figure 28.9.)

- Lower than normal hCG (based on last menstrual period)
- Sonographic findings of a miscarriage
  - Complete abortion—empty uterine cavity
  - Incomplete abortion—parts of the products of conception remain within the uterus
  - Missed abortion—no detectable fetal heart motion with abnormal fetal shape
  - Inevitable abortion—low-lying gestational sac with an open internal cervical os
- Subchorionic hemorrhage–a bleed between the endometrium and the gestational sac
  - Clinical findings of a subchorionic hemorrhage
    - Vaginal bleeding or spotting
    - Uterine cramping
    - Closed cervix
  - Sonographic findings of a subchorionic hemorrhage **(Fig. 6-40)**
    - Crescent-shaped anechoic or hypoechoic region adjacent to the gestational sac
    - May be large and resemble a second gestational sac

REFERENCES

1. AIUM-ACR-ACOG-SMFM-SRU. Practice parameter for the performance of standard diagnostic obstetric ultrasound examinations. *J Ultrasound Med*. 2018;37:E13-E24.
2. Penny SM. *Examination Review for Ultrasound: Abdomen & Obstetrics and Gynecology*. 3rd ed. Wolters Kluwer; 2022:Section III.

3. Stephenson SR, Dmitrieva J. *Diagnostic Medical Sonography: Obstetrics and Gynecology*. 5th ed. Wolters Kluwer; 2023:339-394.
4. AIUM. Practice parameter for documentation of an ultrasound examination. *J Ultrasound Med*. 2020;39:E1-E4.
5. Guidelines for Cleaning and Preparing External- and Internal-Use Ultrasound Transducers and Equipment Between Patients as Well as Safe Handling and Use of Ultrasound Coupling Gel. Accessed November 12, 2023. https://www.aium.org/resources/official-statements/view/guidelines-for-cleaning-and-preparing-external-and-internal-use-ultrasound-transducers-and-equipment-between-patients-as-well-as-safe-handling-and-use-of-ultrasound-coupling-gel
6. AIUM Routine Quality Assurance of Clinical Ultrasound Equipment version 2.0. Accessed November 12, 2023. http://aium.s3.amazonaws.com/resourceLibrary/rqa2.pdf
7. Kline-Fath BM, Bulas DI, Lee W. *Fundamental and Advanced Fetal Imaging: Ultrasound and MRI*. 2nd ed. Wolters Kluwer; 2021:Appendix 9.81-1034.

CHAPTER 7

Detailed First-Trimester Sonography

INTRODUCTION

This chapter will provide some information regarding the detailed first-trimester sonogram described by the AIUM. The detailed first-trimester sonographic examination is performed between 12 weeks 0 days and 13 weeks 6 days and is usually an adjunct to the standard examination. Early detection of major anomalies allows the patient to seek further resources, including genetic testing and counseling.

SPECIFICATIONS OF THE DETAILED FIRST-TRIMESTER SONOGRAM[1]

- A combined transabdominal and transvaginal imaging may prove most beneficial for detecting fetal anomalies.
- Magnification, adjusting the depth appropriately, sector size, and correct focal zone placement at the area of interest are important.
- Other image optimization tools such as harmonics, compounding, and speckle reduction may enhance the image to improve diagnosis.
- Power and color Doppler imaging can be used at times to complement grayscale imaging.

SCANNING PLANES AND STRUCTURES REQUIRED FOR A DETAILED FIRST-TRIMESTER SONOGRAM[1,2]

- General assessment
  - Required
    - The output display standard is based on a thermal index for bone ratio which is less than or equal to 0.7.
    - Embryo/fetal cardiac activity must be documented.

- Cardiac activity can be demonstrated with M-mode or with a cine loop.
- Beats per minute, which is the heart rate, should be obtained.
- Number of fetuses and gestational sacs
  - Amnionicity and chorionicity should be documented if multiple gestations are observed (see Chapter 9 for more details on multiple gestations).
- Fetal biometry
  - Required
    - Crown–rump length
      - At least three measurements should be obtained, and the mean reported.
      - Fetus should fill at least two-thirds of the image space available.
      - The long axis of the fetus should be perpendicular to the ultrasound beam.
      - The fetus should be in a neutral position with fluid between the fetal chin and anterior neck.
        - The angle between the chin and anterior neck should not be greater than 90 degrees.
      - The fetus should be in the midsagittal position, with the profile, spine, and rump visible.
      - The caliper crossbars should be placed on the outer border of the skin on the fetal head and rump. The caudal caliper should not be on the distal spine or posterior thigh or include the limbs.
      - The maximum length of the fetus from the cranial to caudal calipers should be measured in a straight line, parallel to the long axis of the fetus.
  - If indicated or suspicious
    - Biparietal diameter (BPD) and head circumference (HC)
      - An axial scan of the fetal head with the ultrasound beam perpendicular to the midline falx should be obtained and magnified to fill most of the image space without compromising image quality.
      - The fetal calvarium should not be distorted by transducer pressure or adjacent structures.
      - The brain and calvarium should appear symmetric with the midline falx centrally located.

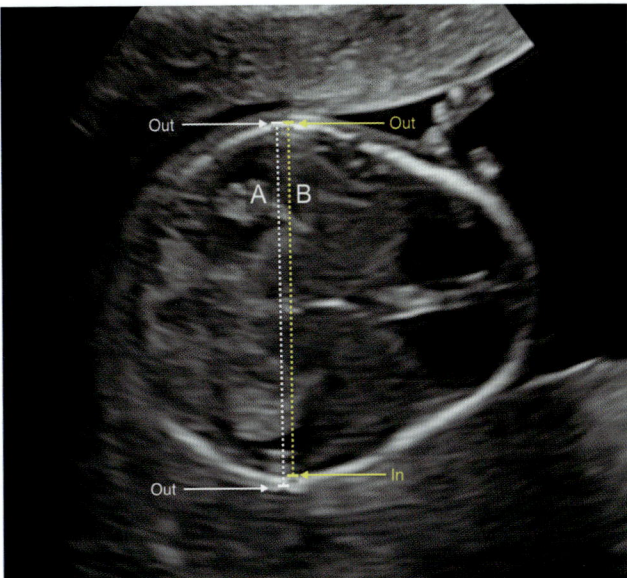

Figure 7-1. First-trimester biparietal diameter. Biparietal diameter (BPD) measurement of a fetus at 13 weeks of gestation. According to the setting used, the measurement is achieved either outside to outside (A) or outside to inside (B). (Reprinted with permission from Abuhamad A, Chaoui R. *First Trimester Ultrasound Diagnosis of Fetal Abnormalities.* Wolters Kluwer; 2018. Figure 4.14.)

- The thalami should be seen, and the third ventricle is typically visible.
- Measurements are made at the widest diameter of the calvarium, perpendicular to the midline falx.
- The skin should not be included in the measurement.
- For BPD, the crossbar of the "near" caliper should be placed on the outside edge of the bone.
- The crossbar of the "far" caliper may be placed on the inside edge of the bone (outer to inner) or on the outer edge of the bone (outer to outer) depending on the nomogram used **(Fig. 7-1)**.
- For HC, the measurement is made by placing an ellipse on the outer surface of the calvarium excluding skin **(Fig. 7-2)**.

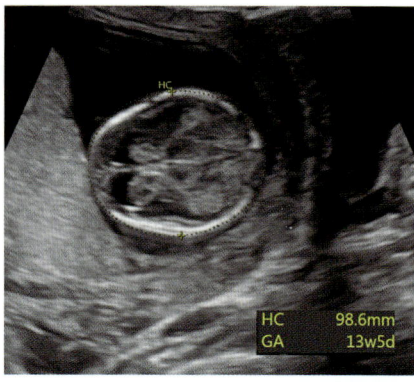

Figure 7-2. First-trimester head circumference. Head circumference (*HC*) measurement of a fetus at 13 + 5 weeks of gestation. Note that the calipers are placed outside to outside for HC measurement. GA, gestational age. (Reprinted with permission from Abuhamad A, Chaoui R. *First Trimester Ultrasound Diagnosis of Fetal Abnormalities*. Wolters Kluwer; 2018. Figure 4.15.)

- Abdominal circumference
  - An axial scan of the fetal abdomen is obtained and magnified to fill most of the available image space without compromising image quality.
  - The fetal stomach and, if possible, the intrahepatic portion of the portal vein should be seen.
  - The kidneys and umbilical cord insertion into the fetus should not be in the image.
  - One vertebral body should be identified, and a single rib on each side lateral to the spine should be seen to ensure that the abdomen is in a true axial plane and not oblique.
  - Optimally, the cross-section of the spine is at 3 or 9 o'clock.
  - Measurements should be made along the outer skin edge. This can be done by an ellipse or two perpendicular diameters **(Fig. 7-3)**.
- Femoral length
  - The femoral diaphysis should be magnified to fill most of the image space without compromising imaging quality.
  - The ultrasound beam is perpendicular to the long axis of the femur.

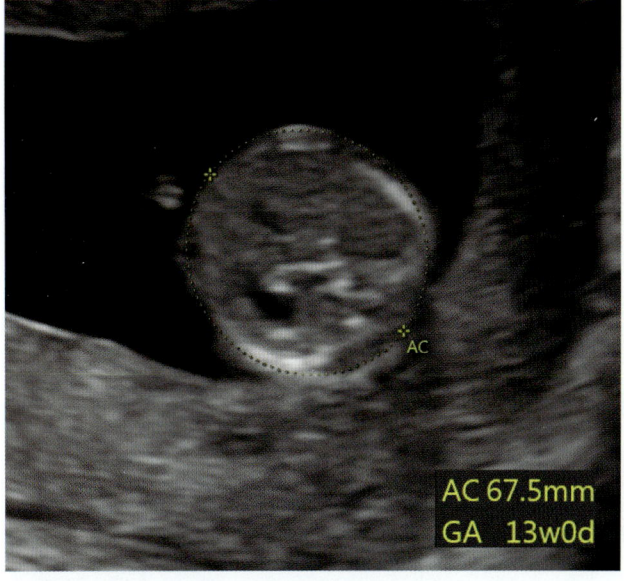

Figure 7-3. First-trimester abdominal circumference. Abdominal circumference (*AC*) measurement of a fetus at 13 weeks of gestation. **GA,** gestational age. (Reprinted with permission from Abuhamad A, Chaoui R. *First Trimester Ultrasound Diagnosis of Fetal Abnormalities.* Wolters Kluwer; 2018. Figure 4.16.)

- ○ The calipers are placed at the proximal and distal ends of the ossified diaphysis **(Fig. 7-4)**.
- ○ Spur artifacts at the end of the femur should not be included.
- ○ The longest visible diaphysis is measured.
- Fetal head
  - Required—axial images
    - Transventricular images (see 6-15, 6-16 and 6-22)
      - ○ Cranial bones
        - Evaluate the cranium for proper oval shape, no bulges, and appropriate ossification.
      - ○ Falx cerebri
        - Evaluate the falx cerebri for symmetric cerebral hemispheres and that the falx travels completely from anterior to posterior.
        - Choroid plexus

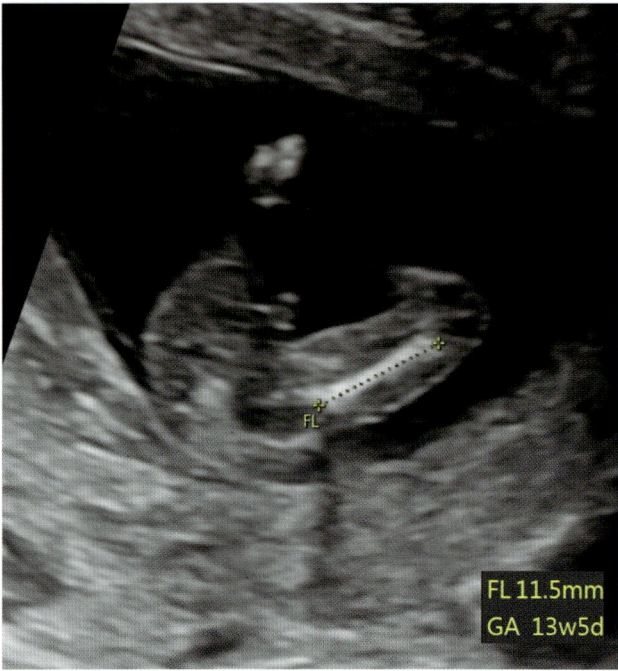

Figure 7-4. First-trimester femur length. Femur length (*FL*) measurement of a fetus at 13 weeks of gestation. (Reprinted with permission from Abuhamad A, Chaoui R. *First Trimester Ultrasound Diagnosis of Fetal Abnormalities.* Wolters Kluwer; 2018. Figure 4.17.)

- Ensure that the choroid plexus fills the majority of the lateral ventricles.
- If indicated or suspicious—axial
  - Lateral ventricles
    - Evaluate the lateral ventricles for symmetry.
  - Cerebral cortex
    - The normal cortex will be thin and seen mostly anteriorly.
- Required—transthalamic (see Fig. 6-22)
  - The transthalamic plane demonstrates the thalami, the cerebral peduncles, and typically the third ventricle and aqueduct of Sylvius.
    - Falx cerebri
      - Echogenic structure in the midline.

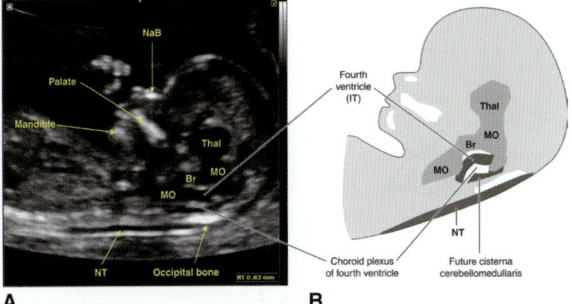

Figure 7-5. Anatomy of the face, brain, and posterior fossa on an early sonogram (A) and diagram (B). Sonogram and diagram showing the intracranial translucency in a normal fetus. Midsagittal plane view of the fetal face showing the nasal bone (*NaB*), palate, mandible, nuchal translucency (*NT*), thalamus (*Thal*), midbrain (*Mb*), brain stem (*Br*), and medulla oblongata (*MO*). The fourth ventricle presents as an intracranial translucency (*NT*) between the brain stem and the choroid plexus. The intracranial translucency is absent if spina bifida is present. (Reprinted with permission from Woletz P. The use of ultrasound in the first trimester. In: Stephenson SR, Dmitrieva J, eds. *Diagnostic Medical Sonography: Obstetrics & Gynecology*. 4th ed. Wolters Kluwer; 2018. Figure 15-20.)

- Thalami
  - Bilateral, hypoechoic structures adjacent to the midline of the brain.
- Posterior fossa (see Fig. 6-23)
  - To image the posterior fossa one needs to angle posterior-inferiorly.
- If indicated or suspicious—transthalamic
  - The third ventricle is located between the two lobes of the thalamus.
- Required—sagittal **(Fig. 7-5)**
  - The following structures should be noted:
    - Thalami
    - Midbrain
    - Brain stem
    - Fourth ventricle (intracranial translucency)
    - Cisterna magna
- Facial structures
  - If indicated or suspicious—axial
    - Orbits

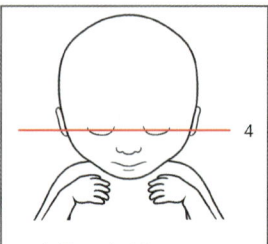
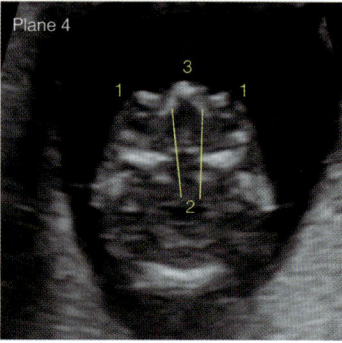

1. Eyes/orbits
2. Maxillary processes
3. Nose

A

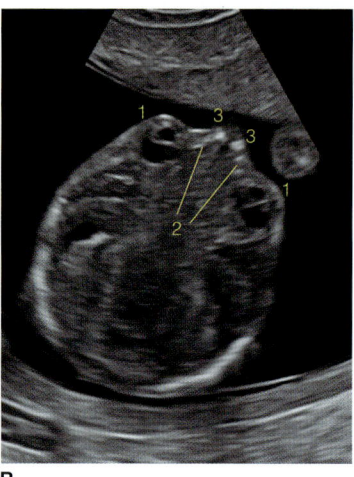

B

Figure 7-6. Fetal orbits. A. Level of the orbits drawing on the left, with a corresponding axial transabdominal sonogram of the orbits demonstrating two orbits (*1*), the eyes, maxillary processes (*2*), and the nose (*3*). B. Transvaginal image demonstrates more detail of the same anatomy in figure A. (Reprinted with permission from Abuhamad A, Chaoui R. *First Trimester Ultrasound Diagnosis of Fetal Abnormalities.* Wolters Kluwer; 2018. Figures 5.9 and 9.8.)

- The size and position of the orbits can be analyzed **(Fig. 7-6)**.
- Close-set eyes denote hypotelorism.
- Wide-spaced eyes denote hypertelorism.

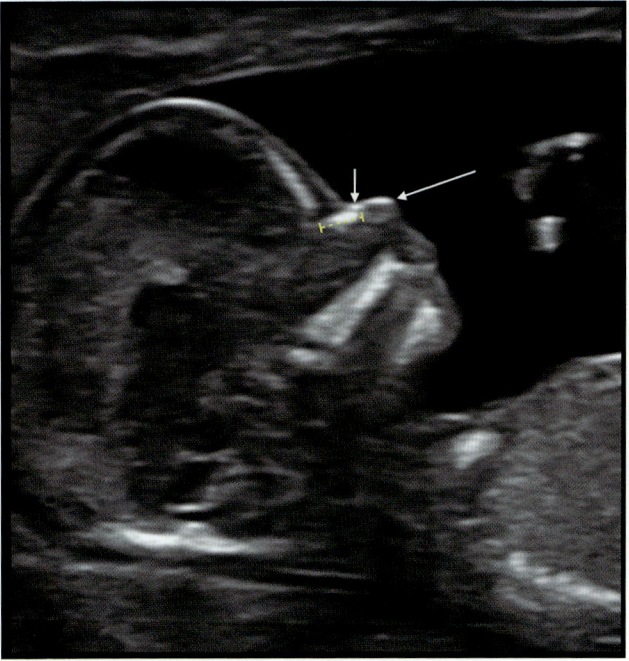

Figure 7-7. Midsagittal view of a fetus at 13 weeks of gestation showing the display of the nasal bone. Yellow calipers measure the nasal bone. Note the presence of two other echogenic lines, superior to the nasal bone, representing the nasal skin (*short arrow*) and the tip of the nose (*long arrow*). (Reprinted with permission from Abuhamad A, Chaoui R. *First Trimester Ultrasound Diagnosis of Fetal Abnormalities.* Wolters Kluwer; 2018. Figure 1.3.)

- Required—sagittal
  - Nasal bones **(Fig. 7-7)**
    - Evaluate the nasal contour.
    - The presence or absence of the nasal bones should be determined **(Fig. 7-8)**.
    - Guidelines for nasal bone assessment[3]
      - The gestational period must be 11 to 13 weeks and 6 days.
      - The magnification of the image should be such that the fetal head and thorax occupy the whole image.
      - A midsagittal view of the face should be obtained.

Nasal Bone Length

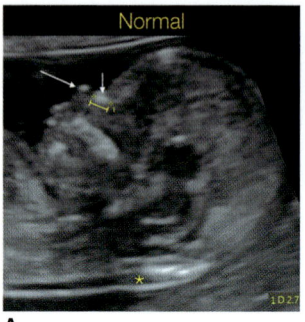
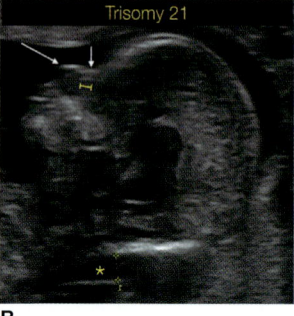

Figure 7-8. Midsagittal views of the fetal face showing the measurement of the nasal bone length in a normal fetus (**A**) and in a fetus with trisomy 21 (**B**). In more than half of the fetuses with trisomy 21, the nasal bone is either completely nonossified or, as in this case, poorly ossified, resulting in a short and thin appearance. *Long arrows* point to the nose tip and *short arrows* to the nasal skin. Nuchal translucency measurement is also seen (*asterisk*).
(Reprinted with permission from Abuhamad A, Chaoui R. *First Trimester Ultrasound Diagnosis of Fetal Abnormalities.* Wolters Kluwer; 2018. Figure 9.15.)

- This is defined by the presence of the echogenic tip of the nose and rectangular shape of the palate anteriorly, the translucent diencephalon in the center, and the nuchal membrane posteriorly.
- Minor deviations from the exact midline plane would cause nonvisualization of the tip of the nose and visibility of the maxilla.
- The transducer should be held parallel to the direction of the nose and should be gently tilted from side to side to ensure that the nasal bone is seen separate from the nasal skin.
- The echogenicity of the nasal bone should be greater than the skin overlying it.
  - In this respect, the correct view of the nasal bone should demonstrate three distinct lines: the first two lines, which are proximal to the forehead, are horizontal and parallel to each other, resembling an "equal sign."

- The top line represents the skin and bottom one, which is thicker and more echogenic than the overlying skin, represents the nasal bone.
- A third line, almost in continuity with the skin, but at a higher level, represents the tip of the nose.
- When the nasal bone line appears as a thin line, less echogenic than the overlying skin, it suggests that the nasal bone is not yet ossified, and it is therefore classified as being absent.
- Profile
  - Forehead
    - Appearance of the forehead should be analyzed.
    - Prefrontal space distance (PSD) can be obtained.
      - Prefrontal space is the distance between the forehead and a line drawn from the anterior aspect of the maxilla and mandible (Fig. 7-9).

Prefrontal Space Distance

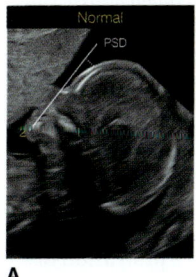
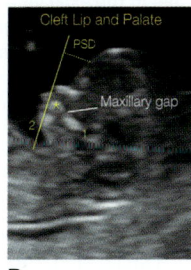
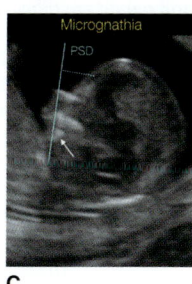

A **B** **C**

Figure 7-9. Midsagittal views of the fetal face showing the measurement of the prefrontal space distance in a normal fetus (A), in a fetus with cleft lip and palate (B), and in a fetus with micrognathia (C). The prefrontal space distance (*PSD*) is the distance between the forehead and a line drawn from the anterior aspect of maxilla (*1*) and mandible (*2*). In the normal fetus (A), the PSD is quite short. In the presence of a facial cleft (fetus B), there is a protrusion of the maxilla (*asterisk*), and the PSD is increased. In the presence of micrognathia (fetus C), the mandible is posteriorly shifted (*arrow*), leading to an increased PSD as well. Note in fetus B the presence of an interrupted maxilla, called maxillary gap, a midsagittal view sign for the presence of cleft lip and palate. (Reprinted with permission from Abuhamad A, Chaoui R. *First Trimester Ultrasound Diagnosis of Fetal Abnormalities*. Wolters Kluwer; 2018. Figure 9.19.)

Unilateral Cleft

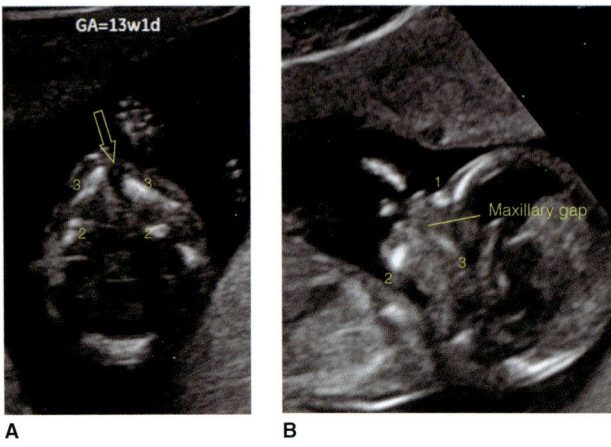

Figure 7-10. Axial (A) and midsagittal (B) views of the face at 13 weeks of gestation in a fetus with a unilateral cleft lip and palate. The cleft lip and palate are demonstrated in the axial view (A) *(open arrow)*. Note the presence of a maxillary gap in the midsagittal view of the face (B). The following facial structures are seen: nasal bone (*1*), mandible (*2*), and maxilla (*3*). (Reprinted with permission from Abuhamad A, Chaoui R. *First Trimester Ultrasound Diagnosis of Fetal Abnormalities.* Wolters Kluwer; 2018. Figure 9.27.)

- In the normal fetus, the PSD is quite short. In the presence of a facial cleft, there is a protrusion of the maxilla, and the PSD is increased.
- In the presence of micrognathia, the mandible is posteriorly shifted, leading to an increased PSD as well.
  ○ Upper lip
    – Evaluate the upper lip to ensure that it is completely intact **(Fig. 7-10)**.
  ○ Mandible **(Fig. 7-11)**
- Maxilla
  ○ Evaluate for a maxillary gap **(Fig. 7-12)**.
    – The normal maxilla will not have a gap.
    – The presence of a maxillary gap is suspicious for a cleft palate.

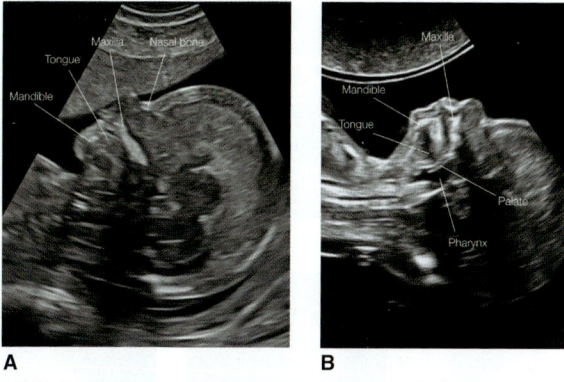

Figure 7-11. Normal mandible. Transvaginal sonogram of the midsagittal plane of the fetal face in two fetuses (A and B) at 13 weeks of gestation. In fetus A, the ultrasound beam is perpendicular to the long axis of the face and clearly displays the nose with nasal bone, the maxilla, and chin with mandible. Note in A the tongue between the maxilla and mandible. In fetus B, the ultrasound beam is inferior below the chin and shows the posterior aspect of the mouth region with the tongue, hard and soft palate, and the pharynx. (Reprinted with permission from Abuhamad A, Chaoui R. *First Trimester Ultrasound Diagnosis of Fetal Abnormalities.* Wolters Kluwer; 2018. Figure 9.5.)

Maxillary Gap

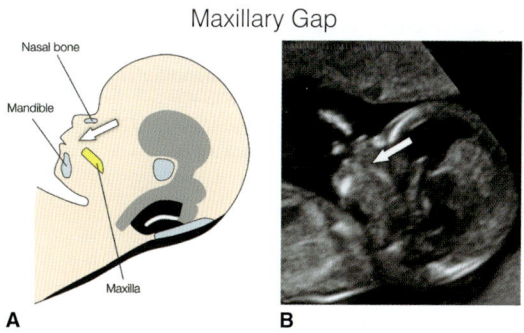

Figure 7-12. Maxillary gap. Schematic drawing of the midsagittal view of the fetal face (A) along with the corresponding sonogram (B) demonstrating the maxillary gap (*white arrows*) in a fetus with cleft lip and palate. In this midsagittal view plane, the entire maxilla should be seen. The size and location of the maxillary gap vary according to the size and type of clefts. (Reprinted with permission from Abuhamad A, Chaoui R. *First Trimester Ultrasound Diagnosis of Fetal Abnormalities.* Wolters Kluwer; 2018. Figure 9.26.)

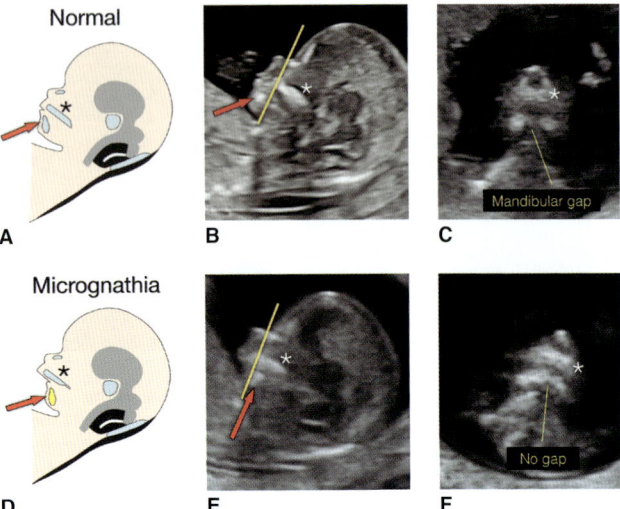

Figure 7-13. Schematic drawing of the midsagittal plane of the fetal face (A, D) along with the corresponding midsagittal (B, E) and retronasal triangle (C, F) views in a normal fetus (A–C) and in a fetus with micrognathia (D–F). Note in the normal fetus that the tip of the mandible (*red arrow*) reaches under the anterior aspect of the maxilla (*asterisk*), as shown in A and B. In the normal fetus, the retronasal triangle (C) demonstrates the normal mandibular gap. In the fetus with micrognathia (D–F), the chin is receded behind the line (*red arrow*) (E), and no mandibular gap is noted in the retronasal triangle view, as shown in F. (Reprinted with permission from Abuhamad A, Chaoui R. *First Trimester Ultrasound Diagnosis of Fetal Abnormalities.* Wolters Kluwer; 2018. Figure 9.35.)

- Required—coronal/tangential
  - Mandible
    - Evaluate for absence of mandibular gap (Fig. 7-13)
      - The absence of the mandibular gap raises a concern for micrognathia (recessed chin).
      - In the normal fetus, the tip of the mandible reaches under the anterior aspect of the maxilla.
      - In the normal fetus, the retronasal triangle demonstrates the normal mandibular gap. In the fetus with micrognathia, the chin is receded, and no mandibular gap is noted in the retronasal triangle view (Fig. 7-14).

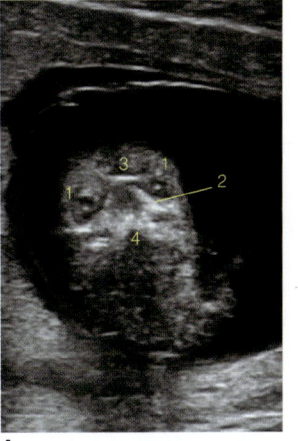 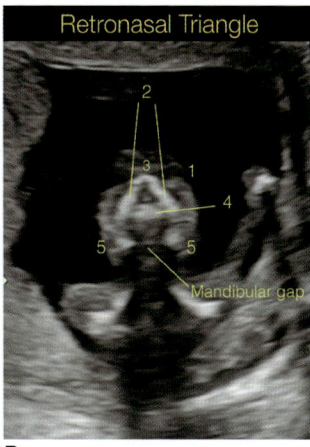

A **B**

Figure 7-14. Retronasal triangle. Coronal planes in two fetuses (A and B) at 12 weeks of gestation, were obtained at the frontal aspects of the bony face. In fetus A, the coronal plane is at the level of the orbits and shows the two eyes (*1*) with orbits and lenses, between the maxillary processes (*2*), the nasal bones (*3*), and the anterior aspect of the maxilla (*4*) with the alveolar ridge. In fetus B, the plane is oblique and demonstrates the retronasal triangle, which is formed by the nasal bones superiorly (*3*), the frontal processes of the maxilla laterally (*2*), and the alveolar ridge (primary palate) inferiorly (*4*). This coronal section (B) is posterior to the tip of the mandible, and therefore the two lateral bodies of the mandible are seen (*5*) with a normal gap between, called the mandibular gap. (Reprinted with permission from Abuhamad A, Chaoui R. *First Trimester Ultrasound Diagnosis of Fetal Abnormalities.* Wolters Kluwer; 2018. Figure 9.7.)

- If Indicated or suspicious—coronal/tangential
  - Retronasal triangle with ancillary bones including the frontal process of the maxilla and alveolar ridge.
    - Nasal bone may be evaluated in this view as well.
  - Upper lip
    - The upper lip should be intact and contiguous.
  - Orbits
    - The lenses should be noted.
  - Ears
    - There should be evidence of both ears and three-dimensional imaging can be helpful **(Fig. 7-15)**.

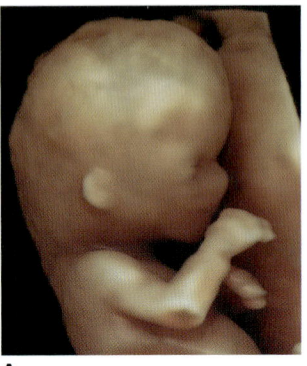
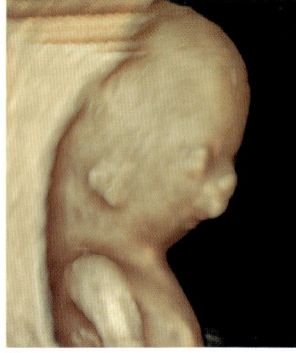

Figure 7-15. Fetal ear in the first trimester. A. Three-dimensional volume in surface mode at 12 weeks of gestation in a normal fetus. B. Abnormal ear and micrognathia are noted in this image. (Reprinted with permission from Abuhamad A, Chaoui R. *First Trimester Ultrasound Diagnosis of Fetal Abnormalities*. Wolters Kluwer; 2018. Figure 3.27.)

- Neck
  - Required—axial, sagittal, coronal
    - Evaluation for cystic hygroma, dilated jugular lymphatic sac, other abnormal fluid collections, and masses.
  - Required—sagittal
    - Nuchal translucency (See *AIUM Guidelines for Nuchal Translucency Measurements between 11 and 14 weeks* in Chapter 6.)
  - If indicated or suspicious—sagittal
    - Nuchal translucency measurement
      - Measurement is required if it appears enlarged or part of a screening protocol for aneuploidy risk assessment.
      - A quality assessment program is recommended.
- Fetal thorax
  - Note: The use of color Doppler should be limited in the first trimester, though color flow is useful to evaluate the fetal heart, great vessels, and circulation. Again, the output display standard should be monitored to keep the TI for bone, which is less than or equal to 0.7.
  - Required—axial
    - Cardiac position and axis **(Fig. 7-16)**

Chapter 7. Detailed First-Trimester Sonography

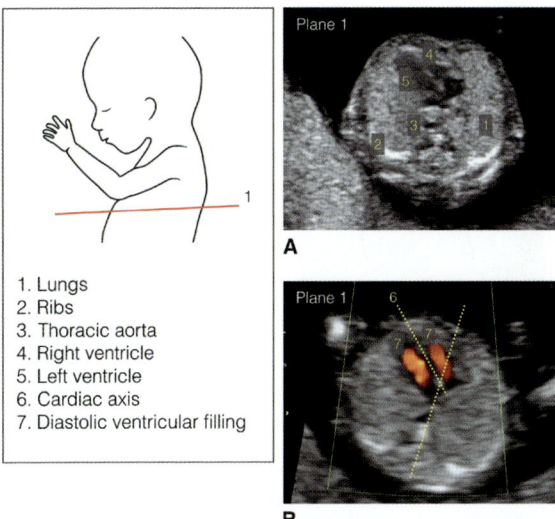

1. Lungs
2. Ribs
3. Thoracic aorta
4. Right ventricle
5. Left ventricle
6. Cardiac axis
7. Diastolic ventricular filling

Figure 7-16. The fetal chest is assessed in two planes: axial plane at the level of the four-chamber view and axial plane at the level of the three-vessel trachea view. This figure shows plane 1, at the level of the four-chamber view. This plane is for the anatomic assessment of the heart, lungs, and the rib cage. Plane 1 is best assessed in grayscale (A) and color Doppler (B) as shown here. Cardiac axis can also be measured in this plane and adding color Doppler facilitates its measurement (B). (Reprinted with permission from Abuhamad A, Chaoui R. *First Trimester Ultrasound Diagnosis of Fetal Abnormalities*. Wolters Kluwer; 2018. Figure 5.11.)

- ○ Subjective assessment
  - The size of the heart should occupy no more than one-third of the fetal chest.
- Four-chamber view without color Doppler
  - ○ Evaluate for symmetric chambers and the presence or absence of pericardial effusion.
  - ○ Evaluate for symmetric atrioventricular valves.
- Four-chamber view with color Doppler (see **Fig. 7-16**)
  - ○ Diastolic filling should be assessed.
- Three-vessel and trachea view with color Doppler **(Fig. 7-17)**
  - ○ Antegrade flow should be assessed.
- Symmetrical lungs
  - ○ The lungs may be evaluated in coronal also.
  - ○ Ensure that there are no chest masses or effusions.

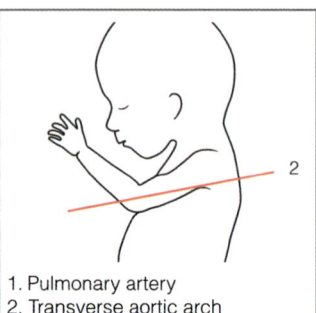 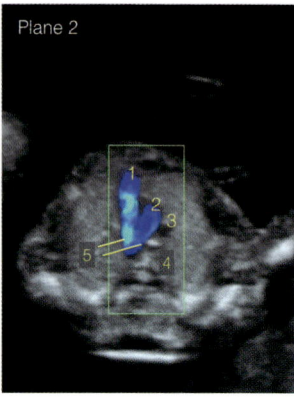

1. Pulmonary artery
2. Transverse aortic arch
3. Superior vena cava
4. Trachea
5. Systolic flow in great vessels

Figure 7-17. The fetal chest is assessed in the axial plane at the level of the three-vessel trachea view (plane 2) shown here. Plane 2 is best obtained in color Doppler showing the pulmonary artery, the aorta, the superior vena cava, and the trachea. This plane allows for the detection of complex cardiac anomalies in the first trimester. (Reprinted with permission from Abuhamad A, Chaoui R. *First Trimester Ultrasound Diagnosis of Fetal Abnormalities.* Wolters Kluwer; 2018. Figure 5.12.)

- If indicated or suspicious—axial
  - Cardiac axis
    - The normal cardiac axis is ≈45 ± 15 degrees and it should be angled leftward.
    - Symmetric chambers should be determined.
    - Pericardial effusions should be ruled out.
  - The ribs should be of normal shape, length, and ossification.
  - Tricuspid valve flow (Fig. 7-18 and 7-19)
    - The sample volume is placed over the valve to cover inflow and regurgitation when present.
    - Tricuspid regurgitation is a sonographic marker of trisomy 21.
- Required—sagittal
  - Diaphragm demarcation (Fig. 7-20)
    - The contour of the diaphragm should be noted as smooth and separating the chest from the abdomen.
    - The slightly hyperechoic lung, as compared to the liver, will be noted with the diaphragm in between. The bowel tends to have the same echogenicity as the lung.

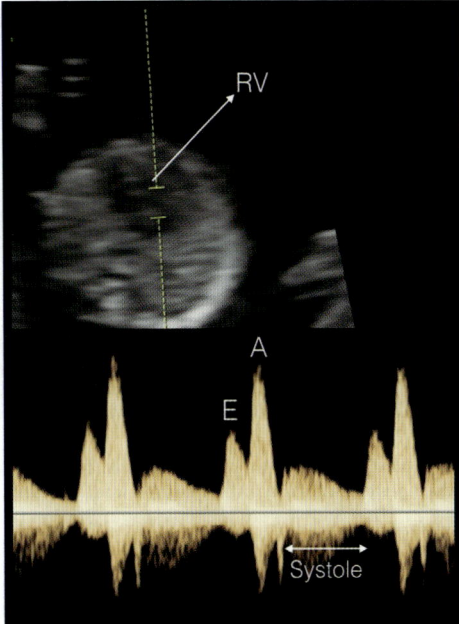

Figure 7-18. Tricuspid valve assessment. A. Axial plane of the fetal chest in a fetus at 13 weeks of gestation showing placement of the pulsed Doppler sample volume for tricuspid Doppler flow assessment. Note that the sample volume is placed over the valve to cover inflow and regurgitation when present. In this example, there is no tricuspid regurgitation in systole (*double arrow*) and the Doppler spectrum is normal with *E* corresponding to early diastole and *A* corresponding to the atrial kick portion of diastole. (Reprinted with permission from Abuhamad A, Chaoui R. *First Trimester Ultrasound Diagnosis of Fetal Abnormalities.* Wolters Kluwer; 2018. Figure 1.5.)

- If indicated or suspicious—sagittal
  - Aortic arch with color Doppler **(Fig. 7-21)**
    - Antegrade flow should be noted.
  - Ductal arch **(Fig. 7-22)**
    - Antegrade flow should be noted.
- Required–coronal **(Fig. 7-23)**
  - Lungs should be clearly noted.
  - Diaphragm demarcation
    - The contour of the diaphragm should be evaluated.

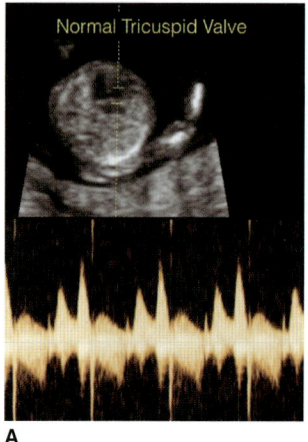
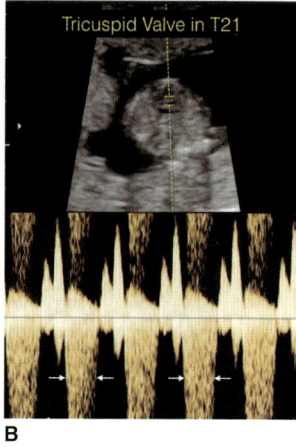

Figure 7-19. Doppler velocity waveforms across the tricuspid valve at 12 weeks of gestation in a normal fetus (A) and in a fetus (B) with trisomy 21 (*T21*) with severe tricuspid regurgitation (*arrows*). (Reprinted with permission from Abuhamad A, Chaoui R. *First Trimester Ultrasound Diagnosis of Fetal Abnormalities*. Wolters Kluwer; 2018. Figure 3.18.)

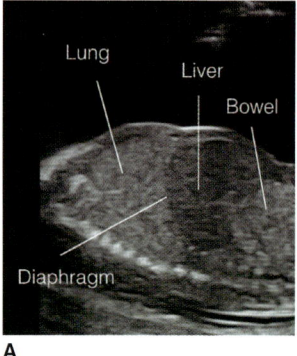
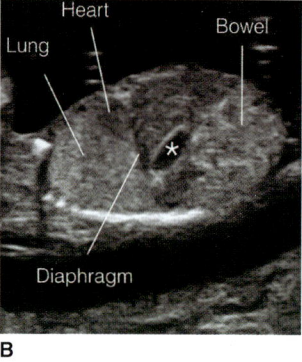

Figure 7-20. Diaphragm. Right (A) and left (B) parasagittal planes of the fetal chest at 13 weeks of gestation. Note in the right thorax (A) the slightly hyperechoic lung as compared to the liver and the diaphragm in between. The bowel has the same echogenicity as the lung. The parasagittal view on the left (B) shows the lung, portion of the heart, the diaphragm, and the stomach (*asterisk*). (Reprinted with permission from Abuhamad A, Chaoui R. *First Trimester Ultrasound Diagnosis of Fetal Abnormalities*. Wolters Kluwer; 2018. Figure 10.5.)

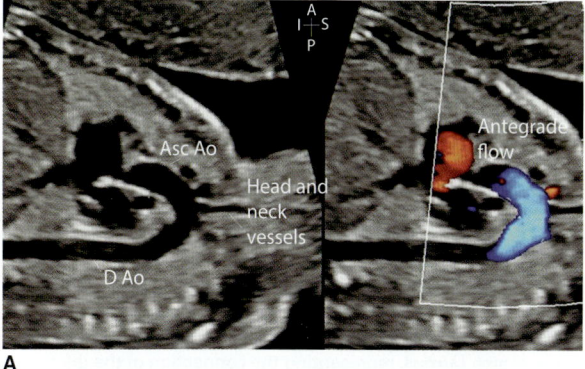

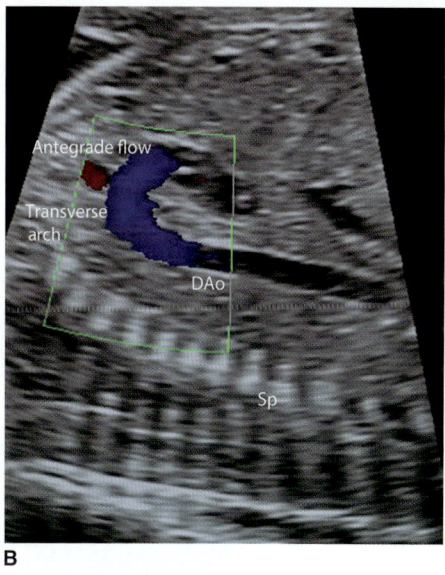

Figure 7-21. Aortic arch. A. Longitudinal view of the aortic arch. Ascending aorta (*Asc Ao*) continues as the transverse arch in a "candy cane" shape. The aorta gives rise to the head and neck vessels and continues as the descending aorta (*DAo*), anterior to the spine (Sp). **B.** Antegrade flow in the aortic arch as demonstrated on color flow Doppler. (Reprinted with permission from Simpson JM, Hunter HE. Fetal echocardiography. In: Eidem BW, Lopez L, Johnson JN, Cetta F, eds. *Echocardiography in Pediatric and Adult Congenital Heart Disease*. 3rd ed. Wolters Kluwer; 2021. Figure 33.15.)

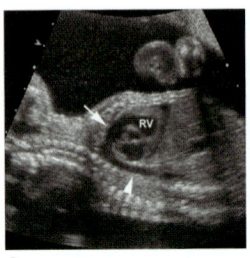 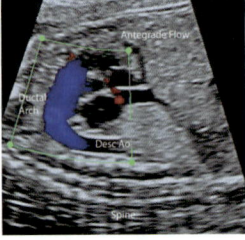

Figure 7-22. Right ventricular outflow tract and ductal arch. A. Right ventricular outflow tract and ductal arch to the descending aorta. Sagittal image demonstrating the right ventricular (*RV*) outflow tract and ductal arch (*arrow*), representing the connection of the ductus arteriosus to the descending thoracic aorta (*arrowhead*). **B.** Longitudinal view of the "hockey stick" ductal arch continuing as the descending aorta (*DescAo*). Antegrade flow in the ductal arch demonstrated on color flow Doppler. (**A.** Reprinted with permission from Doubilet PM, Benson CB. *Atlas of Ultrasound in Obstetrics and Gynecology: A Multimedia Reference.* 2nd ed. Wolters Kluwer Health/Lippincott Williams & Wilkins; 2012. Figure 2.5.6. **B.** Reprinted with permission from Kimball TR. Stress Echocardiography. In: Eidem BW, O'Leary PW, Cetta F, eds. *Echocardiography in Pediatric and Adult Congenital Heart Disease.* 2nd ed. Wolters Kluwer; 2015. Figure 32-16B.)

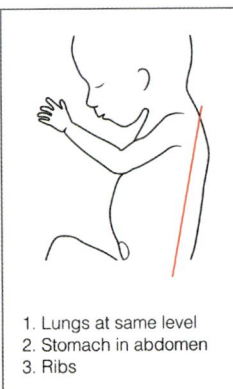 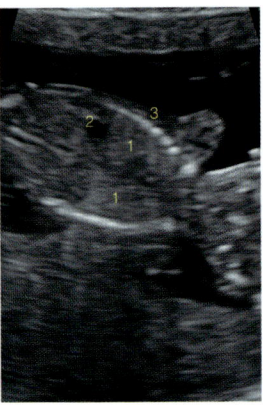

1. Lungs at same level
2. Stomach in abdomen
3. Ribs

Figure 7-23. Coronal plane of the fetal chest and abdomen for the assessment of the diaphragm when there is a suspicion of diaphragmatic hernia. This plane shows both lungs at the same level as the stomach and liver in abdomen. (Reprinted with permission from Abuhamad A, Chaoui R. *First Trimester Ultrasound Diagnosis of Fetal Abnormalities.* Wolters Kluwer; 2018. Figure 5.13.)

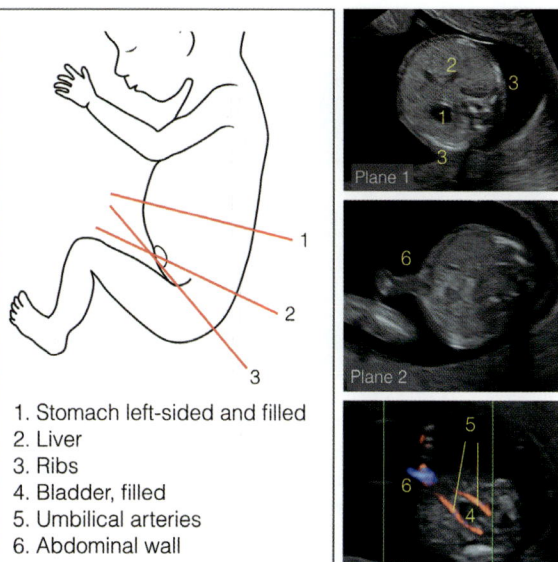

Figure 7-24. Three axial planes (planes 1 to 3) for the anatomic evaluation of the fetal abdomen. Plane 1 is at the level of the stomach and demonstrates the normal position of the stomach and liver. Plane 2 is at the level of the cord insertion in the abdomen and demonstrates an intact anterior abdominal wall and plane 3 is in color Doppler at the level of the bladder confirming its presence along with the presence of two umbilical arteries. (Reprinted with permission from Abuhamad A, Chaoui R. *First Trimester Ultrasound Diagnosis of Fetal Abnormalities.* Wolters Kluwer; 2018. Figure 5.14.)

- Fetal abdomen **(Fig. 7-24)**
  - Required—axial
    - Stomach level
      - The stomach will be seen as a fluid-filled structure within the left side of the abdomen.
    - Liver
      - The liver will have a right-side location.
    - Kidney level **(Fig. 7-25)**
      - Bilateral renal pelvises should be noted.
      - Power or color Doppler will assist in identifying the renal arteries if the kidneys are not well visualized.

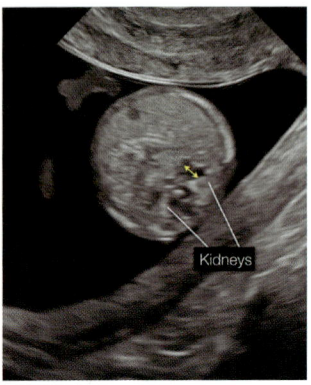 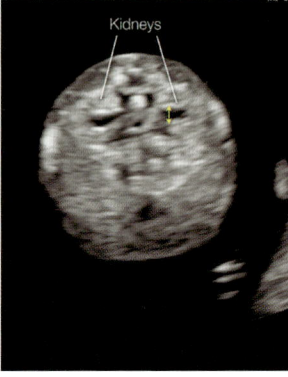

A   **B**

Figure 7-25. Fetal kidneys. Axial planes of the fetal abdomen were obtained transvaginally in two fetuses at 12 (A) and 13 (B) weeks of gestation. Note the presence of fetal kidneys in the posterior aspect of the abdomen. The cross-sectional plane is ideally suited for the assessment of the diameter of the renal pelvis, measured as a vertical diameter (*double-headed arrow*). It is much easier to see the kidneys in a cross-section of the abdomen using the transvaginal approach.
(Reprinted with permission from Abuhamad A, Chaoui R. *First Trimester Ultrasound Diagnosis of Fetal Abnormalities.* Wolters Kluwer; 2018. Figure 13.9.)

- Cord insertion into the abdominal wall level (see Fig. 7-24)
  - Physiologic bowel herniation should not be seen after 12 weeks 6 days.
- Urinary bladder with fluid level
  - A sagittal measurement of the bladder is recommended if suspicious for abnormalities.
  - Enlargement of the urinary bladder can be determined if it exceeds greater than or equal to 7 mm in length in the sagittal plane.
    - Megacystis, or an enlarged urinary bladder, may resolve as the pregnancy progresses **(Fig. 7-26)**.
- Color Doppler of umbilical arteries on each side of the urinary bladder (see Fig. 7-24)
- If indicated or suspicious—axial
  - Portal vein
    - The portal vein should be seen coursing away from the stomach, toward the liver.

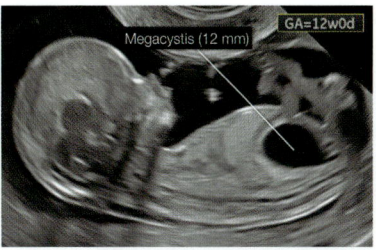
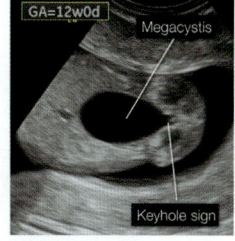
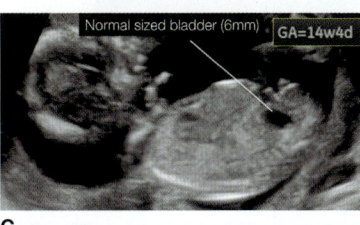
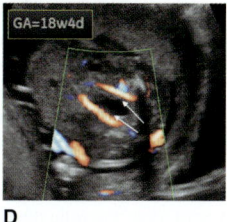

Figure 7-26. Resolution of megacystis (enlarged bladder). **A.** A midline sagittal plane of a fetus at 12 weeks of gestation with megacystis, with a longitudinal bladder diameter of 12 mm. **B.** The corresponding axial plane at the level of the pelvis at 12 weeks of gestation showing the presence of a keyhole sign, suggesting posterior urethral valves. The fetus had no additional anatomic or chromosomal abnormalities. **C.** The follow-up ultrasound at 14 weeks of gestation showing resolution of the megacystis with a longitudinal bladder diameter of 6 mm. **D.** An axial plane of the pelvis in color Doppler at 18 weeks of gestation showing normal bladder and umbilical arteries with no bladder wall hypertrophy, as evidenced by the proximity of the umbilical arteries to the internal bladder wall (*arrows*). Resolution of first-trimester megacystis is a common event. (Reprinted with permission from Abuhamad A, Chaoui R. *First Trimester Ultrasound Diagnosis of Fetal Abnormalities.* Wolters Kluwer; 2018. Figure 13.15.)

- Required—sagittal
  - Contour of anterior wall
    - Assess the fetus for signs of hydrops/masses.
- If indicated or suspicious—sagittal
  - Ductus venosus flow (**Figs. 7-27** and **7-28**)
    - Normal Doppler flow pattern is seen, with continuous flow entering the fetal heart.
    - The ductus venosus restricts the volume of highly oxygenated maternal blood returning to the fetal heart.

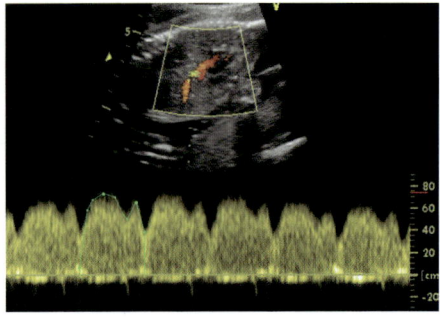

Figure 7-27. Ductus venosus flow. The ductus venosus should be identified and a pulse wave Doppler performed in a fetal echocardiogram. Here, normal Doppler flow pattern is seen, with continuous flow entering the fetal heart. Ductus venosus restricts the volume of highly oxygenated maternal blood returning to the fetal heart. Absence of the ductus venosus can cause right heart volume overload. Reversed flow in the ductus venosus can indicate right ventricular diastolic dysfunction or early atrial contraction/arrhythmia, where the atrium contracts against a closed valve. (Reprinted with permission from Pike JI, Krishnan A, Donofrio MT. Normal fetal heart survey. In: Kline-Fath BM, Bulas DI, Bahado-Singh R, eds. *Fundamental and Advanced Fetal Imaging: Ultrasound and MRI*. Wolters Kluwer; 2015. Figure 4.4.)

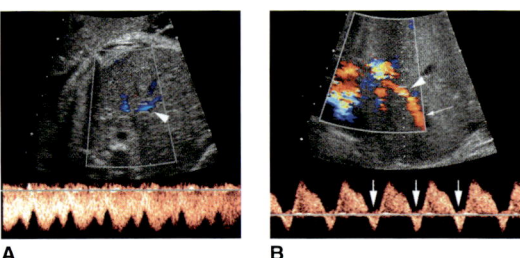

Figure 7-28. Ductus venosus Doppler. A. Normal spectral Doppler waveform acquired from the ductus venosus (*arrowhead*) in the liver, demonstrating continuous flow away from the transducer toward the inferior vena cava and heart. **B.** The Doppler gate has been placed on the ductus venosus (*arrowhead*) which shows a color signal that is more yellow than the umbilical vein (*small arrow*) due to its higher velocity. The waveform is abnormal, in that reversed flow (*arrows*) is seen during a portion of each cycle. (Reprinted with permission from Doubilet PM, Benson CB, Benacerraf BR. *Atlas of Ultrasound in Obstetrics and Gynecology: A Multimedia Reference*. 3rd ed. Wolters Kluwer; 2019. Figure 18.3.2.)

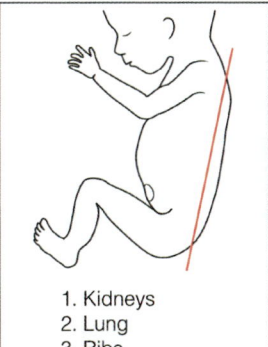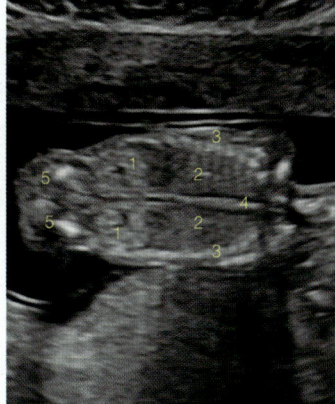

1. Kidneys
2. Lung
3. Ribs
4. Spine
5. Pelvic bones

Figure 7-29. Coronal kidneys in the first trimester. A coronal view at the level of the posterior abdomen allows for the best visualization of the slightly hyperechogenic kidneys in the first trimester. (Reprinted with permission from Abuhamad A, Chaoui R. *First Trimester Ultrasound Diagnosis of Fetal Abnormalities.* Wolters Kluwer; 2018. Figure 5.15.)

- ○ Absence of the ductus venosus can cause right heart volume overload.
- ○ Reversed flow in the ductus venosus is abnormal and can indicate right ventricular diastolic dysfunction or early atrial contraction/arrhythmia, where the atrium contracts against a closed valve.
- Required—coronal
  - Kidneys (Fig. 7-29)
    - ○ Both kidneys should be noted on both sides of the spine in the coronal plane.
- If indicated or suspicious—coronal
  - Color Doppler of the renal vessels can be performed to prove renal agenesis (Fig. 7-30).
- Extremities
  - Required
    - Confirm each of the four extremities.
    - Confirm three long bones within each of the extremities.
      - ○ Each arm should contain the humerus, radius, and ulna (Fig. 7-31).
      - ○ Each leg should contain the femur, tibia, and fibula (Fig. 7-32).

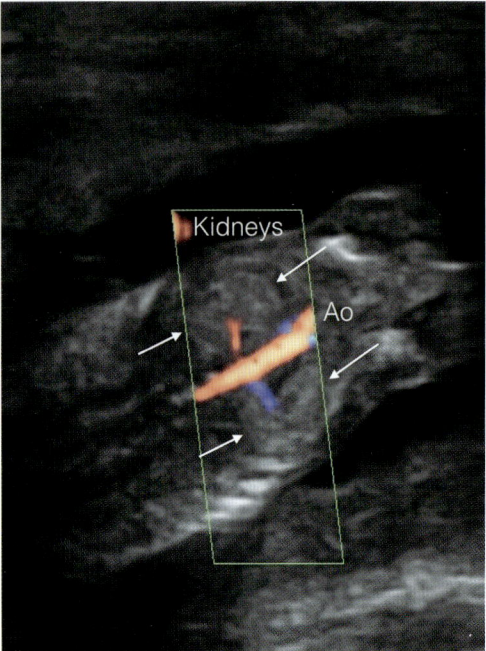

Figure 7-30. Coronal plane in color Doppler of the posterior abdomen and pelvis at 13 weeks of gestation showing the descending aorta (*Ao*) with the left and right renal arteries arising from the Ao and coursing into the kidneys (*arrows*). Absence of one or both of the renal arteries is diagnostic for renal agenesis, unilateral or bilateral respectively.
(Reprinted with permission from Abuhamad A, Chaoui R. *First Trimester Ultrasound Diagnosis of Fetal Abnormalities.* Wolters Kluwer; 2018. Figure 3.13.)

- Confirm presence of hands and feet.
- If indicated or suspicious
  - Confirm the presence of the fingers, thumbs, and toes.
  - Three-dimensional assessment of extremities can be performed.
- Spine
  - Required—axial and longitudinal (**Figs. 7-33** and **7-34**)
    - The vertebral elements should be noted, along with correct alignment.
    - Evaluate the skin edge along the length of the spine for signs of bulges (**Fig. 7-35**).

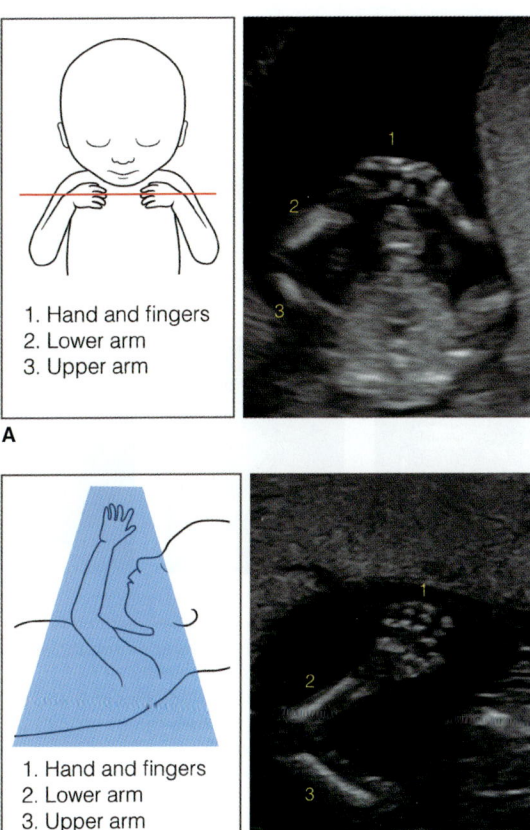

Figure 7-31. Upper extremities. A. The upper extremities in the first trimester can be demonstrated in an axial view at the level of the face, thorax, or upper abdomen as shown here. This view shows both arms and hands. **B.** Parasagittal oblique plane demonstrating the three segments of an upper extremity: upper arm (*3*), lower arm (*2*), and hand with fingers (*1*). The hands with fingers are often better seen in the first trimester than later in gestation. (Reprinted with permission from Abuhamad A, Chaoui R. *First Trimester Ultrasound Diagnosis of Fetal Abnormalities.* Wolters Kluwer; 2018. Figures 5.16 and 5.18.)

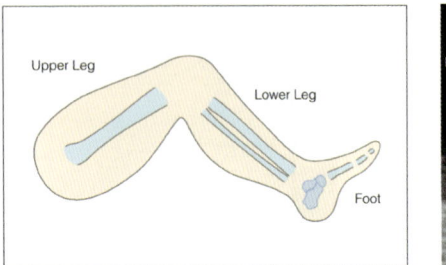
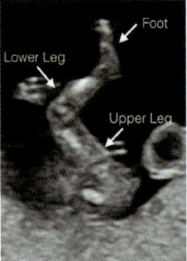
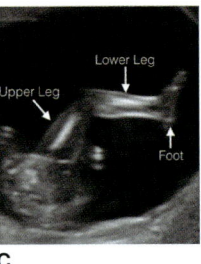
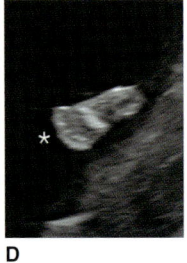
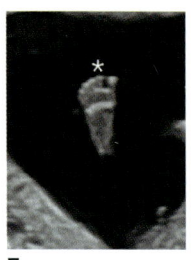

Figure 7-32. Schematic drawing (A) and corresponding two-dimensional sonograms (B and C) of the lower extremity visualized in a parasagittal plane in two fetuses at 13 weeks of gestation. Note the upper leg, lower leg, and foot (all labeled). Planes D and E show a ventral view of the foot. Note that the toes can be visualized at this early gestation (*asterisk*). (Reprinted with permission from Abuhamad A, Chaoui R. *First Trimester Ultrasound Diagnosis of Fetal Abnormalities.* Wolters Kluwer; 2018. Figure 14.8.)

- If indicated or suspicious—axial and longitudinal
  - Scapula **(Fig. 7-36)**
- Placenta
  - Required–axial, sagittal **(Fig. 7-37)**
    - The position of the placenta should be determined in relationship to the lower uterine segment, internal os of the cervix, and cesarean scar site (if applicable).
    - Placental position should be reported if centrally located over the internal cervical os, if the patient has a history of cesarean section, or if there is suspicion for placenta accreta spectrum (PAS).
      - PAS includes placenta accreta, placenta increta, and placenta percreta.

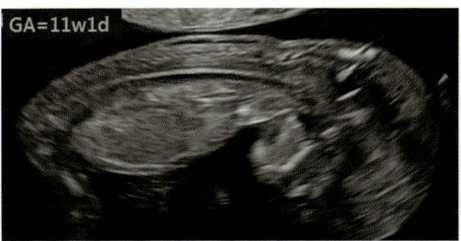

A

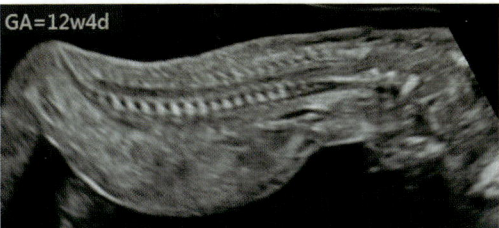

B

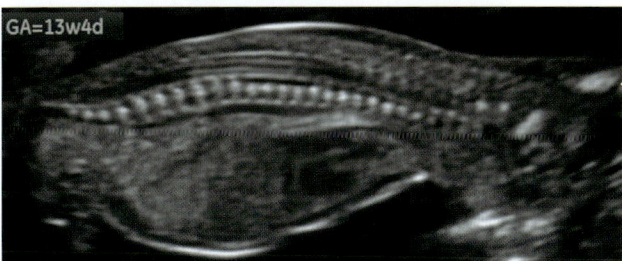

C

Figure 7-33. Midline sagittal planes of the fetal spine in two-dimensional ultrasound in three fetuses at 11 (A), 12 (B), and 13 (C) weeks of gestation. Note the progressive ossification of the spine between 11 (A) and 13 (C) weeks of gestation. (Reprinted with permission from Abuhamad A, Chaoui R. *First Trimester Ultrasound Diagnosis of Fetal Abnormalities.* Wolters Kluwer; 2018. Figure 14.13.)

- ○ All of these abnormalities are associated with an abnormal adherence of the placenta to the myometrium **(Fig. 7-38)**.
- Evaluate the umbilical cord insertion into the placenta.
- Assess the echotexture of the placenta.

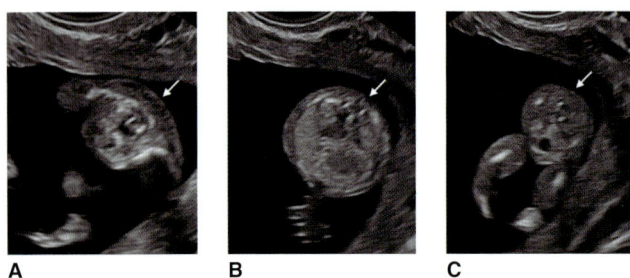

Figure 7-34. Axial spine first trimester. Cervical (A), thoracic (B), and lumbosacral (C) axial planes of the spine in a fetus at 12 weeks of gestation. Note the normal spine and the overlying skin (*arrows*). Along with a sagittal and coronal view of the spine, these planes allow for a comprehensive evaluation of the fetal spine in the first trimester. (Reprinted with permission from Abuhamad A, Chaoui R. *First Trimester Ultrasound Diagnosis of Fetal Abnormalities.* Wolters Kluwer; 2018. Figure 14.14.)

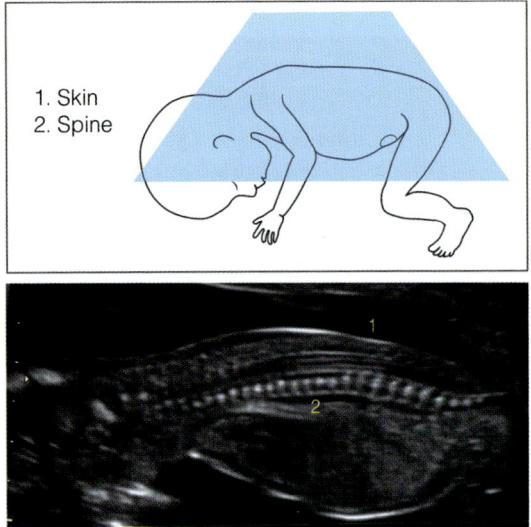

Figure 7-35. Midsagittal view of the fetus in a dorsoposterior position demonstrating the fetal spine. Note the beginning of ossification of vertebral bodies and intact skin covering the back. (Reprinted with permission from Abuhamad A, Chaoui R. *First Trimester Ultrasound Diagnosis of Fetal Abnormalities.* Wolters Kluwer; 2018. Figure 5.22.)

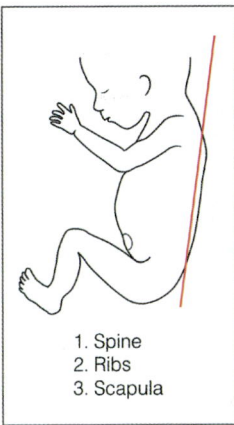
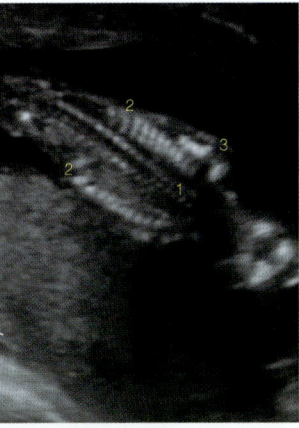

1. Spine
2. Ribs
3. Scapula

Figure 7-36. Fetal spine and scapula. This posterior coronal plane of the fetus demonstrates the spine, scapula, and ribcage. This plane is helpful when spinal deformities are suspected. (Reprinted with permission from Abuhamad A, Chaoui R. *First Trimester Ultrasound Diagnosis of Fetal Abnormalities*. Wolters Kluwer; 2018. Figure 5.23.)

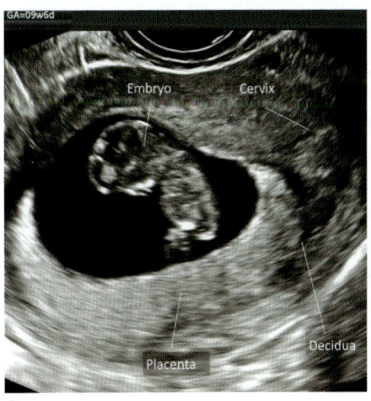
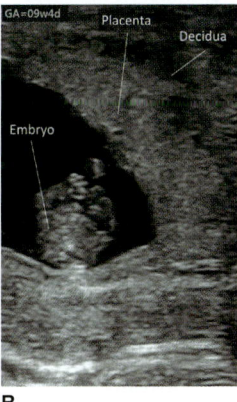

A   B

Figure 7-37. Placenta in the first trimester. Two-dimensional sonogram in two pregnancies (A, B) at 9 weeks of gestation demonstrating the appearance of the placenta. Note that the placenta is slightly more echogenic than the surrounding endometrium. The decidua (endometrium behind the placenta) is hypoechoic in appearance. (Reprinted with permission from Abuhamad A, Chaoui R. *First Trimester Ultrasound Diagnosis of Fetal Abnormalities*. Wolters Kluwer; 2018. Figure 15.3.)

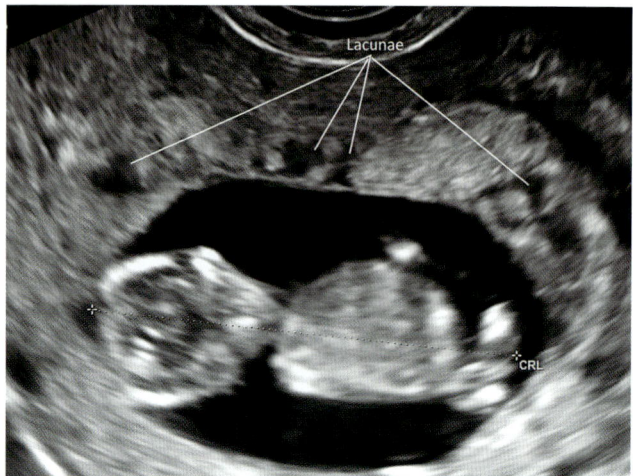

Figure 7-38. Placenta accreta in the first trimester. Transvaginal sonogram of a pregnancy at 11 weeks gestation demonstrating the presence of multiple placental lacunae in a patient with two prior cesarean sections. The presence of placental lacunae in the first trimester increases the risk for placenta accreta, and thus the pregnancy should be mindfully followed. (Reprinted with permission from Abuhamad A, Chaoui R. *First Trimester Ultrasound Diagnosis of Fetal Abnormalities.* Wolters Kluwer; 2018. Figure 15.22.)

- Evaluate the placenta for heterogeneity, masses, cystic spaces, or lacunae.
- If indicated or suspicious—axial, sagittal
  - Color Doppler evaluation is required if PAS is present.
  - Evaluate the basal layer of the placenta for signs of myometrial thinning.
    - With PAS, there is typically a loss of clear retroplacental zone or possibly even a compromised maternal urinary bladder wall interface.
  - The presence of uterine vesical vascularity should be evaluated.
- Uterus, adnexa, cul-de-sac
  - Required
    - Evaluate the uterus for myometrial masses such as leiomyomata (fibroids).
      - When fibroids are discovered, provide the number, size, and location of clinically significant masses.

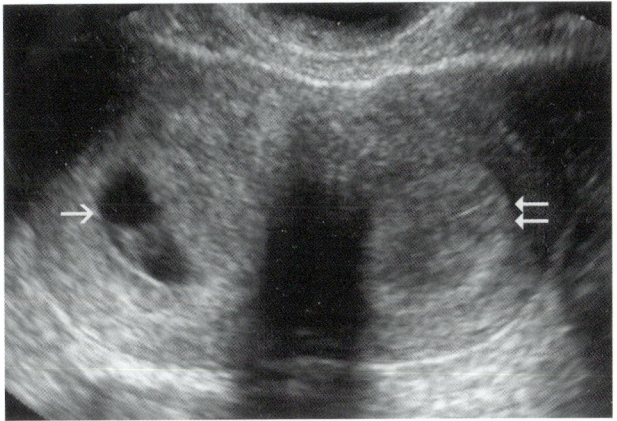

Figure 7-39. Bicornuate pregnancy. Transverse section of a bicornuate uterus in the first trimester. The gestational sac is in the right horn (*single arrow*) and the left horn shows decidual changes (*double arrows*). (Reprinted with permission from Scott JR, Gibbs RS, Karlan BY, Haney AF. *Danforth's Obstetrics and Gynecology*. 9th ed. Lippincott Williams & Wilkins; 2003. Figure 8.10.)

- Müllerian duct anomalies should be recognized and reported **(Fig. 7-39)**. They may be associated with an increased likelihood of early pregnancy loss.
- Intrauterine linear structures
  - The linear structures are likely synechiae or bands which are found with Asherman syndrome.
- Evaluate both ovaries for signs of abnormalities.
- Evaluate the adnexa and cul-de-sac for masses, fluid, and any other abnormalities.

GENITALIA IN THE FIRST TRIMESTER[2]

- Cell-free DNA testing is highly accurate for determining gender.
- The fetal genitalia can be evaluated in the first trimester, though this is not a routine.
- A qualitative evaluation or measurement of the angle between the genital tubercle and the fetal longitudinal axis can be obtained.
  - An angle measuring greater than 30 degrees is more suggestive of a male gender, while an angle less than 30 degrees is more suggestive of a female gender **(Figs. 7-40** and **7-41)**.

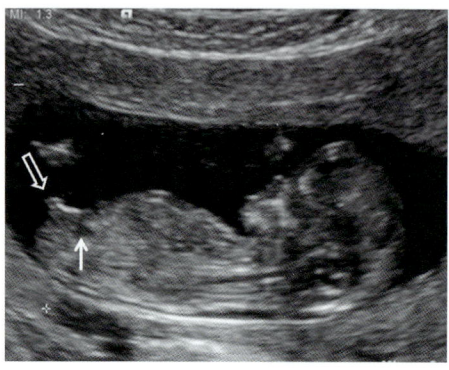

Figure 7-40. Genital tubercle of a male fetus. Sagittal view of a 12- to 13-week fetus demonstrating the presence of a small urinary bladder (*solid arrow*). An angle measuring greater than 30 degrees, as depicted in this image, is more suggestive of a male gender. (Reprinted with permission from Sonek JD, Retzke JD, Hyett J. Normal fetal ultrasound survey. In: Kline-Fath BM, Bulas DI, Bahado-Singh R, eds. *Fundamental and Advanced Fetal Imaging: Ultrasound and MRI*. Wolters Kluwer; 2015. Figure 1.22.)

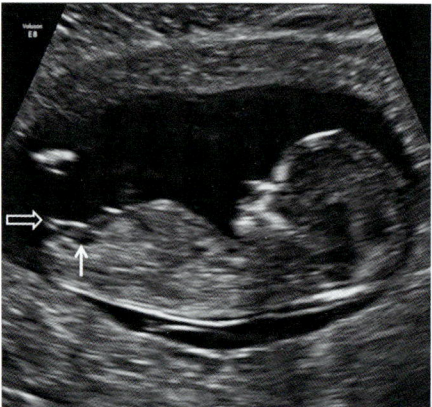

Figure 7-41. Genital tubercle of a female fetus. Sagittal view of a 12- to 13-week fetus demonstrating the presence of a small urinary bladder (*solid arrow*). The genital tubercle (*open arrow*) points in a direction parallel to the longitudinal axis of the fetus, indicating female gender. (Reprinted with permission from Sonek JD, Hiett AK, Hyett J. Normal fetal ultrasound survey. In: Kline-Fath BM, Bulas DI, Lee W, eds. *Fundamental and Advanced Fetal Imaging: Ultrasound and MRI*. 2nd ed. Wolters Kluwer; 2021. Figure 3.21.)

SUGGESTED MINIMAL PROTOCOL FOR A FIRST-TRIMESTER ANOMALY SCAN[2]

- Transabdominal or transvaginal scanning is performed as suitable for the specific examination.
- The minimal examination should include all the following:
  - A transverse section of the skull, midline echo, and the choroid plexuses should be provided.
  - A midsagittal view of the face to demonstrate the nasal bone and maxilla should be obtained.
  - A sagittal section of the spine should be obtained to determine the presence of kyphoscoliosis.
  - The transverse section of the thorax demonstrates the four-chamber view of the heart and record blood flow across the tricuspid valve should be achieved.
  - A transverse and sagittal section of the fetal trunk to demonstrate the stomach, urinary bladder, and abdominal cord insertion.
  - Demonstration of all parts of each extremity, including all long bones, hands, and feet.

TRISOMY SONOGRAPHIC DETECTION IN THE FIRST TRIMESTER

- Sonographic findings of trisomy 21 in the first trimester **(Fig. 7-42)**.
- Sonographic findings of trisomy 18 in the first trimester **(Fig. 7-43)**.
- Sonographic findings of trisomy 13 in the first trimester **(Fig. 7-44)**.

OVERVIEW OF SEVERAL COMMON FETAL ANOMALIES IDENTIFIABLE IN THE FIRST TRIMESTER[2]

- Acrania, anencephaly, and exencephaly **(Fig. 7-45)**
  - Acrania is the absence of the fetal skull.
    - Anencephaly is acrania with the absence of the normal cerebral hemispheres.
    - Exencephaly is acrania with exposed neural tissue.
- Arnold–Chiari malformation and spina bifida
  - Arnold–Chiari malformation may be difficult to diagnose in the first trimester. However, measurements of certain brain structures can assist in the diagnosis of open spina bifida if suspicion exists, such as the brain stem to brain stem-occipital bone ratio (BS/BSOB).
  - BS/BSOB ratio

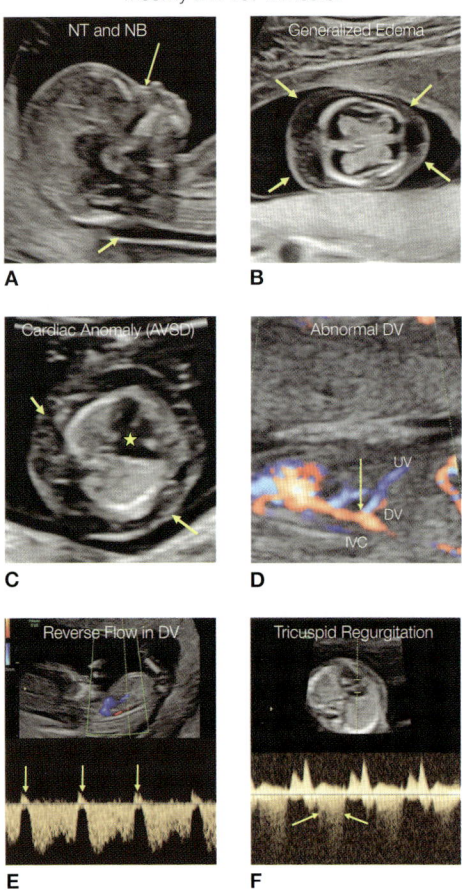

Figure 7-42. First-trimester trisomy 21 (Down syndrome). First-trimester markers of trisomy 21 include thickened nuchal translucency (*NT*) (*A-short arrow*) and absent or hypoplastic nasal bone (*NB*) (*A-long arrow*), generalized edema (B and *C-arrows*), cardiac anomaly (C-star), most commonly an atrioventricular septal defect (AVSD), abnormal course of the umbilical vein (*UV*) with an absent or abnormal connection of the ductus venosus (*DV*), here connecting to the inferior vena cava (*IVC*) (*D-arrow*), reverse flow in the DV (*E-arrows*), and tricuspid regurgitation (*F-arrows*). (Reprinted with permission from Abuhamad A, Chaoui R. *A Practical Guide to Fetal Echocardiography: Normal and Abnormal Hearts*. 4th ed. Wolters Kluwer; 2022. Figure 2.1.)

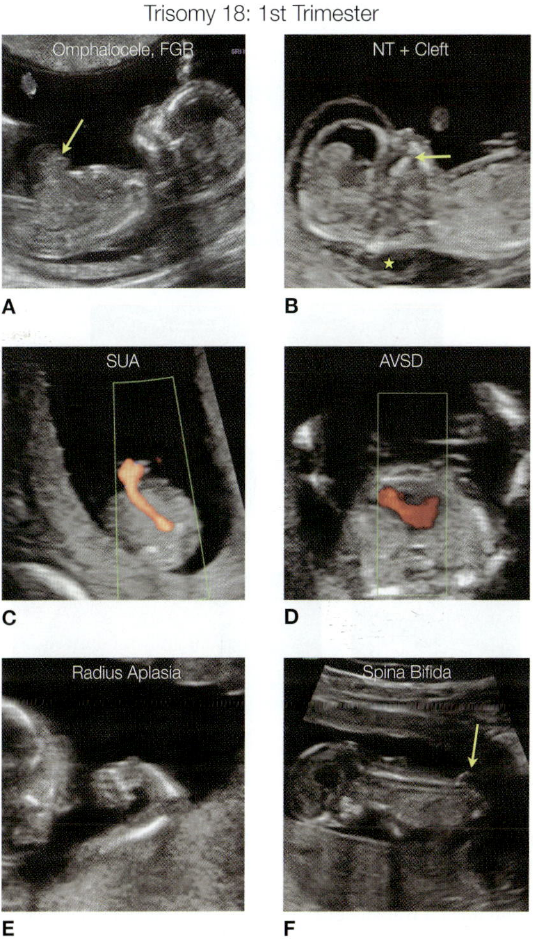

Trisomy 18: 1st Trimester

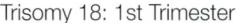

Figure 7-43. First-trimester trisomy 18. Fetuses with trisomy 18 (Edwards syndrome) may present in the first trimester with multiple and often severe anomalies including fetal growth restriction (A), omphalocele (A, *arrow*), thickened nuchal translucency (NT) (B, *star*), facial cleft, shown here with the maxillary gap (B, *arrow*), single umbilical artery (SUA) (C), cardiac anomalies, such as atrioventricular septal defect (AVSD) (D), or skeletal abnormalities with radial aplasia (E) or open spina bifida (F), among others. (Reprinted with permission from Abuhamad A, Chaoui R. *A Practical Guide to Fetal Echocardiography: Normal and Abnormal Hearts*. 4th ed. Wolters Kluwer; 2022. Figure 2.6.)

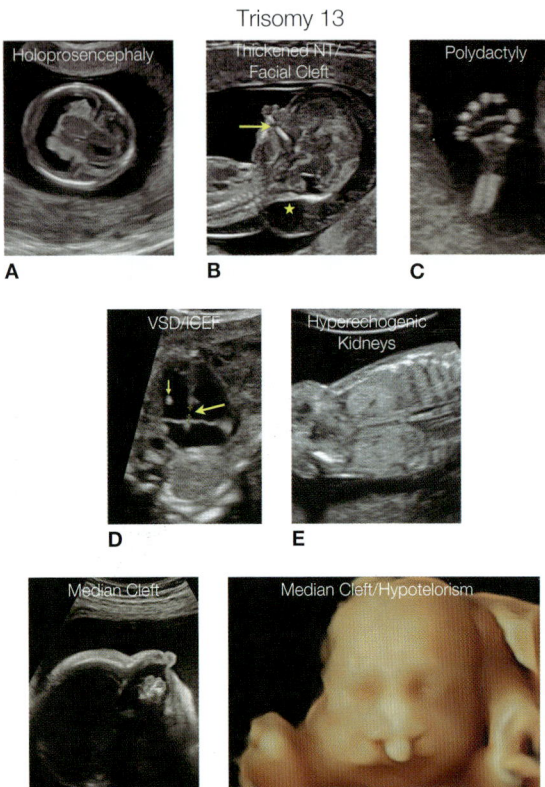

Figure 7-44. Fetuses with trisomy 13 (Patau syndrome) very commonly have severe anomalies in the first and second trimesters of pregnancy. Typical anomalies include holoprosencephaly (A), thickened nuchal translucency (*NT*) (B, *star*), facial cleft, shown with maxillary gap (B, *arrow*), and polydactyly (C). Cardiac abnormalities may present as tachycardia in the first trimester and in the second trimester include intracardiac echogenic focus (*ICEF*) (D, *small arrow*), ventricular septal defect (*VSD*) (D, *big arrow*), left ventricular outflow tract obstruction with aortic coarctation, or even hypoplastic left heart syndrome, among others. Renal anomalies include hyperechogenic dysplastic kidneys (E). Facial dysmorphism includes facial median clefts (F, G), eye anomalies with hypotelorism (G), and cyclopia. (Reprinted with permission from Abuhamad A, Chaoui R. *A Practical Guide to Fetal Echocardiography: Normal and Abnormal Hearts.* 4th ed. Wolters Kluwer; 2022. Figure 2.8.)

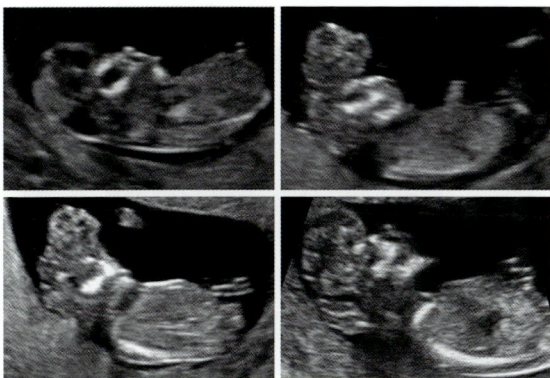

Figure 7-45. Acrania in the first trimester. Acrania with varying degrees of distortion and disruption of the brain at 11 to 13 weeks gestation. (Reprinted with permission from Nucci M, Sciorio C, Nicolaides KH. First trimester evaluation. In: Kline-Fath BM, Bulas DI, Bahado-Singh R, eds. *Fundamental and Advanced Fetal Imaging: Ultrasound and MRI.* Wolters Kluwer; 2015. Figure 8.8.)

- In the standard sagittal view of the fetal skull/face used to obtain the nuchal translucency, several distinct intracranial structures can be seen **(Fig. 7-46)**.
- The first anteroposterior measurement obtained is of the brain stem (BS), which begins at the interface between the posterior edge of the brain stem and the floor of the fourth ventricle.
- The second anteroposterior measurement is from the interface between the posterior edge of the brain stem to the inner edge of the occipital bone. This includes the fourth ventricle and the cisterna magna—termed the brain stem to occipital bone measurement or BSOB.
- The BS/BSOB ratio should be less than 1.0. A BS/BSOB ratio greater than 1.0 is associated with a high risk for open neural tube defects.
- Omphalocele and gastroschisis
  - Omphalocele **(Fig. 7-47)**
    - An omphalocele is the herniation of abdominal contents into the base of the umbilical cord.
    - Omphalocele can be difficult to diagnose in the first trimester due to the normal occurrence of physiologic bowel herniation.

Normal

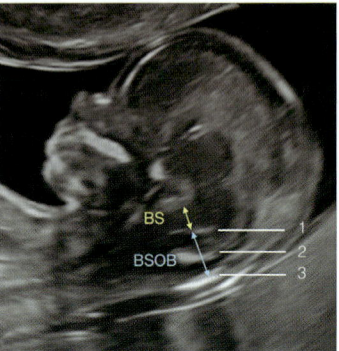

A

Open Spina Bifida

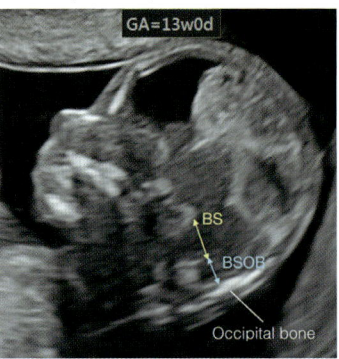

B

Figure 7-46. Obtaining the BS/BSOB measurements. Transvaginal sonogram of the midsagittal plane of the face and posterior brain in a normal fetus (A) and in a fetus with open spina bifida (B) at 13 weeks of gestation. The three echogenic lines in A correspond to the posterior border of the brainstem (*1*), the choroid plexus of the fourth ventricle (*2*), and the occipital bone (*3*). Quantification of the posterior fossa can be achieved by measuring the brainstem diameter (*BS*) (*yellow double-headed arrow*) and the distance from the BS to the occipital bone (*BSOB*) (*blue double-headed arrow*). In normal fetuses (A) the BS is smaller than the BSOB and the ratio of both is smaller than 1. In open spina bifida (B) BS is larger and BSOB is shorter which leads to a **ratio** >**1**. (Reprinted with permission from Abuhamad A, Chaoui R. *First Trimester Ultrasound Diagnosis of Fetal Abnormalities*. Wolters Kluwer; 2018. Figure 8.42.)

Chapter 7. Detailed First-Trimester Sonography 243

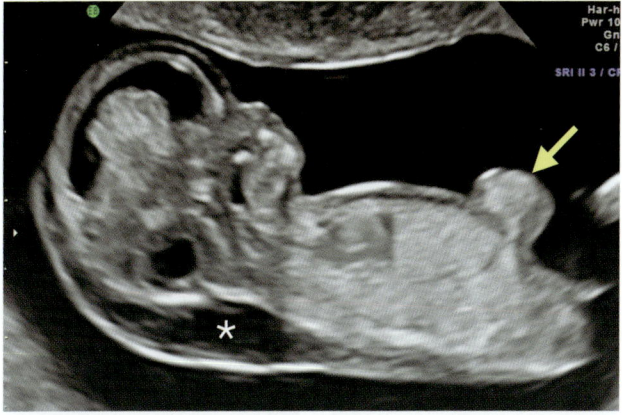

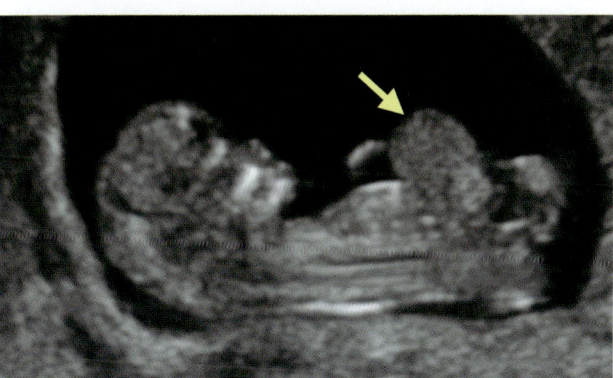

Figure 7-47. Omphalocele in the first trimester. Midline sagittal plane in two fetuses with small (A) and large (B) omphalocele (*arrows*) at 12 weeks of gestation. In fetus A, the omphalocele is small and contains bowel only, whereas in fetus B, the omphalocele is relatively large and contains liver and bowel. Note the presence of an enlarged nuchal translucency (*asterisk*) in fetus A and workup revealed trisomy 18 in this fetus. (Reprinted with permission from Abuhamad A, Chaoui R. *First Trimester Ultrasound Diagnosis of Fetal Abnormalities*. Wolters Kluwer; 2018. Figure 12.13.)

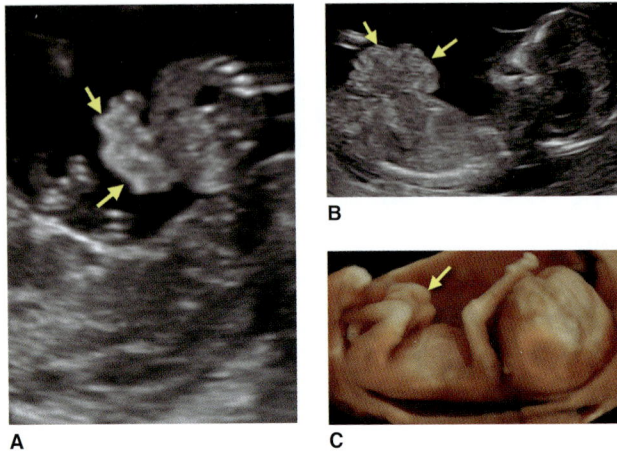

Figure 7-48. Gastroschisis in the first trimester. Axial (A), sagittal (B) views in two-dimensional sonogram and corresponding three-dimensional surface mode (C) of a fetus at 13 weeks of gestation with gastroschisis. Note the irregular surface appearance of the herniated bowel loops (*arrows*), which is typical for gastroschisis. (Reprinted with permission from Abuhamad A, Chaoui R. *First Trimester Ultrasound Diagnosis of Fetal Abnormalities*. Wolters Kluwer; 2018. Figure 12.22.)

- Omphalocele is often associated with Trisomy 18 (Edward syndrome).
- Gastroschisis **(Fig. 7-48)**
  - Gastroschisis is the herniation of the bowel outside of the abdomen, typically through an opening located just right lateral to the umbilical cord insertion site in the abdomen.
  - Cord insertion is typically normal, while the association with chromosomal anomalies is lower for gastroschisis compared to omphalocele.

REFERENCES

1. AIUM practice parameter for the performance of detailed diagnostic obstetric ultrasound examinations between 12 weeks 0 days and 13 weeks 6 days. *J Ultrasound Med*. 2021;40:E1–E16.
2. Kline-Fath BM, Bulas DI, Lee W. *Fundamental and Advanced Fetal Imaging: Ultrasound and MRI*. 2nd ed. Wolters Kluwer; 2021:1–156.
3. The Fetal Medicine Foundation. Accessed November 12, 2023. FMF Certification Nasal Bone. https://fetalmedicine.org/nasal-bone

Standard Second- or Third-Trimester Sonography

CHAPTER 8

INTRODUCTION

This chapter will provide fetal and maternal anatomy that should be included in the second- or third-trimester sonogram. This examination is typically performed after 18 weeks gestational age. A protocol is provided and normal measurements for fetal structures that are typically evaluated during a routine sonogram, and thus these are provided as well. Though biophysical profile scoring (BPP) may vary per institution, the basic assessment is provided at the conclusion of this chapter.

AIUM RECOMMENDATIONS FOR A STANDARD SECOND- OR THIRD-TRIMESTER SONOGRAM[1,2]

- Fetal number
  - Multiple gestations require further documentation (see Chapter 9)
    - Chorionicity
    - Amnionicity
    - Comparison of fetal size
    - Evaluation of amniotic fluid per gestational sac
    - Fetal genitalia (when visualized)
- Cardiac activity
  - M-mode to obtain fetal heart rate (beats per minute) **(Fig. 8-1)**
  - Video clips can also be used.
- Fetal presentation
  - Understanding fetal lie is important.

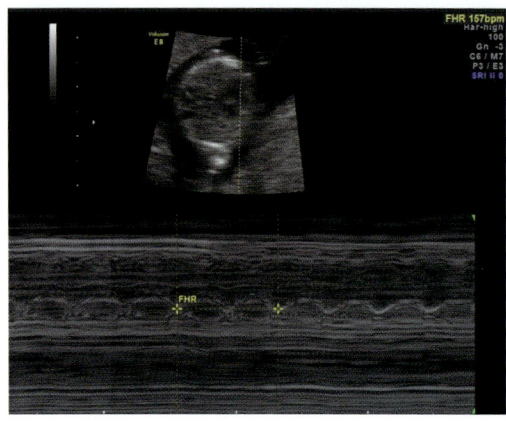

Figure 8-1. M-mode. This is a normal M-mode of the fetal heart in a fetus at 12 weeks of gestation. Note that the M-mode line intersects the heart, and the cardiac activity is displayed on the M-mode spectrum. Note that the fetal heart rate is measured at 157 beats per minute. (Reprinted with permission from Abuhamad A, Chaoui R. *First Trimester Ultrasound Diagnosis of Fetal Abnormalities.* Wolters Kluwer; 2018. Figure 2.3.)

- Fetal presentation is identified by what part of the fetus is nearest to the maternal internal cervical os (e.g., cephalic, breech, transverse, etc.) **(Fig. 8-2)**.

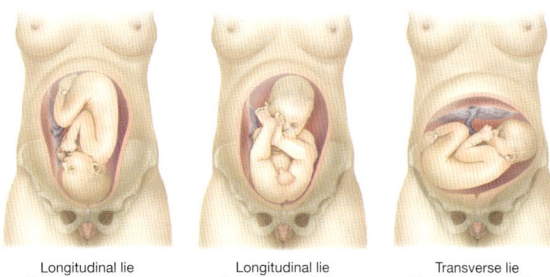

Longitudinal lie
Vertex presentation

Longitudinal lie
Breech presentation

Transverse lie
Shoulder presentation

Figure 8-2. Types of fetal lie and presentation. Fetal lie is likely longitudinal, transverse, or oblique, while fetal presentation may described as cephalic, breech, or by what fetal part is presenting or closest to the internal os. (Reprinted with permission from Gullett J, Pigott DC. Second and third trimester pregnancy. In: Cosby KS, Kendall JL, eds. *Practical Guide to Emergency Ultrasound.* 2nd ed. Wolters Kluwer Health/Lippincott Williams & Wilkins; 2014. Figure 16.14.)

Chapter 8. Standard Second- or Third-Trimester Sonography

- Amniotic fluid volume
  - There are three semiquantitative methods.
    - Amniotic fluid index (AFI) **(Fig. 8-3)**
    - Single deepest pocket
    - Two-diameter pocket

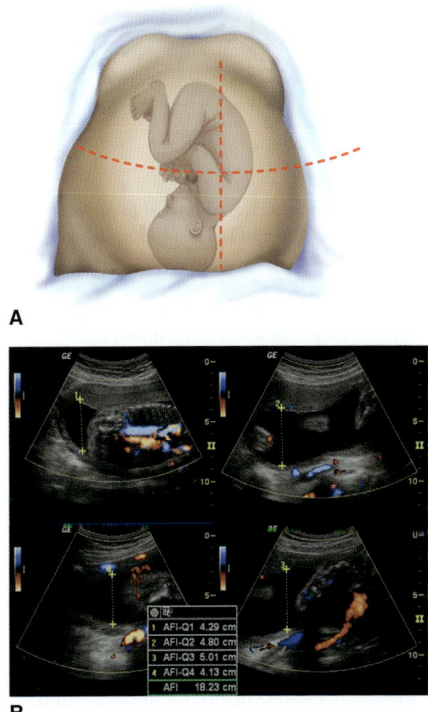

Figure 8-3. Amniotic fluid index (AFI). A. Diagram shows the division of the pregnant abdomen into four quadrants for obtaining the amniotic fluid index (*AFI*). B. Four sonogram images showing measurements of maximum vertical pockets of amniotic fluid in each of the four quadrants of the uterus with the sum of the measurements equaling the AFI, as shown in the box. (**A.** Reprinted with permission from Quigley K. Intrauterine Growth Restriction. In: Stephenson SR, Dmitrieva J, eds. *Diagnostic Medical Sonography: Obstetrics & Gynecology*. 4th ed. Wolters Kluwer; 2018. Figure 30-17. **B.** Reprinted with permission from Davidson CM. Antenatal fetal assessment, therapy, and outcomes. In: Suresh MS, Segal BS, Preston R, Fernando R, LaToya Mason C, eds. *Shnider and Levinson's Anesthesia for Obstetrics*. 5th ed. Wolters Kluwer Health/Lippincott Williams & Wilkins; 2013. Figure 4-7.)

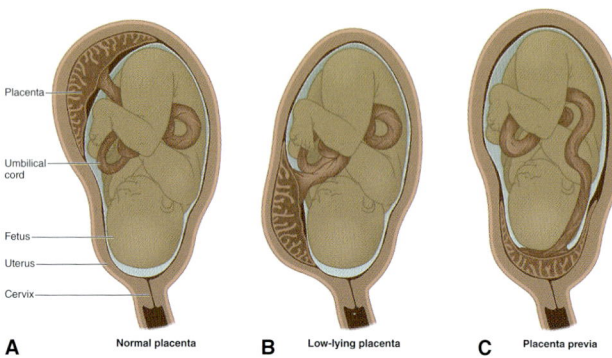

Figure 8-4. Placental locations. A. Normal placenta. B. Low lying. C. Placenta previa. Not pictured here is the marginal placenta, which technically ends at the edge of the internal os (<2 cm). (Reprinted with permission from Salmanian B, Belfort MA, Shamshirsaz AA. Placenta previa. In: Belfort MA, Shamshirsaz AA, Clark SL, Fox KA, eds. *Operative Techniques in Obstetric Surgery*. Wolters Kluwer; 2023. Figure 4.8.1.)

- Placenta
  - Placental location, appearance, and relationship to the internal os should be documented **(Fig. 8-4)**.
    - Placental location can be anterior, posterior, fundal, right or left lateral, and inferior (previa). A combination of these can be present as well (e.g., anterior, right lateral)
  - Transvaginal or transperineal examination should be performed if the relationship between the cervix and the placenta cannot be evaluated transabdominally.
- Umbilical cord
  - The number of vessels should be documented.
    - Umbilical cord should have three vessels (two arteries and one vein).
  - Placental cord insertion site should be documented when technically possible **(Fig. 8-5)**.
  - Velamentous cord insertion should be further evaluated for further evidence of vasa previa or abnormal placental cord insertion. Color and pulsed Doppler should be used.
- Fetal biometry
  - Biparietal diameter
    - Measured at the level of the thalami and cavum septum pellucidum (CSP) **(Fig. 8-6)**.

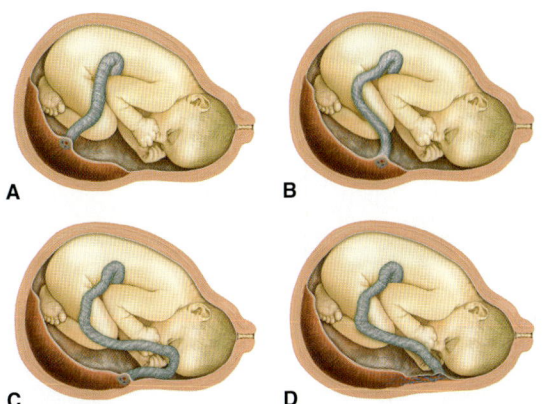

Figure 8-5. Cord insertion into the placenta. **A.** Central cord insertion. **B.** Eccentric cord insertion. **C.** Marginal cord insertion (battledore placenta). **D. Velamentous cord insertion.** (Reprinted with permission from Allen LM. Abnormalities of the placenta and umbilical cord. In: Stephenson SR, ed. *Diagnostic Medical Sonography: Obstetrics & Gynecology*. 3rd ed. Wolters Kluwer Health/Lippincott Williams & Wilkins; 2012. Figure 18-38.)

- Measurement is typically taken from the outer edge of the proximal skull to the inner edge of the distal skull.
- Another way to describe this measurement is from the outside of the upper parietal bone to the inside of the lower parietal bone.
- Cerebellum should not be in the image.
- Abnormal head shapes can alter the accuracy of this measurement.
  - Brachycephaly—round skull
  - Dolichocephaly—narrow, elongated skull
- Head circumference
  - Measured at the level of the thalami and CSP.
  - Measurement is taken around the outer edge of the bony calvarium **(Fig. 8-7)**.
  - Abnormal head shape does not typically alter the accuracy of this measurement.
  - Exclude the subcutaneous tissue of the skull.
- Abdominal circumference
  - Measured at the skin line on an accurate transverse view of the abdomen at the level of the junction of the umbilical vein and portal sinus **(Fig. 8-8)**.

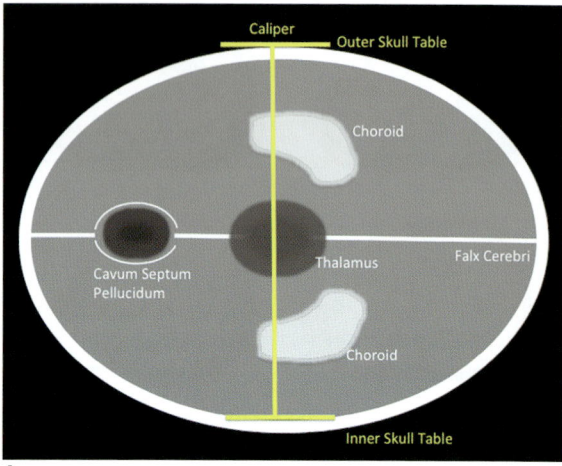

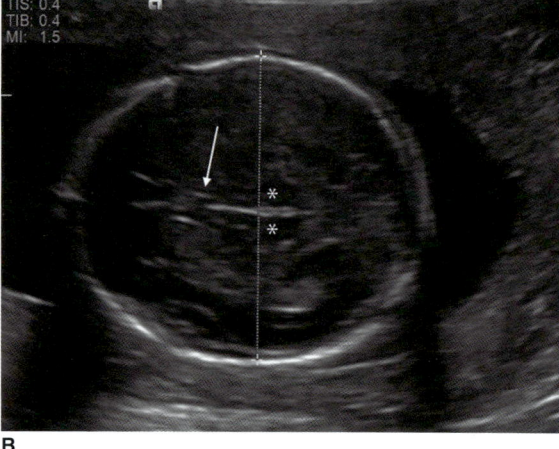

Figure 8-6. Biparietal diameter. A. Drawing of the level of the biparietal diameter. **B.** This measurement is obtained on an axial image of the fetal head at the level of the thalami (asterisk) and cavum septum pellucidum (*arrow*). (**A.** Reprinted with permission from Gullett J, Pigott DC. Second and third trimester pregnancy. In: Cosby KS, Kendall JL, eds. *Practical Guide to Emergency Ultrasound*. 2nd ed. Wolters Kluwer Health/Lippincott Williams & Wilkins; 2014. Figure 16.9. **B.** Cosby KS, Kendall JL. *Practical Guide to Emergency Ultrasound*. 2nd ed. Wolters Kluwer; 2015. Figure 16-9.)

Chapter 8. Standard Second- or Third-Trimester Sonography

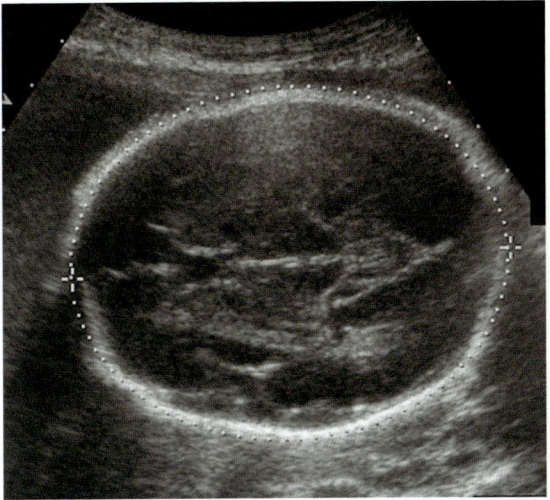

Figure 8-7. Head circumference. Head circumference measurement. On an image at the same level as the biparietal diameter, the head circumference is measured with electronic ellipse calipers (+ ⋯ +) around the outer rim of the ossified cranium. (Reprinted with permission from Doublet PM, Benson CB. *Atlas of Ultrasound in Obstetrics and Gynecology: A Multimedia Reference.* 2nd ed. Wolters Kluwer Health/Lippincott Williams & Wilkins; 2012. Figure 2.1.2.)

- The fetal stomach should be visible.
- Abdominal diameter may be requested by some institutions (see Fig. 8-8).
- Femur length
  - The femoral diaphysis length is obtained when the long axis of the femoral shaft is perpendicular to the sound beam **(Fig. 8-9)**.
  - The distal femoral epiphysis should not be included in the measurement.
- The following assessment areas represent the minimal elements of a standard examination of fetal anatomy. A more detailed examination would ensue if abnormalities were noted during this examination (see Chapter 9).
  - Fetal head, face, and neck:
    - Lateral cerebral ventricles **(Fig. 8-10)**
    - Choroid plexus
    - Midline falx (see Fig. 8-6)

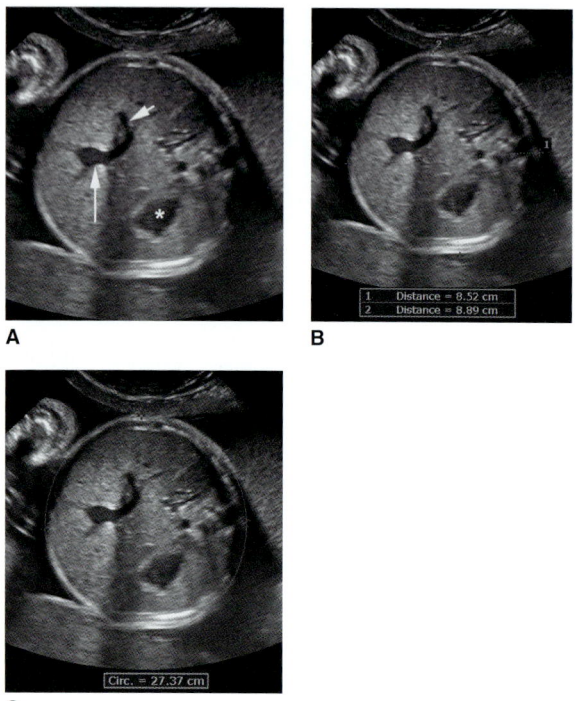

Figure 8-8. Abdominal circumference and abdominal diameter. A. Transverse image of the fetal abdomen at 28 weeks gestation at the correct level and plane for obtaining measurements. The junction of the umbilical vein (*long arrow*) and left portal vein (*short arrow*) is seen, as is the stomach (*asterisk*). B. Anteroposterior diameter (*calipers 1*) is measured from the anterior skin surface to the posterior skin surface. Transverse diameter (*calipers 2*) is measured from one lateral skin surface to the opposite. C. Abdominal circumference (*elliptical calipers*) is measured around the outer perimeter of the abdomen. (Reprinted with permission from Doubilet PM, Benson CB, Benacerraf BR. *Atlas of Ultrasound in Obstetrics and Gynecology: A Multimedia Reference.* 3rd ed. Wolters Kluwer; 2019. Figure 18.1.2.)

- CSP (see Fig. 8-6)
- Cerebellum (Fig. 8-11)
- Cisterna magna (Fig. 8-12)
- Upper lip (Fig. 8-13)
- Nuchal fold (measured between 16 and 20 weeks) (Fig. 8-14)

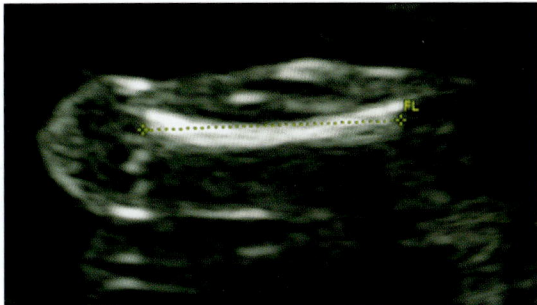

Figure 8-9. Femur length. The femur length is measured with the longest portion of the bone perpendicular to the transducer. The calipers are placed in the center of the femur and measured to the end of the bright edges, ensuring not to include the femoral tip. (Reprinted with permission from Galan HL, Reeves S. Growth, Doppler, and fetal assessment. In: Kline-Fath BM, Bulas DI, Bahado-Singh R, eds. *Fundamental and Advanced Fetal Imaging: Ultrasound and MRI*. Wolters Kluwer; 2015. Figure 3.7.)

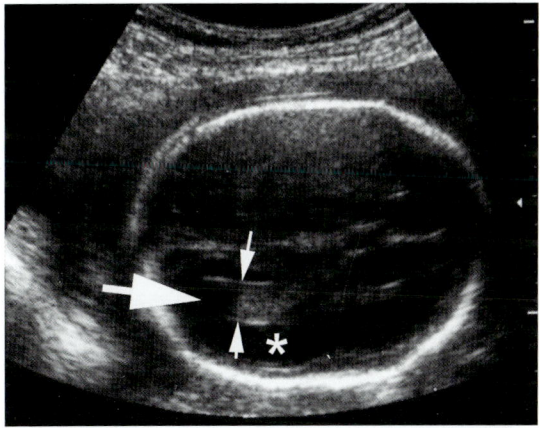

Figure 8-10. Lateral ventricle measurement. Standard axial view of the lateral ventricle (*large arrow*) showing the atrial (also referred to as the trigone) location where measurements of lateral ventricular width are made (*small arrows*). Do not mistake the anechoic area lateral to the lateral ventricle (*asterisk*) for an enlarged lateral ventricle. Note that the lateral ventricle on the transducer side of the head cannot be seen due to a reverberation artifact from the skull. (Reprinted with permission from Sanders RC. Possible Fetal anomalies. In: Sanders RC, Hall-Terracciano B, eds. *Clinical Sonography: A Practical Guide*. 5th ed. Wolters Kluwer; 2016. Figure 27-5A.)

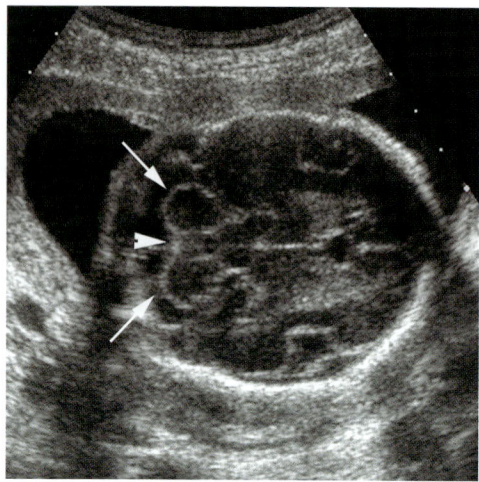

Figure 8-11. Cerebellum. Axial view of the posterior fossa demonstrating the normal contour of the cerebellum, with rounded cerebellar hemispheres (*arrows*) on either side of the more echogenic cerebellar vermis (*arrowhead*). (Reprinted with permission from Doubilet PM, Benson CB. *Atlas of Ultrasound in Obstetrics and Gynecology: A Multimedia Reference.* 2nd ed. Wolters Kluwer Health/Lippincott Williams & Wilkins; 2012. Figure 2.1.4.)

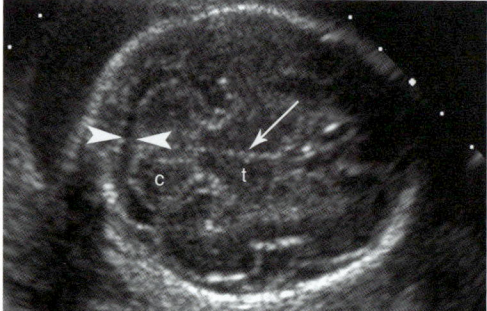

Figure 8-12. Cisterna Magna measurement. Landmarks for the transcerebellar plane are the thalami (*t*), third ventricle (*arrow*), and cerebellar hemispheres (*c*). The cisterna magna (*between arrowheads*) is measured from the vermis to the occiput. (Reprinted with permission from Brant WE. Obstetric ultrasound. In: Brant WE, Helms CA, eds. *Fundamentals of Diagnostic Radiology.* 4th ed. Wolters Kluwer Health/Lippincott Williams & Wilkins; 2012. Figure 37.29.)

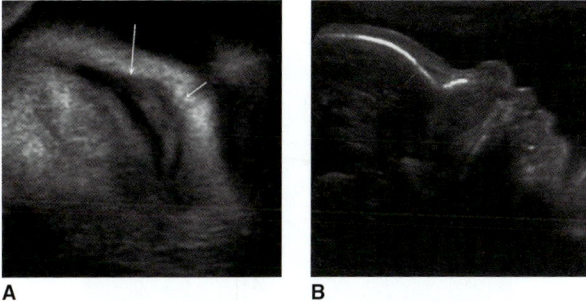

Figure 8-13. Fetal lip. A. Two-dimensional sonogram of a normal fetal lip at 31 weeks showing the white roll, vermillion border (*long arrow*), and Cupid bow (*short arrow*). B. Normal 2D sagittal face profile. (Reprinted with permission from Estroff JA. Face: Anomalies of nose, mouth, lip and tongue. In: Kline-Fath BM, Bulas DI, Lee W, eds. *Fundamental and Advanced Fetal Imaging: Ultrasound and MRI.* 2nd ed. Wolters Kluwer; 2021. Figure 19.3A,C.)

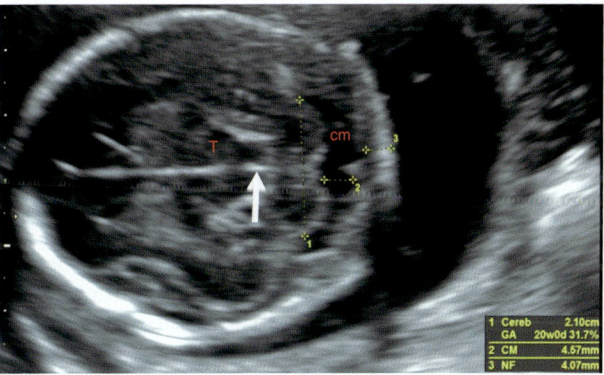

Figure 8-14. Nuchal fold. Transcerebellar plane—nuchal fold. The landmarks of the transcerebellar plane are the thalamus (*TX*), the inferior portion of the third ventricle (*arrow*) near where it joins the aqueduct, and the cisterna magna (*cm*). Measurements, which are routinely made at this level, include the transverse cerebellum (*1*), which in mm approximates the gestational age, the anteroposterior dimension of the cisterna magna (*2*), and the thickness of the nuchal fold (*3*) in the second trimester, which is normal at less than 6 mm. (Reprinted with permission from Brant WE. Obstetric ultrasound. In: Klein JS, Brant WE, Helms CA, Vinson EN, eds. *Brant and Helms' Fundamentals of Diagnostic Radiology.* 5th ed. Wolters Kluwer; 2019. Figure 52.34.)

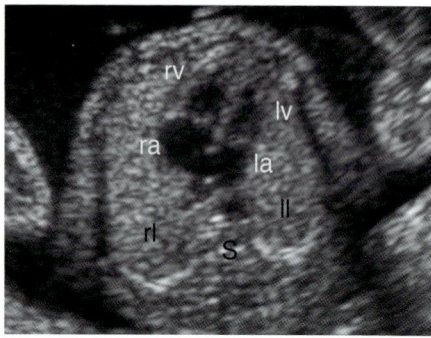

Figure 8-15. Normal Four-Chamber Heart View. Axial sonogram through the fetal chest demonstrates the normal heart and fluid-filled lungs in an 18-week fetus. The right ventricle (*rv*) and the left ventricle (*lv*) are approximately equal in size, as are the right atrium (*ra*) and the left atrium (*la*). The heart normally occupies about one-third of the cross-sectional area of the thorax. The developing lungs are echogenic. The spine (*S*) is seen posteriorly. rl, right lung; ll, left lung. (Reprinted with permission from Brant WE. Obstetric ultrasound. In: Brant WE, Helms CA, eds. *Fundamentals of Diagnostic Radiology*. 4th ed. Wolters Kluwer Health/Lippincott Williams & Wilkins; 2012. Figure 37.42.)

- Fetal chest
  - Heart
    - Four-chamber view, heart size, and position (Fig. 8-15)
    - The normal fetal heart will not take up more than one-third of the fetal chest.
    - Under normal conditions, the cardiac axis is 45 degrees.
    - The ventricular septum should be intact with no openings.
    - The normal foramen ovale will be noted at the level of the atrial septum.
    - Outflow tracts (Fig. 8-16)
      - The normal outflow tracts will travel perpendicularly or crisscross each other (Fig. 8-17).
        - Left ventricle outflow tract
          - The aortic outflow tract originates from the left ventricle.
        - Right ventricular outflow tract
          - The pulmonary outflow tract originates from the right ventricle.
      - Three-vessel view and three-vessel trachea view (if technically feasible) (see Chapter 9)

Chapter 8. Standard Second- or Third-Trimester Sonography

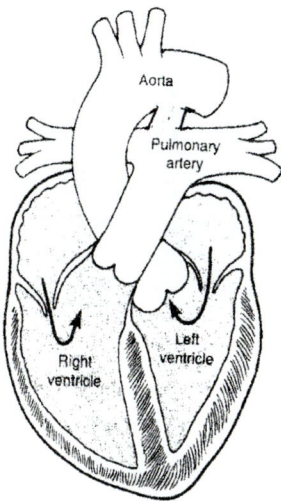

Figure 8-16. The normal crisscrossing of the outflow tracts. Diagram of the heart demonstrating the normal crossing of the pulmonary artery and aorta. The pulmonary artery should be located more anterior than the aorta and be noted crossing over the aorta to originate at the right ventricle. (Reprinted with permission from Penny SM. *Examination Review for Ultrasound: Abdomen & Obstetrics and Gynecology.* 3rd ed. Wolters Kluwer; 2023. Figure 27-6.)

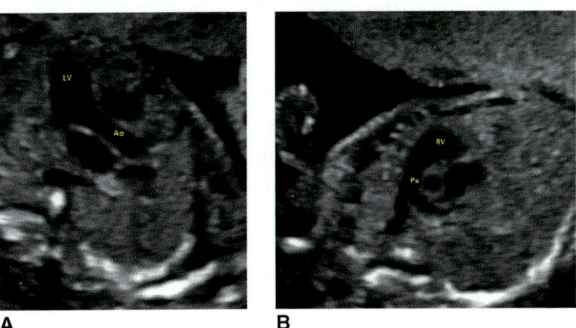

Figure 8-17. Outflow tracts. Left ventricular outflow tract (A) and right ventricular outflow tract (B) of the fetal heart. Ao, aorta; LV, left ventricle; Pa, pulmonary artery; RV, right ventricle. (Reprinted with permission from Stone J, Peña JA. Basic principles of ultrasound. In: Reece EA, Leguizamón GF, Macones GA, Wiznitzer A, eds. *Clinical Obstetrics: The Fetus & Mother.* 4th ed. Wolters Kluwer; 2022. Figure 12.7.)

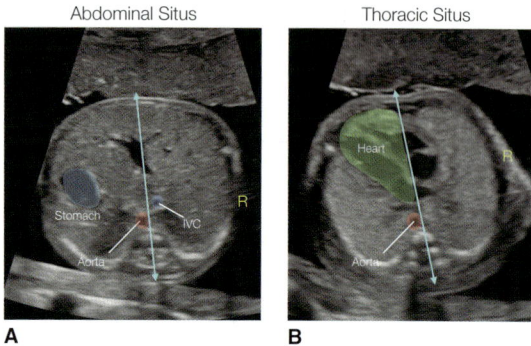

Figure 8-18. Correct fetal situs. Note that in **(A)**, the stomach is located on the left side of the abdomen. In **(B)**, the apex of the heart is pointing to the left side of the fetus. This confirms correct situs.
(Reprinted with permission from Abuhamad A, Chaoui R. *A Practical Guide to Fetal Echocardiography: Normal and Abnormal Hearts.* 4th ed. Wolters Kluwer; 2022. Figure 6.7.)

- Fetal abdomen
  - Stomach (presence, size, and situs)
    - The stomach should be within the left side of the abdomen, just under the apex of the heart, which should be pointed to the left side of the fetus **(Fig. 8-18)**. Back-to-back images should be obtained to prove this fact.
    - Note the shape of the stomach, there should not be two cystic structures at the level of the stomach. This could be evidence of duodenal atresia (double-bubble sign), which is associated with Trisomy 21.
  - Kidneys **(Fig. 8-19)**
    - Both kidneys should be noted at the same level in the transverse plane adjacent to the thoracic spine.
    - If a renal pelvis or both renal pelvi are dilated (pelviectasis), a posteroanterior measurement should be obtained **(Fig. 8-20)**.
  - Umbilical cord insertion site into the fetal abdomen **(Fig. 8-21)**
  - Umbilical cord vessel number **(Fig. 8-22)**
    - The normal umbilical cord contains two arteries and one vein.
    - A three vessel umbilical cord can be demonstrated in a transverse section of the umbilical cord or by demonstrating the two umbilical arteries coursing around the urinary bladder with color or power Doppler.

Chapter 8. Standard Second- or Third-Trimester Sonography

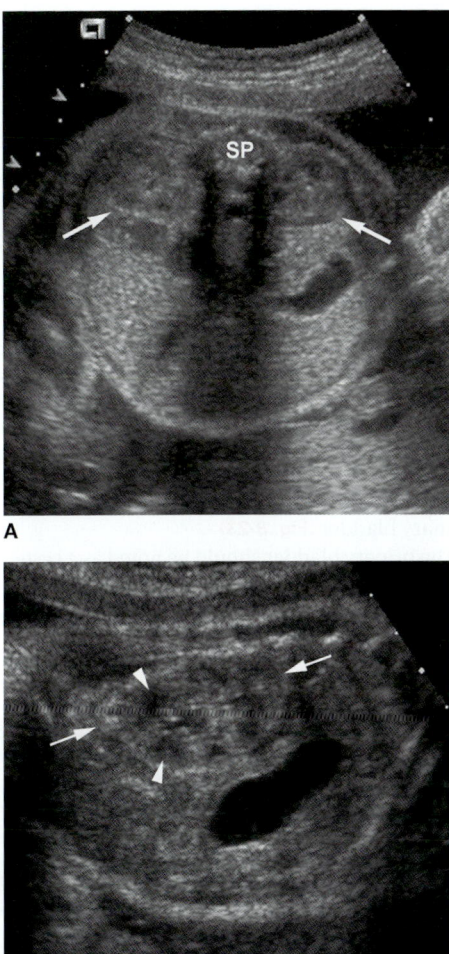

Figure 8-19. Fetal kidneys. A. Transverse view of the fetal abdomen revealing the kidneys (*arrows*) on both sides of the spine (*SP*). **B.** Longitudinal image of the fetal kidney (*between arrows*) revealing corticomedullary differentiation, with several identifiable medullary pyramids (*arrowheads*). (Reprinted with permission from Doubilet PM, Benson CB. *Atlas of Ultrasound in Obstetrics and Gynecology: A Multimedia Reference*. 2nd ed. Wolters Kluwer Health/Lippincott Williams & Wilkins; 2012. Figures 2.6.6 and 2.6.7.)

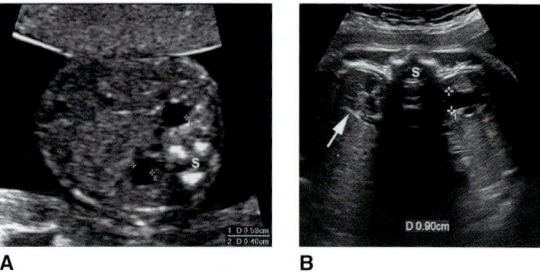

Figure 8-20. Mildly dilated renal pelvis. A. Transverse image of 18-week fetal kidneys, both with mildly dilated renal pelvi (*calipers*) that measured anteroposterior as 4.0 mm on one side and 5.3 mm on the other. S, spine. **B.** Transverse image of 40-week fetal kidneys showing mildly dilated renal pelvis (*calipers*) on one side measuring 9.0 mm and a normal contralateral kidney (*arrow*). (Reprinted with permission from Doubilet PM, Benson CB, Benacerraf BR. *Atlas of Ultrasound in Obstetrics and Gynecology: A Multimedia Reference.* 3rd ed. Wolters Kluwer; 2019. Figure 14.2.3.)

- Urinary bladder **(Fig. 8-23)**
  - The urinary bladder should be noted as a cystic structure in the center of the pelvis.
  - It will fill once and empty about every 30 to 45 minutes.
  - Enlargement of the urinary bladder can be associated with several fetal abnormalities and chromosomal anomalies.

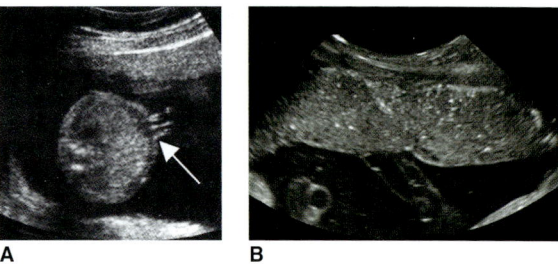

Figure 8-21. Cord insertion. A. Normal cord insertion (*arrow*) into the fetal abdomen. **B.** Normal cord insertion centrally located within the placenta. (**A.** Reprinted with permission from Sanders RC. Possible fetal anomalies. In: Sanders RC, Hall-Terracciano B, eds. *Clinical Sonography: A Practical Guide.* 5th ed. Wolters Kluwer; 2016. Figure 27-15. **B.** Reprinted with permission from Hernandez-Andrade E, Soto Torres EE, Tirosh D. Ultrasound evaluation of the placenta, amniotic fluid, umbilical cord, and amniotic membranes. In: Kline-Fath BM, Bulas DI, Lee W, eds. *Fundamental and Advanced Fetal Imaging: Ultrasound and MRI.* 2nd ed. Wolters Kluwer; 2021. Figure 13.1-30.)

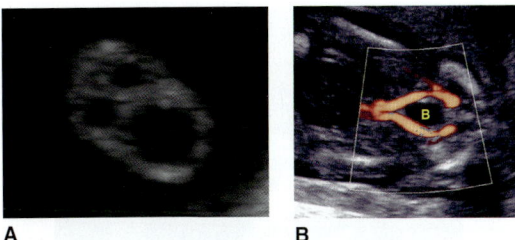

Figure 8-22. Normal three-vessel cord. A. A transverse section of a three-vessel cord demonstrates the normal two smaller umbilical arteries and one large umbilical vein. **B.** Two umbilical arteries can be seen coursing around the fetal urinary bladder using power Doppler, confirming the presence of a three-vessel umbilical cord as well. (**A.** Reprinted with permission from Allen LM. Abnormalities of the placenta and umbilical cord. In: Stephenson SR, ed. *Diagnostic Medical Sonography: Obstetrics & Gynecology.* 3rd ed. Wolters Kluwer Health/Lippincott Williams & Wilkins; 2012. Figure 18-28. **B.** Reprinted with permission from Allen L. Abnormalities of the placenta and umbilical cord. In: Stephenson SR, Dmitrieva J, eds. *Diagnostic Medical Sonography: Obstetrics & Gynecology.* 4th ed. Wolters Kluwer; 2018. Figure 20-30.)

- External genitalia **(Fig. 8-24)**
  - Demonstrating external genitalia is especially important in the presence of multiple gestations and when medically indicated.
  - There are some sex linked fetal anomalies.

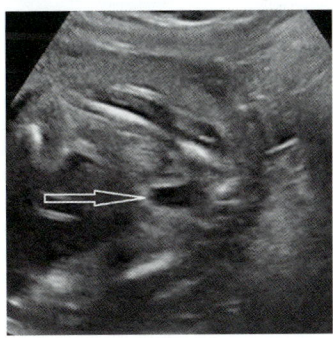

Figure 8-23. Normal fetal bladder. Axial view of the lower pelvis and bladder (*arrow*). (Reprinted with permission from Avni FE. Renal and adrenal abnormalities. In: Kline-Fath BM, Bulas DI, Bahado-Singh R, eds. *Fundamental and Advanced Fetal Imaging: Ultrasound and MRI.* Wolters Kluwer; 2015. Figure 19.1-6C.)

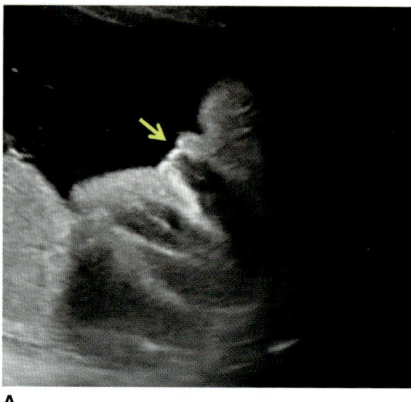

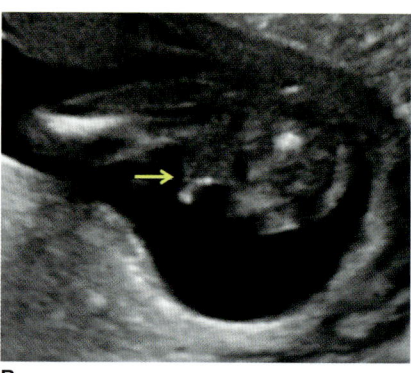

Figure 8-24. Normal appearance of external genitalia. A. Normal female external genitalia representing the labia majora and labia minora (*arrow*). B. Normal male external genitalia demonstrating the scrotum and penis (*arrow*). (Reprinted with permission from Amarillas L. Sonographic assessment of the fetal genitourinary system and fetal pelvis. In: Stephenson SR, Dmitrieva J, eds. *Diagnostic Medical Sonography: Obstetrics & Gynecology*. 4th ed. Wolters Kluwer; 2018. Figures 26-35 and 26-36.)

- Spine
  - The fetal spine consists of:
    - Cervical
    - Thoracic
    - Lumbar
    - Sacrum

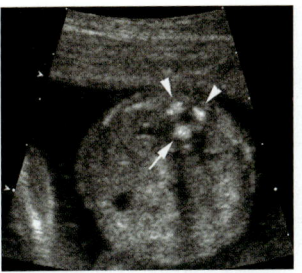 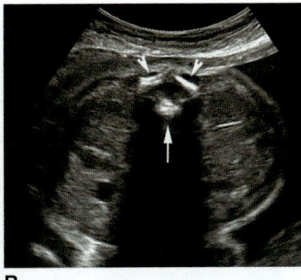

Figure 8-25. Transverse fetal spine. A. Transverse fetal spine at 18 weeks demonstrating the three ossification centers: two posterior elements (*arrowheads*) and one anterior element (*arrow*). Skin can be seen clearly covering the spine posteriorly. B. Transverse fetal spine at 30 weeks demonstrating more clearly the posterior (*arrowheads*) and anterior (*arrow*) ossification centers. (Reprinted with permission from Doubilet PM, Benson CB. *Atlas of Ultrasound in Obstetrics and Gynecology: A Multimedia Reference.* 2nd ed. Wolters Kluwer Health/Lippincott Williams & Wilkins; 2012. Figure 2.3.1.)

- Demonstrate the fetal spine in at least two planes (transverse, longitudinal, and/or coronal) (**Figs. 8-25** to **8-27**).
- Extremities (**Fig. 8-28**)
  - Presence of legs and arms
  - Presence of hands and feet
- Fetal weight estimate (provided by calculation package)
- The following assessment areas represent the minimal elements of a standard examination of maternal anatomy. A more detailed examination would ensue if abnormalities were noted during this examination (see Chapter 9).
  - Evaluation of the uterus, adnexal structures, and cervix.
    - Presence of uterine fibroids (leiomyomata), their location and size, and potential for clinical impact.
    - Presence, location, and size of adnexal masses.
      - The maternal ovaries and ovarian masses may be noted in the second trimester, though the ovaries may not be identifiable in the later stage of pregnancy.
  - The cervix should be evaluated (**Fig. 8-29**).
    - Shortening or funneling of the cervix should be noted.
    - The optimal imaging method for obtaining cervical length is transvaginal imaging.

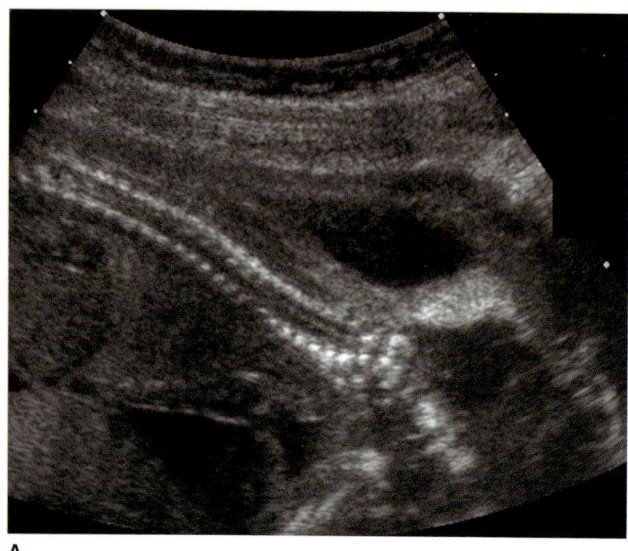

A

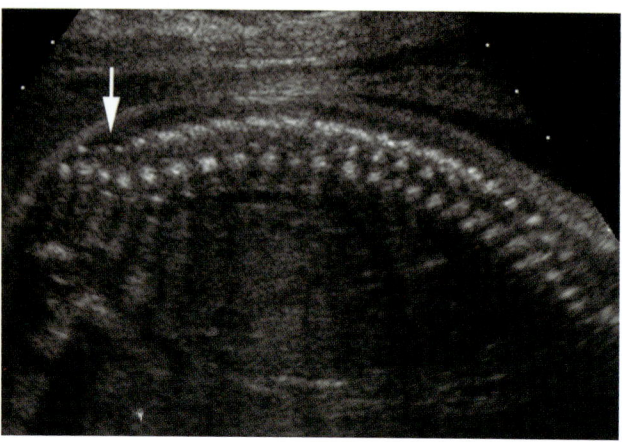

B

Figure 8-26. Longitudinal fetal spine. A. Longitudinal image of the cervical and thoracic spine. **B.** Longitudinal image of the thoracic, lumbar, and sacral spine (*arrow*). (Reprinted with permission from Doubilet PM, Benson CB. *Atlas of Ultrasound in Obstetrics and Gynecology: A Multimedia Reference*. 2nd ed. Wolters Kluwer Health/Lippincott Williams & Wilkins; 2012. Figure 2.3.2.)

Chapter 8. Standard Second- or Third-Trimester Sonography

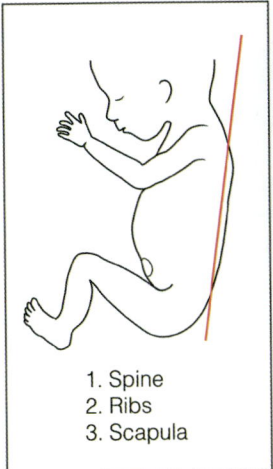
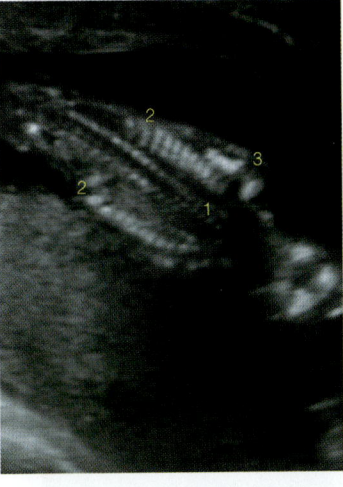

1. Spine
2. Ribs
3. Scapula

Figure 8-27. Coronal fetal spine. Posterior coronal plane of the fetus demonstrating the spine, scapula, and ribcage. This plane is helpful when spinal deformities are suspected. (Reprinted with permission from Abuhamad A, Chaoui R. *First Trimester Ultrasound Diagnosis of Fetal Abnormalities.* Wolters Kluwer; 2018. Figure 5.23.)

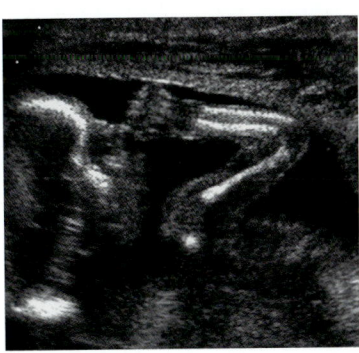
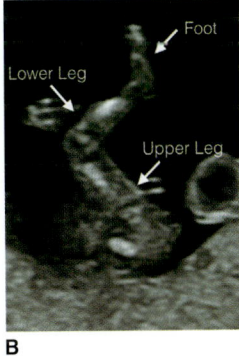

A   B

Figure 8-28. Normal fetal arm and leg. A. Normal upper extremity, including the hand, forearm, and humerus. B. Normal upper and lower leg and foot in sagittal. (**A.** Reprinted with permission from Doubilet PM, Benson CB, Benacerraf BR. *Atlas of Ultrasound in Obstetrics and Gynecology: A Multimedia Reference.* 3rd ed. Wolters Kluwer; 2019. Figure 18.2.1. **B.** Reprinted with permission from Abuhamad A, Chaoui R. *First Trimester Ultrasound Diagnosis of Fetal Abnormalities.* Wolters Kluwer; 2018. Figure 14.8.)

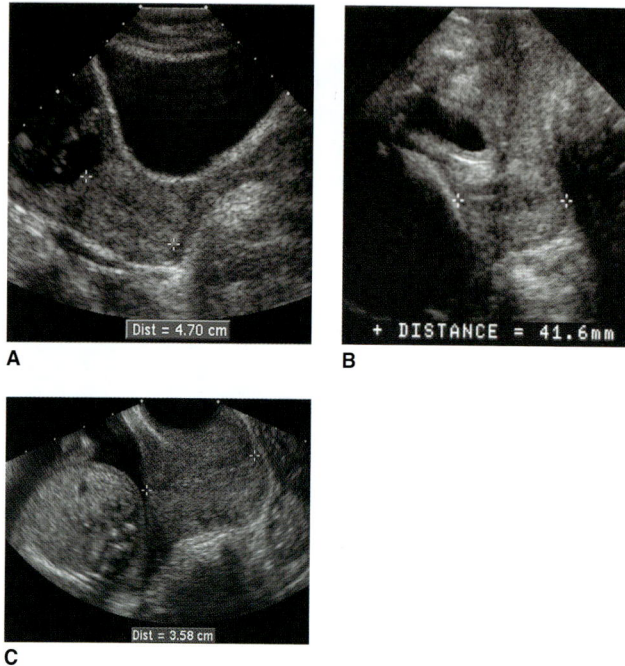

Figure 8-29. Normal cervix. The cervix is normal in configuration and length (*calipers*) on transabdominal (A), translabial (B), and transvaginal (C) sonograms, measuring at least 3 cm on each of these sagittal images. (Reprinted with permission from Doubilet PM, Benson CB. *Atlas of Ultrasound in Obstetrics and Gynecology: A Multimedia Reference.* 2nd ed. Wolters Kluwer Health/Lippincott Williams & Wilkins; 2012. Figure 3.2.1.)

- Transperineal (translabial) can also be used as well.
- The transabdominal view of the cervix is not as accurate as transvaginal and transvaginal due to the variable distention of the bladder and the additional distance from the transducer to the cervix which may both distort the normal anatomy.
- If shortening or funneling of the cervix is suspected transabdominally, then translabial or transvaginal analysis should be considered (**Figs. 8-30** and **8-31**).
- The optimal duration of time for an examination of the cervix is at least 5 minutes.

Chapter 8. Standard Second- or Third-Trimester Sonography

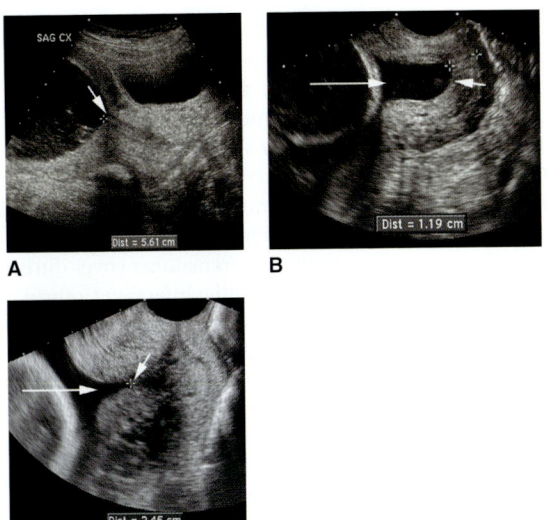

Figure 8-30. Normal cervix and incompetent cervix. A. Transabdominal measurement (*calipers*) when the internal os (*arrow*) is closed (i.e., no funneling). **B.** Transvaginal measurement (*calipers*) when the internal os (*long arrow*) is open and there is U-shaped funneling (*short arrow*). **C.** Transvaginal measurement (*calipers*) when the internal os (*long arrow*) is open and there is V-shaped funneling (*short arrow*). (Reprinted with permission from Doubilet PM, Benson CB. *Atlas of Ultrasound in Obstetrics and Gynecology: A Multimedia Reference*. 2nd ed. Wolters Kluwer Health/Lippincott Williams & Wilkins; 2012. Figure 17.1.1.)

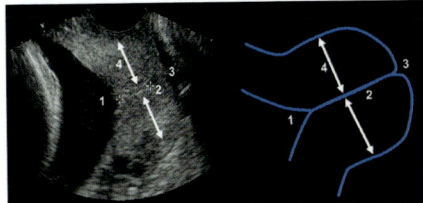

Figure 8-31. Clear visualization of (*1*) the internal cervical os, (*2*) the endocervical canal, (*3*) the external cervical os, and (*4*) similar thickness of the anterior and posterior cervical lips. (Reprinted with permission from Hernandez-Andrade E, Yeo L, Lo AJ, Hassan SS, Romero R. Ultrasound imaging of the uterine cervix. In: Kline-Fath BM, Bulas DI, Lee W, eds. *Fundamental and Advanced Fetal Imaging: Ultrasound and MRI*. 2nd ed. Wolters Kluwer; 2021. Figure 14.8.)

PATIENT PREPARATION

- Transabdominal second/third-trimester sonogram
  - The patient's urinary bladder should be emptied.
- Transvaginal second/third-Trimester Sonogram
  - The patient's urinary bladder should be empty for a transvaginal pelvic sonogram.
  - Preparation of transvaginal transducers between patients requires routine mandatory high-level disinfection and the use of a high-quality single-use transducer cover during each examination. (See the heading Infection Control and Equipment Maintenance in Chapter 6.)
  - The patient, the sonographer, or the physician may introduce the vaginal transducer, preferably under real-time monitoring.
  - Consideration of having a chaperone present should follow local policy.

SUGGESTED EQUIPMENT[1,2]

- The female pelvis should be examined sonographically with a real-time scanner, preferably a 3.5-MHz or higher curved linear array or sector transducer for transabdominal fetal imaging.
- Transvaginal imaging offers an improved resolution of both maternal pelvic and fetal structures in the early second trimester. The transvaginal transducer is typically 5 MHz or higher.
- As with other sonographic imaging, the frequency utilized depends upon the approach as well. Furthermore, the ultrasound equipment will offer differing operating frequencies. The sonographic practitioner should ensure that the highest frequency is always utilized, appreciating the fact that as operating frequency increases, there is a trade-off between resolution and beam penetration.
- Quality control and improvement, safety, infection control, patient education, and equipment performance monitoring should be developed and implemented in accordance with the AIUM Standards and Guidelines for the Accreditation of Ultrasound Practices found at https://www.aium.org/accreditation/accreditation.aspx

PATIENT POSITIONING

- Transabdominal second/third-trimester sonogram
  - The patient is typically placed in the supine position.

- Transvaginal second/third-trimester sonogram
  - The patient is typically placed in the lithotomy position.
  - The patient may be placed in the supine position with the hips elevated up from the examining table with the use of a positioning pad as well.
  - This position would be optimal for imaging the cervix transvaginally.

LABELING OF SONOGRAPHIC EXAMINATIONS[3]

- All sonographic images, whether still-frame images or video should include the following:
  - Patient's name and other identifying information (e.g., medical record number)
  - Facility's identification information
  - Date and time of the examination
  - Output display standard (thermal index and mechanical index)
  - Label the anatomic location and which side of the body, when appropriate
  - Image orientation when appropriate

INFECTION CONTROL AND EQUIPMENT MAINTENANCE[4]

- Infection control
  - Institutional guidelines should be in place for transducer disinfection to reduce the risk of iatrogenic and nosocomial infections.
  - Always follow your facility's established protocol for infection control.
  - The following is a summation of the AIUM's Guidelines for Cleaning and Preparing External- *and Internal-Use Ultrasound Transducers and Equipment Between Patients as well as Safe Handling and Use of Ultrasound Coupling Gel.*
    - Transabdominal transducers
      - Preparation of transabdominal transducers between patients requires a low-level disinfection process.
      - Nonsterile gel is used.
      - No transducer cover is required unless there is contaminated intact skin or nonintact skin, in which case both a cover and sterile gel are recommended.

- Transvaginal transducers
  - Barriers (probe covers) used for transvaginal transducers must be single-use transducer covers that meet the sterility requirements of the procedure.
  - Use sterile or bacteriostatic gel.
  - Consult the manufacturer's instructions for disinfecting devices.
  - After the procedure, perform high-level disinfection. Commercially available wall or table-top disinfectant units are available for endocavity transducers.
  - A complete list of Food and Drug Administration (FDA)-cleared liquid sterilants and high-level disinfectants is available online.
  - Rinse the transducer with water to remove disinfectant.

EQUIPMENT MAINTENANCE[5]

- Regular interval inspection of equipment and transducers (connector, cable, housing, acoustic lens) is recommended to ensure performance. Imaging with a tissue-mimicking phantom may help reveal imaging degradation.
- A record of quality assurance activities must be maintained and kept current. The ultrasound equipment must meet all state and federal guidelines and testing must be maintained in good operating condition and undergo routine quality assurance at least once a year or more frequently if problems arise.
- Always report machine or equipment malfunction to facility management and remove such equipment from use.

CLINICAL INVESTIGATION

- If accessible, evaluate the patient's laboratory findings associated with pregnancy. *These are provided in Chapter 5 of this text.*
- Why did your doctor order this sonogram? *This is especially important for follow-up obstetric exams. Though some patients may be poor historians, others may be capable of providing much beneficial information regarding their current and past clinical records.*
- Have you had a sonogram for this pregnancy already? *If the patient has had a previous sonogram during the current pregnancy, the findings would be most useful, especially for dating the pregnancy if the patient had a first-trimester*

sonogram. The earlier measurements of a crown-rump length would be more accurate for dating than a second/third-trimester sonogram. If a report can be provided, prior sonographic findings should be analyzed so that you are completely informed.

- When was the first day of your last menstrual period? *Obtaining this data can be useful, but do keep in mind that many patients are unsure. If the patient is sure, then the date can be entered into the calculation package of the ultrasound machine. The machine will provide an estimated gestational age.*
- Gravidity and parity score? *Gravidity refers to the number of pregnancies, parity refers to the number of pregnancies that led to birth at or beyond 20 weeks gestational age or of an infant weighing more than 500 grams. Some institutions may utilize TPAL (term, preterm, abortions, and living children) to further describe the patient's history.*
- Were there any complications for live births (living children)? *This question is useful, with follow-up questions. For example, if the patient had a miscarriage, one can inquire about how early the miscarriage occurred. If the patient had full-term pregnancies, one can inquire about if there were any complications or congenital abnormalities.*
- If pain, where is your pain? *If possible, have the patient point—with one finger—to the most painful region. Assessing the area of the complaint before an obstetric sonogram can provide some beneficial insight. Right lower quadrant can be associated with appendicitis, bowel, and ovarian masses, or ovarian torsion.*
- How long have you had pain? *This question can reveal a chronic or acute situation.*
- Are you having any vaginal bleeding? *In the second/third trimesters, vaginal bleeding may be associated with placenta previa, placental abruption, early delivery, or premature rupture of membranes.*
- Are you diabetic or have high blood pressure? *Diabetics and those suffering from high blood pressure can have related pregnancy issues. This is a good question to assess the overall health of the patient. For example, patients with preexisting diabetes are at an increased risk for fetal anomalies. Hypertension during pregnancy can lead to a poor outcome for both the mother and fetus.*

- Are you taking any drugs or using any drugs? *Drugs taken during the second/third trimesters may be used for various reasons, though due to the potential side effects of some drugs on the fetus, they are often advised against during pregnancy.*
- Do you have any history of taking any fertility drugs for this pregnancy? *Fertility drugs can lead to multiple gestations and heterotopic pregnancies. There may also be multiple ovarian follicles discovered sonographically.*
- Is there a family history of chromosomal abnormalities? *This would be useful, especially if the patient has a personal history of children with known chromosomal abnormalities. Ask this question before the examination ensues.*
- Is there a family history of multiple gestations? *A family history of multiple gestations increases the risk for multiple gestations.*
- Have you had any pelvic/obstetric surgeries, such as a Cesarean section (C-section)? *This is a general question to assess the patient for general pelvic issues and prior complaints that could affect the current pregnancy. A prior C-section increases the risk for placenta previa, placenta accreta spectrum (PAS), and vasa-previa.*

SUGGESTED PROTOCOL FOR A STANDARD SECOND- OR THIRD-TRIMESTER SONOGRAM[6-8]

- Basic initial survey
  - A basic survey will include the following objectives:
    - Assess the number of fetuses.
    - If multiple gestations are present, Chapter 9 of this text will be helpful.
    - Visualize fetal heart motion.
    - If multiple gestations, confirm heart motion in each fetus.
    - Visualize the fetal skull.
    - Perform a global view of the amniotic fluid amount.
    - If possible, perform a quick assessment of the cervix for funneling, especially if clinically indicated (e.g., vaginal bleeding, premature rupture of membranes, cramping, etc.).
- Obtain a midline sagittal image of the gestation, revealing initial fetal presentation/lie.
- Maternal anatomy and fetal environment assessment
  - Maternal anatomy assessment
    - Maternal uterus

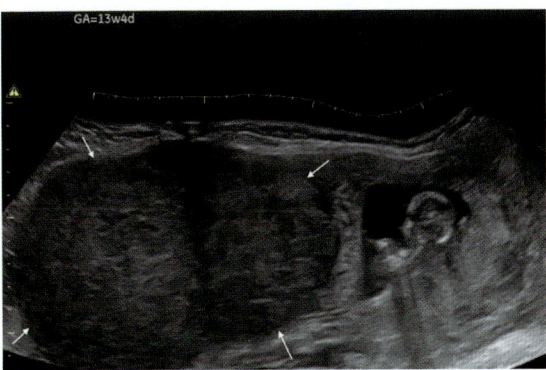

Figure 8-32. Fibroid during pregnancy. A large fibroid is demonstrated using extended field-of-view imaging (*arrows*). The pregnancy would most likely be measuring larger than expected for the gestational age. (Reprinted with permission from Abuhamad A, Chaoui R. *First Trimester Ultrasound Diagnosis of Fetal Abnormalities*. Wolters Kluwer; 2018. Figure 5.26.)

- ○ Evaluate the uterus in sagittal and transverse for signs of a fibroid tumor (leiomyoma) or other uterine masses **(Fig. 8-32)**.
- ○ Myometrial contractions may be confused for fibroids. It is important to note that contractions will resolve with time, typically by the end of the examination, while fibroids will maintain the same size and shape **(Fig. 8-33)**.
- Maternal ovaries and adnexal regions
  - ○ The ovaries and adnexa should be assessed especially when clinically indicated.
  - ○ If identified, measure the ovaries in both sagittal and transverse planes.
  - ○ In the second trimester, the ovaries may be readily identifiable, while in the third trimester, the ovaries may not be visualized.
    - Ovarian torsion and ovarian masses, especially large cysts, can lead to pain during pregnancy.
    - Ovarian torsion findings are discussed in Chapter 2.
  - ○ The adnexa should be evaluated for masses, specifically when pain is a clinical symptom.
    - Right lower quadrant pain should be carefully evaluated because this could be a sign of appendicitis (see Chapter 2).

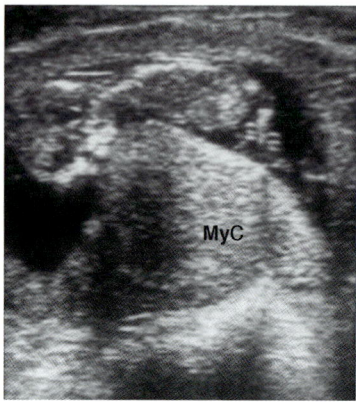

Figure 8-33. A huge myometrial contraction (*MyC*) involves much of the posterior aspect of the uterus, including a portion of the cervix mimicking a placenta previa. The contraction disappeared 30 minutes later. (Reprinted with permission from Sanders RC. Second- and third-trimester bleeding. In: Sanders RC, Hall-Terracciano B, eds. *Clinical Sonography: A Practical Guide.* 5th ed. Wolters Kluwer; 2016. Figure 24-12.)

- The appendix may be displaced during pregnancy and lead to pain in other locations in the lower abdomen and pelvis (Fig. 8-34).
- Fetal environment assessment
  - Placenta
    - The location of the placenta should be documented in both sagittal and transverse and is described by its location relative to the maternal uterine anatomy.
    - Therefore, the placenta may be anterior, posterior, right lateral, left lateral, fundal, or inferior (placenta previa).
    - There can also be a combination of these (e.g., anterior, right lateral; posterior, left lateral; etc.).
  - A detailed view of the cervix can be performed at the end of the exam.
    - Placenta previa should be noted and described based on the location of the placental edge and the internal os (see Fig. 8-4). Note what type of placenta previa is present, such as complete, partial, or low-lying.
    - In the second/third trimester, the sonographic analysis of the cervix for signs of previa can be performed transabdominally, translabially, or transvaginally (Fig. 8-35).

Chapter 8. Standard Second- or Third-Trimester Sonography

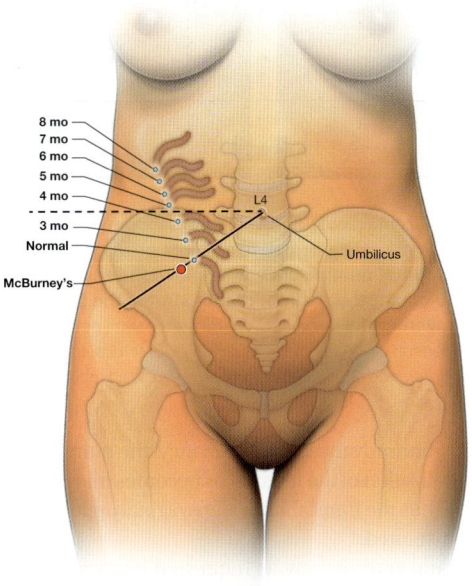

A

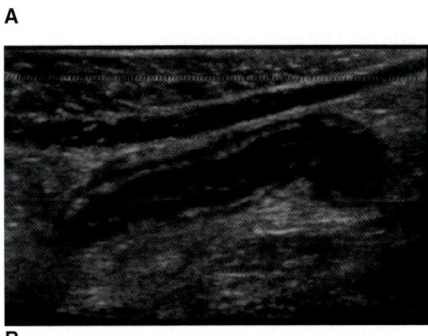

B

Figure 8-34. Changing locations of the appendix with pregnancy and appendicitis appearance. **A.** The normal and postpartum positions of the base of the appendix are medial to McBurney point. In the fifth month, the appendix is at the level of the umbilicus and iliac crest. **B.** Acute appendicitis. The tubular structure in the middle of the image represents the dilated appendix, consistent with acute appendicitis. (**B.** Reprinted with permission from Smith EA, Smith WL. Pediatric imaging. In: Farrell TA, ed. *Radiology 101: The Basics and Fundamentals of Imaging*. 5th ed. Wolters Kluwer; 2020. Figure 5.47.)

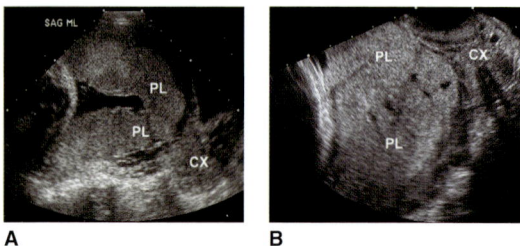

Figure 8-35. Placenta previa. A. Sagittal transabdominal examination of the cervix (*CX*) revealing complete placenta previa (*PL*) in the second trimester. **B.** Sagittal midline view of the lower uterus performed transvaginally on another patient demonstrates the placenta (*PL*) completely covering the cervix (*CX*). (Reprinted with permission from Doubilet PM, Benson CB. *Atlas of Ultrasound in Obstetrics and Gynecology: A Multimedia Reference.* 2nd ed. Wolters Kluwer Health/Lippincott Williams & Wilkins; 2012. Figure 16.1.1.)

- The more advanced the pregnancy, the more difficult the visualization of the internal os becomes transabdominally, and thus the translabial or transvaginal approach should be instituted.
- Placental grading may be requested by some institutions **(Fig. 8-36)**.
  - Grade 0 = Unbroken chorionic plate and the placental should be homogeneous
  - Grade I = Subtle indentations within the chorionic plate and the placenta may contain some small calcifications
  - Grade II = Moderate indentation within the chorionic plate and "comma-like" calcifications within the placenta
  - Grade III = Prominent indentations within the chorionic plate, continuing to the basal layer, with a diffusely heterogeneous placenta containing multiple calcifications and maternal lakes
- The placental attachment to the myometrium should be examined carefully for signs of PAS, especially in patients with a history of previous Cesarean sections, as there is an increased risk for this disorder **(Fig. 8-37)**.
  - In many situations, PAS may be clinically silent, except for those where the placenta penetrates beyond the uterus and invades adjacent organs—placenta percreta. With percreta, patients can have associated urinary symptoms, such as hematuria, or gastrointestinal symptoms.

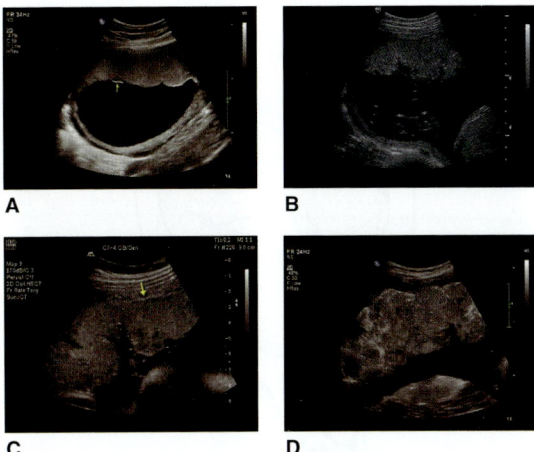

Figure 8-36. Placental grading. **A.** Anterior grade 0 placenta demonstrating the characteristic smooth, homogeneous texture. The perpendicular angle of incidence allows for imaging of the chorionic plate (*arrow*). **B.** This grade I placenta contains scattered calcifications with the beginning of lobulations developing on the fetal side. **C.** In the grade II placenta, lobulations increase with the basal layer (*arrow*) appearing irregular due to small calcifications. **D.** The grade III placenta demonstrates interlobar and septal calcifications. (Reprinted with permission from Dmitrieva J. Normal placenta and umbilical cord. In: Stephenson SR, Dmitrieva J, eds. *Diagnostic Medical Sonography: Obstetrics & Gynecology*. 4th ed. Wolters Kluwer; 2018. Figure 19-8.)

- Placenta accreta is the firm adherence of the placenta to the myometrium.
- Placenta increta is the invasion of the placenta within the myometrium.
- Placenta percreta is the penetration of the placenta beyond the myometrium and possibly into adjacent organs (e.g., urinary bladder invasion, bowel invasion, etc.).
- Evaluate the placental/myometrium interface to ensure that there is a substantial, identifiable boundary (Nitabuch layer), with an adequate myometrial border noted adjacent to the placenta **(Fig. 8-38)**.
- Assess the placenta for signs of placental abruption. Again, the border between the placenta and myometrium should be analyzed for signs of premature separation.

278   **Chapter 8.** Standard Second- or Third-Trimester Sonography

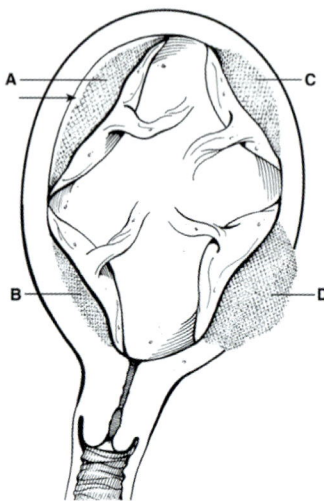

Figure 8-37. Placenta accreta spectrum. A. Normal placenta. Nitabuch layer is the clear space indicated by the arrow. B. Placenta accretes; note the lack of the Nitabuch layer. C. Placenta increta, with deeper invasion into the myometrium. D. Placenta percreta, penetrating the uterine serosa. (Reprinted with permission from Lee RH, Grover J. Placenta accreta. In: Beall MH, Ross MG. *Lippincott's Obstetrics Case-Based Review*. Wolters Kluwer Health/Lippincott Williams & Wilkins; 2011. Figure 30.1.)

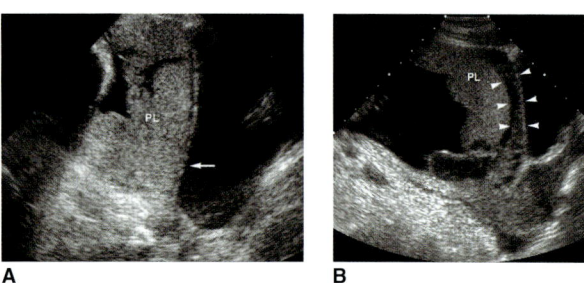

Figure 8-38. Sonographic appearance of placenta accreta in the second trimester. A. Sagittal view of the lower uterus demonstrating marked thinning of the myometrium (*arrow*) beneath the placenta (*PL*). B. A normal sagittal scan of the lower uterus for comparison, with the myometrium (*arrowheads*) appearing as a hypoechoic band under the placenta (*PL*). (Reprinted with permission from Doubilet PM, Benson CB. *Atlas of Ultrasound in Obstetrics and Gynecology: A Multimedia Reference*. 2nd ed. Wolters Kluwer Health/Lippincott Williams & Wilkins; 2012. Figure 16.3.1.)

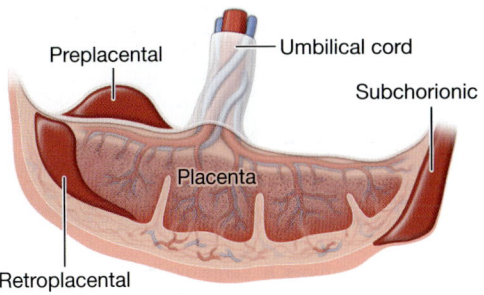

Figure 8-39. Sites of placental abruption.

- Patients may present with abdominal pain, possible vaginal bleeding, uterine contractions, and uterine tenderness.
- Forms of placental abruption include partial, marginal, and complete. Also, the locations of the hemorrhage may be described as preplacental, retroplacental, and subchorionic (**Figs. 8-39** and **8-40**).

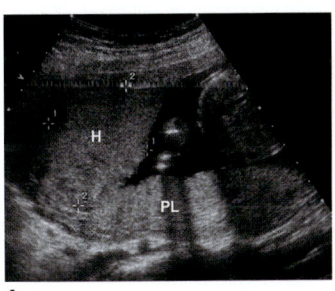
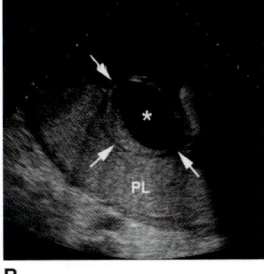

A **B**

Figure 8-40. Placental abruption in the second/third trimester. A. Sonogram showing large isoechoic hematoma (*H, calipers*) adjacent to the placenta (*PL*). **B.** Complex lesion (*arrows*) on the amniotic surface of the placenta (*PL*) represents a preplacental hematoma. The central part of the hematoma (*asterisk*) appears more cystic than the wall. (**A.** Reprinted with permission from Doublet PM, Benson CB. *Atlas of Ultrasound in Obstetrics and Gynecology: A Multimedia Reference*. 2nd ed. Wolters Kluwer Health/Lippincott Williams & Wilkins; 2012. Figure 16.2.4. **B.** Reprinted with permission from Doublet PM, Benson CB, Benacerraf BR. *Atlas of Ultrasound in Obstetrics and Gynecology: A Multimedia Reference*. 3rd ed. Wolters Kluwer; 2019. Figure 19.2.3.)

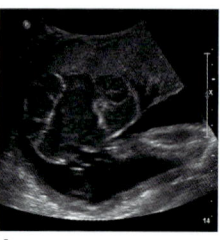 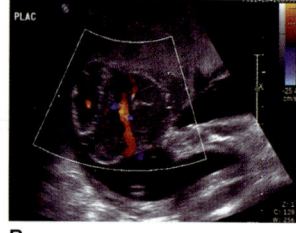

Figure 8-41. Chorioangioma. A. Large ovoid mass protruding from fetal surface of the placenta with internal calcifications consistent with a chorioangioma. B. As a vascular tumor of the placenta, the chorioangioma demonstrates multiple vascular channels within the mass on color Doppler sonography. (Reprinted with permission from Allen L. Abnormalities of the placenta and umbilical cord. In: Stephenson SR, Dmitrieva J, eds. *Diagnostic Medical Sonography: Obstetrics & Gynecology*. 4th ed. Wolters Kluwer; 2018. Figure 20-18.)

- It is important to note that blood will change in echogenicity, and thus while fresh blood may be anechoic, clotted blood may appear, at times, isoechoic to placental tissue **(Fig. 8-41)**. Color Doppler may be useful to evaluate for active bleeding.
- Clinical correlation is vital.
- Evaluate the placenta for signs of intraplacental masses.
  - Placental or maternal lakes are common and are typically clinically insignificant. These pools of blood will appear hypoechoic or anechoic.
  - Solid tumors, such as chorioangiomas, should be identified and measured. Color Doppler should be applied to these lesions (Fig. 8-41).
- Assessment of the umbilical cord
  - Cord insertion into the placenta should be central and demonstrated.
  - Cord insertion into the fetus should be demonstrated unobstructed and in a normal location.
  - If possible, the length of the cord should be evaluated for masses and/or knots.
  - The determination of three vessels should be confirmed with either a transverse image of the cord or color Doppler around the urinary bladder (see Fig. 8-22).
  - Pulsed wave Doppler may be performed on the umbilical artery and a systolic/diastolic ratio (S/D ratio) can be obtained.

- The S/D ratio of the umbilical cord is an assessment of placental function and should always demonstrate increasing diastolic flow and never reversed flow, as this can be related to fetal growth restriction because of placental insufficiency **(Fig. 8-42)**.
- A normal S/D ratio of the umbilical cord declines with advancing gestation.

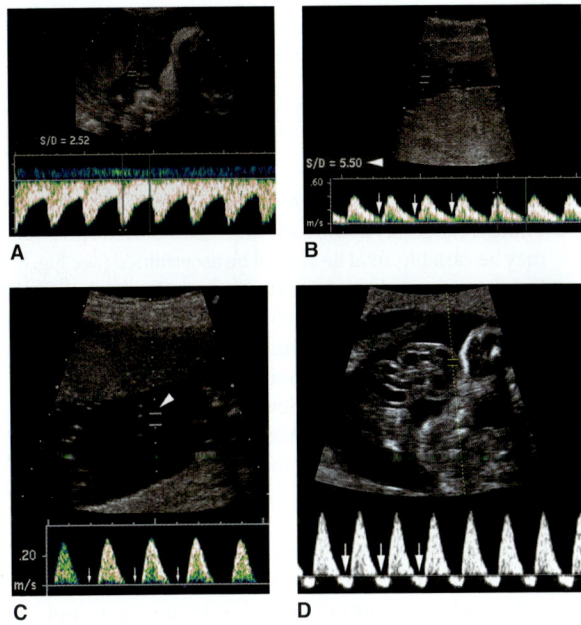

Figure 8-42. Normal and abnormal umbilical cord S/D ratios. A. Spectral Doppler of umbilical artery in a 34-week fetus demonstrating a normal waveform with normal end-diastolic flow and normal S/D ratio (*calipers*) of 2.52. **B.** Doppler waveform of an umbilical artery with elevated S/D ratio to 5.50 (*arrowhead, calipers*), indicating diminished end-diastolic flow (*arrows*). **C.** Doppler interrogation of umbilical artery (*arrowhead*) demonstrating absent end-diastolic flow (*arrows*) on the spectral waveform. **D.** Spectral Doppler of umbilical artery demonstrating reversed end-diastolic flow (*arrows*), with systolic peaks seen as flow above the baseline and end-diastolic flow below the baseline. (Reprinted with permission from Doubilet PM, Benson CB, Benacerraf BR. *Atlas of Ultrasound in Obstetrics and Gynecology: A Multimedia Reference.* 3rd ed. Wolters Kluwer; 2019. Figure 18.3.1.)

- Choosing an appropriate segment of the cord, place the Doppler gate over one of the umbilical cord arteries.
- Obtain the peak systolic and end-diastolic points.
- Velamentous cord insertion should be further evaluated for evidence of vasa previa or abnormal placental cord insertion. Color and pulsed Doppler should be used.
  - Assessment of the amniotic fluid
- Obtain one of the following:
  - AFI
    - Measure each quadrant, entering the measuring each empty pocket into the calculation pocket (see Fig. 8-3).
  - Single deepest pocket
  - Two-diameter pocket
- Fetal Assessment
  - Determine fetal lie and presentation
    - Though especially in the early first trimester, fetal position may be variable, fetal lie should be ascertained (see Fig. 8-2).
    - Head down may be referred to in general as cephalic, while head up may be referred to in general as breech.
    - Vertex is most specifically indicating the vertex of the skull is closest to the internal os, while cephalic is less specific, indicating head down.
    - There are even more specific forms of breech as well, such as footling breech, frank breech, and complete breech (legs crossed).
  - Fetal head
    - Axial plane to the fetal head
      - Assess head shape for normalcy (mesocephaly).
      - Assess lateral ventricles for ventriculomegaly and symmetry.
      - Evaluate the choroid plexus.
      - Assess for signs of cysts.
      - Assess for signs of the "dangling choroid" sign associated with ventriculomegaly.
      - Assess the falx cerebri for continuity from anterior to posterior.
      - Verify the presence of the CSP.
        - If a CSP is not seen in axial, rotate the transducer to a plane consistent with a sagittal midline image of the brain, and then evaluate the midline of the brain for signs of agenesis of the corpus callosum (e.g., absent

CSP, absent corpus callosum, elevated and dilated third ventricle, "sunburst" appearance of sulci, etc.)
- ○ Assess the cerebellum.
  - – Evaluate the shape of the cerebellum, which should be dumbbell shaped.
  - – Ensure the presence of cerebellar vermis.
  - – Ensure that the cerebellar lobes are symmetric.
  - – If appropriate, obtain the diameter measurement of the cerebellum (see Fig. 8-14).
- ○ Evaluate the cisterna magna.
  - – Assess the cistern magna for enlargement.
  - – If appropriate, measure the anteroposterior dimension of cisterna magna to obtain an objective measurement (see Fig. 8-14).
- ○ Nuchal fold (between 16 and 20 weeks)
  - – Assess the nuchal fold for increased thickness.
  - – Measure the anteroposterior dimension of nuchal fold (see Fig. 8-14).
- ○ Obtain appropriate BPD measurement.
- ○ Obtain appropriate HC measurement.
  - – Coronal plane to the fetal head
- ○ Assess the fetal upper lip for clefting (see Fig. 8-13).
  - – Sagittal plane to the fetal head (profile image)
- ○ Assess the fetal profile for normalcy (see Fig. 8-13).
  - – Evaluate for bulging of the forehead, which is termed frontal bossing.
  - – Evaluate for the presence of a small jaw, which is termed micrognathia.
  - – Evaluate for the presence of a hard palate.
  - – Evaluate the presence of nasal bones.
- Fetal spine
  - Demonstrate, as needed to establish symmetry, several longitudinal and transverse fetal spine images of each of the following sections:
    - ○ Cervical
      - – In transverse, it may behoove the practitioner to evaluate the fetus for signs of a nuchal cord with color Doppler (Fig. 8-43).
    - ○ Thoracic
    - ○ Lumbar
      - – Most spina bifida open defects are found within the lumbosacral region.

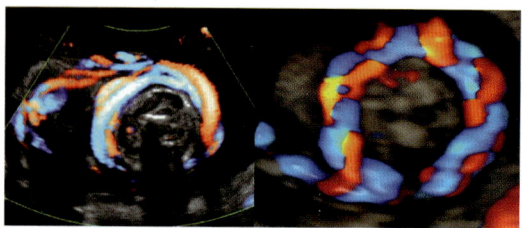

Figure 8-43. Nuchal cord. Transverse views of the fetal neck, and visualization of the nuchal cord with color Doppler. (Reprinted with permission from Hernandez-Andrade E, Soto Torres EE, Tirosh D. Ultrasound evaluation of the placenta, amniotic fluid, umbilical cord, and amniotic membranes. In: Kline-Fath BM, Bulas DI, Lee W, eds. *Fundamental and Advanced Fetal Imaging: Ultrasound and MRI*. 2nd ed. Wolters Kluwer; 2021. Figure 13.1-35.)

- Sacrum
  - Try to obtain an adequate image of the tip of the most distal spine.
- Ensure that the entire spine is completely covered with a skin layer, with no openings.
- Coronal spine images can be useful as well, especially if scoliosis or spina bifida is suspected.
- Fetal chest
  - Transverse heart
  - Obtain an M-mode measurement of the heart.
    - Measure from the beginning of one beat to the beginning of the next to obtain the beats per minute (defer to machine manufacturer as this measurement may be different).
    - A video clip can also be obtained.
    - Obtain a four-chamber view of the heart.
  - Evaluate the size of the fetal heart.
    - Subjectively, a normal heart will not take up more than one-third of the fetal chest.
    - Evaluate the ventricular septum for openings.
      - The normal foramen ovale will be noted at the level of the atrial septum.
    - Evaluate the heart for normal position and cardiac axis.
      - Subjectively, the cardiac axis is 45 degrees, pointing to the left side of the fetus.
    - Obtain an image of the fetal stomach just below the heart to prove situs.
      - A dual image may be most helpful (see Fig. 8-18).

Chapter 8. Standard Second- or Third-Trimester Sonography

- Transverse heart (with angulation)
  - Obtain outflow tract images by angling the transducer slightly cephalad.
    - The normal outflow tracts will travel perpendicularly or crisscross each other (see Fig. 8-17).
      - The left ventricle outflow tract
      - The aortic outflow tract originates from the left ventricle.
      - Right ventricular outflow tract
      - The pulmonary outflow tract originates from the right ventricle.
  - Obtain a three-vessel view and three-vessel trachea view (if technically feasible) **(Fig. 8-44)**.
- Evaluate the chest for masses, especially if an abnormal cardiac axis is noted, as this can be associated with a diaphragmatic hernia **(Fig. 8-45)**.
  - A sagittal image of the fetal thorax and fetal abdomen, including the diaphragm, heart, and stomach, can confirm this diagnosis.
- Fetal abdomen
  - Demonstrate the stomach and obtain the abdominal circumference measurement.
    - Note the size and shape of the stomach.
  - Demonstrate the kidneys.
    - Both kidneys should be noted at the same level in the transverse plane adjacent to the thoracic spine.
  - Demonstrate the umbilical cord insertion site into the fetal abdomen.
  - Fetal pelvis
    - Demonstrate the urinary bladder.
    - Demonstrate external genitalia.
  - Extremities
    - Demonstrate the presence of legs and arms.
    - Obtain femur length measurement.
    - Demonstrate the presence of hands and feet.
  - Transabdominal examination of the cervix in the maternal sagittal midline plane.
    - The urinary bladder should not be distended while examining the cervix.
    - To better examine the cervix, a transvaginal examination can be performed (see Fig. 8-29).

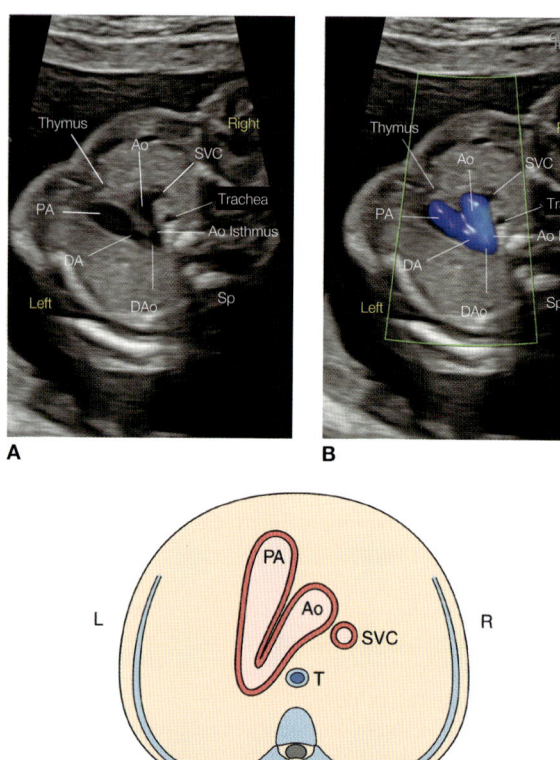

Figure 8-44. Three-vessel trachea view. A. Note anterior location of pulmonary artery (*PA*), with ductus arteriosus (*DA*) connecting with descending aorta (*DAo*). The aorta (*Ao*) and Ao isthmus are also seen connecting with DAo. Superior vena cava (*SVC*) is seen in cross-section to the right side of Ao. Note that DA and Ao isthmus are to the left side of trachea, confirming the presence of normal left Ao and DA. Spine (*Sp*) is seen posteriorly. **B.** Three-vessel trachea view in color Doppler. **C.** Schematic drawings of the three-vessel trachea view in a normal fetus, where the transverse aortic arch (*Ao*) and isthmus merge with the pulmonary artery (*PA*) and ductus arteriosus (*DA*) into the descending aorta in a "V-shape" configuration to the left of the trachea (*T*). (**A**, **B.** Reprinted with permission from Abuhamad A, Chaoui R. *A Practical Guide to Fetal Echocardiography: Normal and Abnormal Hearts*. 4th ed. Wolters Kluwer; 2022. Figure 5.5. **C.** Reprinted with permission from Abuhamad A, Chaoui R. *A Practical Guide to Fetal Echocardiography: Normal and Abnormal Hearts*. 3rd ed. Wolters Kluwer; 2016. Figure 29.2.)

Chapter 8. Standard Second- or Third-Trimester Sonography

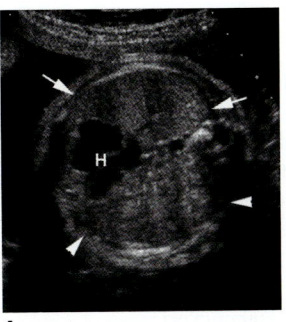
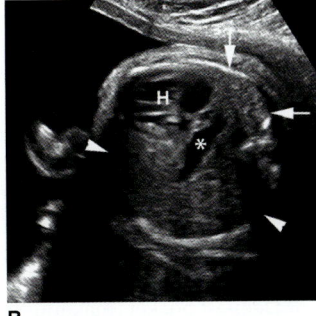

Figure 8-45. Diaphragmatic hernia. Appearance of right lung tissue with left diaphragmatic hernias. **A.** Transverse image of thorax showing moderate-sized left diaphragmatic hernia (*arrowheads*) with a considerable amount of right lung present (*arrows*) posterior to the heart (*H*). **B.** Transverse image of the thorax in a different fetus showing a large left diaphragmatic hernia (*arrowheads*) containing liver and stomach (*asterisk*), with only a small amount of right lung present (*arrows*) behind the heart (*H*) in the posterior right chest.
(Reprinted with permission from Doubilet PM, Benson CB, Benacerraf BR. *Atlas of Ultrasound in Obstetrics and Gynecology: A Multimedia Reference.* 3rd ed. Wolters Kluwer; 2019. Figure 10.4.6.)

SCANNING TIPS

- If fetal anatomy is not identifiable, document the issue within the imaging report. Never assume that something is normal if it is not attestable.
- If the ultrasound machine equipment package contains a list of necessary protocol images, include the package as a resource to help guide the examination and to ensure that no images are omitted. Newer equipment have protocol managers established and these are also often editable.
- For the fetal spine, carefully adjust the gain to ensure that the overlying skin of the spine is clearly seen.
- To evaluate the cervix, and the fetal head is obscuring the internal os, place the patient in the Trendelenburg position (maternal head lower than her feet) and/or have the patient support the fetal head superiorly slightly.
- Place the patient in decubitus positions as needed to better assess fetal anatomy.
- Occasionally, the patient may need to walk around a bit in order for the fetus to change positions.

NORMAL MEASUREMENTS[6,7,8]

- Amniotic fluid
  - Amniotic fluid can be measured using several techniques.
  - Amniotic fluid index
    - Four quadrants are measured in the anteroposterior plane with the patient in supine, perpendicular to the floor.
    - The four quadrants are added together to obtain the AFI.
    - Varies per gestational age
    - Oligohydramnios ≤5 cm
    - Polyhydramnios ≥24 cm
  - Deepest pocket (maximum vertical pocket)
    - Preferred over AFI
    - Oligohydramnios ≤2 cm
    - Polyhydramnios ≥8 cm
- Cervical length (see Fig. 8-31)
  - The cervix can measure between 2.5 cm and 5 cm at 14 to 30 weeks' gestation.
  - Cervical length should be screened between 18 and 22 weeks' gestation.
  - A measurement of less than 2.5 cm is considered short and between 16 and 24 weeks is a strong predictor of preterm birth.
  - However, it is important to note that some authors agree that it should measure at least 3 cm in length.
  - Follow-up examinations may be warranted, as the cervix is a dynamic structure, especially for those in the high-risk population.
- Lateral ventricle
  - The lateral ventricle should be measured at the trigone (atrium) of the lateral ventricle.
  - The diameter of the lateral ventricle should not exceed 1 cm between 15 and 40 weeks' gestation.
- Cisterna magna
  - The cisterna magna should not exceed 1 cm in the anteroposterior dimension.
- Nuchal fold
  - The nuchal fold is typically measured at the level of the biparietal diameter.
  - The measurement is taken from the outer skull to the outer skin.
  - The nuchal fold should not exceed 6 mm.

- Kidneys
  - The renal pelvis is measured in the anteroposterior dimension and it should not exceed 4 mm before 32 weeks' gestation.

BIOPHYSICAL PROFILE[9]

- BPP is performed on fetuses with an increased risk for fetal demise.
- BPP scoring can be found in Table 8-1. The maximum assigned due to the sonographic observations is 8 points (10 total with the nonstress test).

Table 8-1 BIOPHYSICAL PROFILE SCORING

OBSERVATION	2 POINTS	0 POINTS
Fetal breathing	At least 1 episode of sustained breathing at least 30-s of duration within a 30-min period	Absence of fetal breathing or absence of 1 episode of sustained breathing of at least 30-s of duration within a 30-min period
Fetal movement	Three or more gross discrete body or limb movements in a 30-min period	Two or less gross body movements in a 30-min period
Fetal tone	One or more episodes of extension of a fetal extremity with return to flexion, or opening or closing of a hand	Extremities in position of extension or partial flexion with no return to flexion
Qualitative amniotic fluid volume	Largest vertical pocket of amniotic fluid ≥2 cm or an amniotic fluid index of ≥5 cm	Largest vertical pocket of amniotic fluid ≤2 cm or amniotic fluid index ≤4 cm
Nonstress test (nonimaging)	Presence of two or more fetal heart rate accelerations of at least 15 beats per minute lasting a minimum of 15 s with fetal movement in 40 min	No fetal heart rate acceleration or less than 2 accelerations in 40 min

Reprinted with permission from Stephenson SR, Dmitrieva J. *Obstetrics and Gynecology*. 5th ed. Wolters Kluwer; 2023. Table 30-1.

- The lower the score the more likely fetal complications and compromise are present.

WHERE ELSE TO LOOK

- It is apparent that although isolated fetal abnormalities can exist, it is the obligation of the sonographers to pursue connections that work to establish a more conclusive, or at a minimum, better appreciation of overall fetal well-being.
  - Examples of this include the various syndromes. For example, VACTERL association includes the connection between vertebral anomalies, anal atresia, cardiac defects, transesophageal fistula, renal, and limb anomalies (Fig. 8-46).
- This is to say, that when one identifies an anomaly in a fetus, further investigation for linked anomalies should ensue.

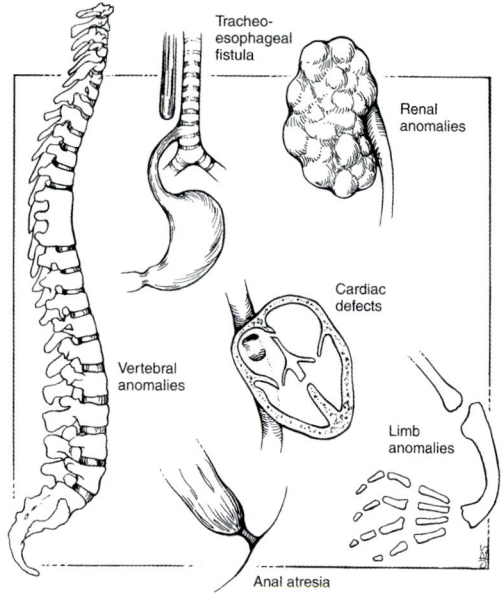

Figure 8-46. The VACTERL association: vertebral anomalies, anal atresia, cardiac defects, TE fistula, renal and limb anomalies. (Reprinted with permission from Trombly JF, Stephenson SR. Patterns of fetal anomalies. In: Stephenson SR, ed. *Diagnostic Medical Sonography: Obstetrics & Gynecology*. 3rd ed. Wolters Kluwer Health/Lippincott Williams & Wilkins; 2012. Figure 28-32.)

- The maternal anatomy, including the entire pelvic region if appropriate to the clinical history, must be carefully analyzed for potential devastating future events.
  - Examples include ovarian masses, uterine masses, bowel problems, and urinary tract disorders.
- Back and pelvic pain are common maternal complaints. Though the causative factor may not be identifiable sonographically, as in the case of muscular contractions or ligament pain, the sonographer must be aware that there may be some pathologies that can lead to such complaints that sonography can provide aid in diagnosis, such as urinary tract stones, hydronephrosis, and cystitis.

REFERENCES

1. AIUM. Practice parameter for the performance of detailed second- and third-trimester diagnostic obstetric ultrasound examinations. *J Ultrasound Med*. 2019;38:3093–3100.
2. AIUM–ACR–ACOG–SMFM–SRU. Practice parameter for the performance of standard diagnostic obstetric ultrasound examinations. *J Ultrasound Med*. 2018;37:E13–E24.
3. AIUM. Practice parameter for documentation of an ultrasound examination. *J Ultrasound Med*. 2020;39:E1–E4.
4. Guidelines for Cleaning and Preparing. External- and Internal- Use Ultrasound Transducers and Equipment Between Patients as Well as Safe Handling and Use of Ultrasound Coupling Gel. Accessed November 12, 2023. https://www.aium.org/resources/official-statements/view/guidelines-for-cleaning-and-preparing-external-and-internal-use-ultrasound transducers-and-equipment-between-patients-as-well-as-safe-handling-and-use-of-ultrasound-coupling-gel
5. AIUM. Routine Quality Assurance of Clinical Ultrasound Equipment version 2.0. Accessed November 12, 2023. http://aium.s3.amazonaws.com/resourceLibrary/rqa2.pdf
6. Norton ME, Scoutt LM, Feldstein VA. *Callen's Ultrasonography in Obstetrics and Gynecology*. 6th ed. Elsevier; 2017.
7. Kline-Fath BM, Bulus DI, Lee W. *Fundamental and Advanced Fetal Imaging*. 2nd ed. Wolters Kluwer; 2021.
8. Penny SM. *Examination Review for Ultrasound: Abdomen & Obstetrics and Gynecology*. 3rd ed. Wolters Kluwer; 2022.
9. Stephenson SR, Dmitrieva J. *Diagnostic Medical Sonography: Obstetrics and Gynecology*. 5th ed. Wolters Kluwer; 2023:Chapter 30.

CHAPTER 9

Detailed Second- or Third-Trimester Sonography and Multiple Gestations

INTRODUCTION

The detailed second- or third-trimester sonographic exam is prescriptive and includes routine examination images as well as some further detailed images of the fetus. A list of these additional items will be provided in this chapter, including some representative sonographic images. A brief overview and the sonographic appearance of multiple gestations are provided in this chapter as well.

WHAT IS A DETAILED SECOND- OR THIRD-TRIMESTER SONOGRAM?[1]

- The detailed second- or third-trimester sonogram includes all the components of a standard second- or third-trimester sonographic examination (see Chapter 8) and additional analysis of indication-driven specific content.

POTENTIAL COMPONENTS OF THE DETAILED SECOND- OR THIRD-TRIMESTER SONOGRAM[1–3]

- All the following elements may not be indicated in every detailed obstetric ultrasound examination. Furthermore, obtaining additional elements not listed may be warranted:
  - Third ventricle (Fig. 9-1)
    - The third ventricle is located within the brain's midline, between the two lobes of the thalamus.

Chapter 9. Detailed Second- or Third-Trimester Sonography   **293**

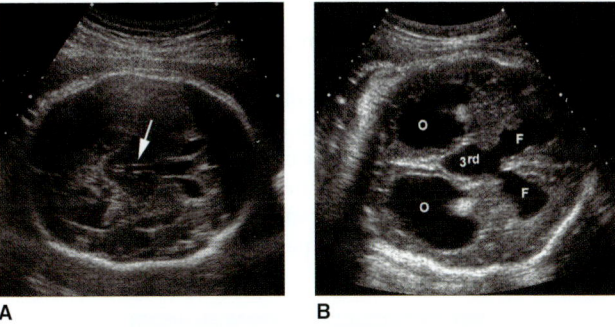

Figure 9-1. Third ventricle. A. Prominent third ventricle. B. Ventriculomegaly image demonstrating a dilated third (3rd) ventricle as well as frontal (*F*) and occipital (*O*) horns of the lateral ventricles. (Reprinted with permission from Doubilet PM, Benson CB. *Atlas of Ultrasound in Obstetrics and Gynecology: A Multimedia Reference.* 2nd ed. Wolters Kluwer Health/Lippincott Williams & Wilkins; 2012. Figure 4.1.4.)

- Fourth ventricle **(Fig. 9-2)**
  - The fourth ventricle is located anterior to the cerebellar vermis.

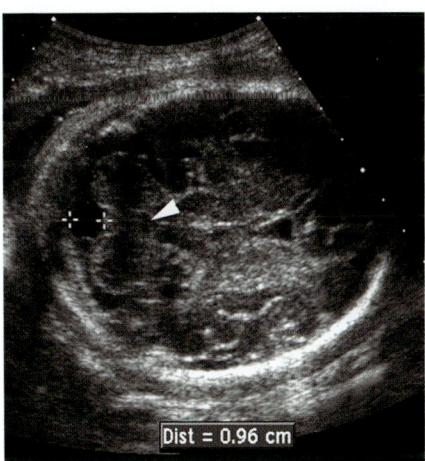

Figure 9-2. Fourth ventricle and cisterna magna. The *calipers* are being used to measure the anteroposterior dimension of the cisterna magna. The *arrowhead* indicates the area of the fourth ventricle. (Reprinted with permission from Doubilet PM, Benson CB. *Atlas of Ultrasound in Obstetrics and Gynecology: A Multimedia Reference.* 2nd ed. Wolters Kluwer Health/Lippincott Williams & Wilkins; 2012. Figure 2.1.5.)

- Lateral ventricular
  - Analyze wall integrity, contour, and the ependymal lining.
- Cerebellar lobes
  - Evaluate for the presence of the cerebellar vermis and for symmetry of the cerebellar lobes (see Fig. 9-2).
  - Evaluate and measure the cisterna magna for enlargement, which may be seen with mega cisterna magna or Dandy–Walker variants, or obliteration, which may be associated with open spina-bifida.
- Corpus callosum (Fig. 9-3)

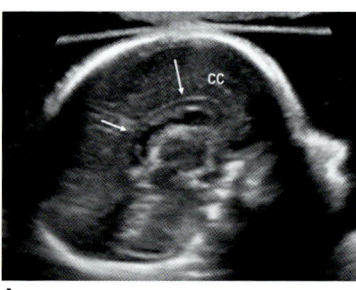

A

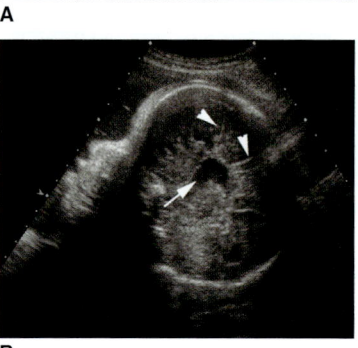

B

Figure 9-3. Corpus callosum. A. The *arrows* indicate the normal corpus callosum (*cc*) in this sagittal image of the fetal brain. **B.** The abnormal appearance of agenesis of the corpus callosum in the sagittal plane demonstrates a dilated and elevated third ventricle (*arrow*) and sunburst appearance of the sulci (*arrowheads*). (**A.** Reprinted with permission from Kline-Fath BM. Supratentorial anomalies. In: Kline-Fath BM, Bulas DI, Lee W, eds. *Fundamental and Advanced Fetal Imaging: Ultrasound and MRI*. 2nd ed. Wolters Kluwer; 2021. Figure 17.1-24. **B.** Reprinted with permission from Doubilet PM, Benson CB. *Atlas of Ultrasound in Obstetrics and Gynecology: A Multimedia Reference*. 2nd ed. Wolters Kluwer Health/Lippincott Williams & Wilkins; 2012. Figure 4.17.2.)

- The corpus callosum can be best seen in the sagittal plane to the midline of fetal brain.
- Absence of the corpus callosum is not only a sign of agenesis of the corpus callosum but may be seen with many brain abnormalities, including Apert syndrome and Dandy–Walker malformation.
- Integrity and shape of the cranial vault
  - Abnormal head shape should be noted **(Fig. 9-4)**.
    - Brachycephaly is a round skull and is often associated with trisomy 21, trisomy 18, and craniosynostosis **(Fig. 9-5)**.
    - Dolichocephaly, which is also referred to as scaphocephaly, is a long, narrow skull. It is associated with craniosynostosis (see Fig. 9-5).
    - A cloverleaf-shaped skull is associated with skeletal dysplasia, including thanatophoric dysplasia (fatal dwarfism) **(Fig. 9-6)**.
    - A lemon-shaped skull is associated with open spina-bifida and a banana-shaped cerebellum.
    - A strawberry-shaped skull is associated with trisomy 18 and other anomalies.
- Brain parenchyma
  - The sonographic appearance of normal fetal brain parenchyma will vary based on the gestational age.
- Neck
  - The posterior neck can be evaluated for signs of a cystic hygroma and skin thickening.

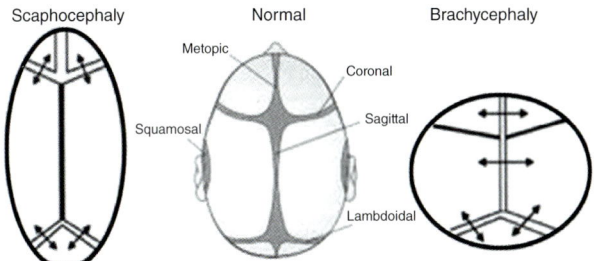

Figure 9-4. Head shapes. Scaphocephaly, which is also referred to as dolichocephaly, is considered to be elongated and narrow. Brachycephaly is described as a round and short head shape. (Reprinted with permission from Meier MP, Goobie SM. Craniofacial surgery—pediatric considerations. In: Mongan PD, Soriano S, Sloan TB, eds. *A Practical Approach to Neuroanesthesia*. Wolters Kluwer Health/Lippincott Williams & Wilkins; 2013:245. Figure 18.1.)

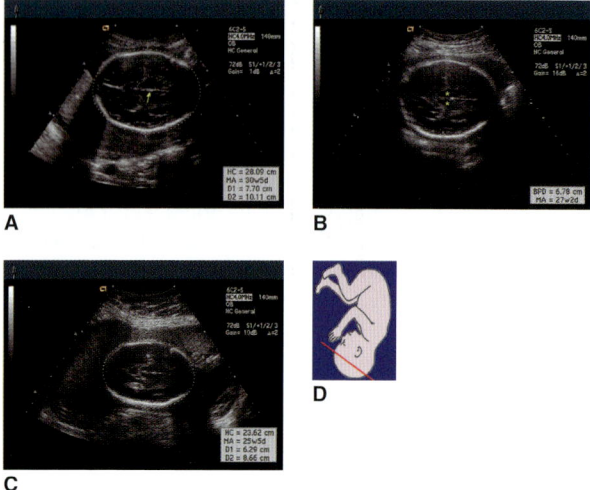

Figure 9-5. Brachycephaly, Normal, and Dolichocephaly. A. The brachycephalic fetal head has a shortened occipital-frontal distance and a larger BPD. The slit-like third ventricle (*arrow*) images between the anterior portion of the two thalami. **B.** The normal-shaped head demonstrating the hypoechoic thalamus (*stars*). This is the main indicator for the BPD and HC measurement level. **C.** The long narrow head, dolichocephaly, would result in a smaller than gestational age BPD measurement and a lengthened occipital-frontal distance. **D.** Proper level of the skull to obtain measurements seen in A-C. (Reprinted with permission from Dmitrieva J. Sonographic assessment of the fetal head. In: Stephenson SR, Dmitrieva J, eds. *Diagnostic Medical Sonography: Obstetrics & Gynecology.* 4th ed. Wolters Kluwer; 2018. Figure 21-4.)

- The anterior neck can be evaluated for an enlargement of the fetal thyroid (goiter).
- Profile
  - The profile image can reveal abnormalities of the face.
    - Micrognathia is the posterior position of the mandible.
    - Evaluate for absent or small nasal bones (between 15 and 22 weeks).
      - Absent or small nasal bones are associated with Down syndrome.
    - Evaluate for abnormal or missing palate.
- Coronal face (nose/lips, lens) **(Fig. 9-7)**
  - The lenses of the eyes should be noted as hyperechoic circular structures within the globe of the eyes.

Chapter 9. Detailed Second- or Third-Trimester Sonography **297**

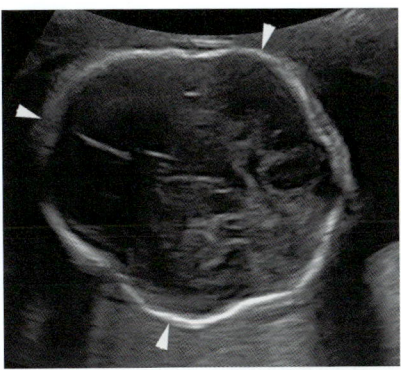

Figure 9-6. Cloverleaf skull. Axial image of fetal malformed head showing bulging anteriorly and laterally (*arrowheads*), characteristic of a skull developing the cloverleaf deformity. (Reprinted with permission from Doubilet PM, Benson CB, Benacerraf BR. *Atlas of Ultrasound in Obstetrics and Gynecology: A Multimedia Reference.* 3rd ed. Wolters Kluwer; 2019. Figure 16.1.1.)

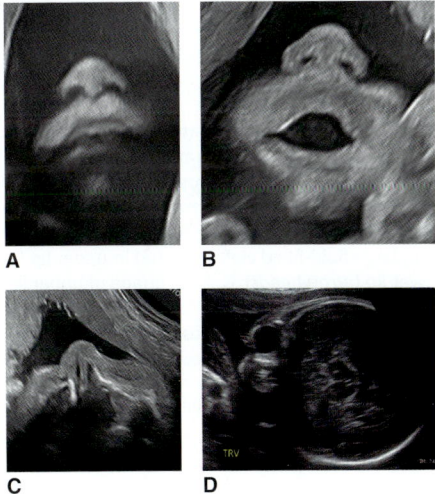

Figure 9-7. Fetal face. The normal fetal face in a 28-week fetus. A. Coronal 2D image of nose and vermillion border of the upper lip. B. Coronal 2D image with mouth open. C. Axial 2D image of nasal vomer and the tip of the nose. D. Axial 2D image of fetal eyelashes in a different 29-week fetus. (Reprinted with permission from Estroff JA. Face: Anomalies of nose, mouth, lip and tongue. In: Kline-Fath BM, Bulas DI, Lee W, eds. *Fundamental and Advanced Fetal Imaging: Ultrasound and MRI.* 2nd ed. Wolters Kluwer; 2021. Figure 19.2.)

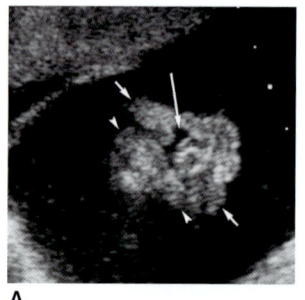
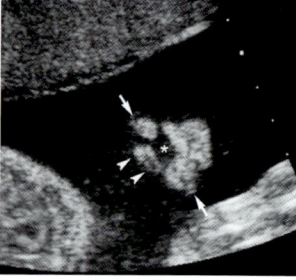
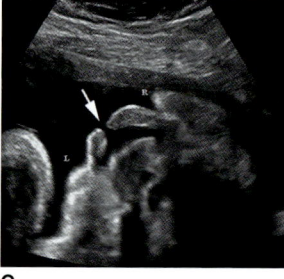

Figure 9-8. Unilateral cleft lip and palate on grayscale sonogram. **A.** Coronal image of lower face demonstrating a large unilateral defect (*long arrow*) in the upper lip (*short arrows*) extending into the palate and ipsilateral nostril. The lower lip (*arrowheads*) is seen inferior to the cleft. **B.** Coronal image of the same fetus slightly more anterior demonstrating large fluid-filled cleft (*asterisk*) in upper lip (*arrows*) above the lower lip (*arrowheads*). **C.** Axial image of upper lip showing defect (*arrow*) on the left (*R,* right; *L,* left). (Reprinted with permission from Doubilet PM, Benson CB, Benacerraf BR. *Atlas of Ultrasound in Obstetrics and Gynecology: A Multimedia Reference.* 3rd ed. Wolters Kluwer; 2019. Figure 8.1.1.)

- The nose/lips image can reveal cleft lip/palate signs **(Fig. 9-8)**.
  - Unilateral cleft palate
  - Bilateral cleft palate
  - Median cleft palate
- The hard palate can be noted as well.
- Palate, maxilla, mandible, and tongue
  - The palate can be evaluated in sagittal and coronal.
  - The maxilla can be evaluated in the sagittal plane and coronal plane **(Fig. 9-9)**.

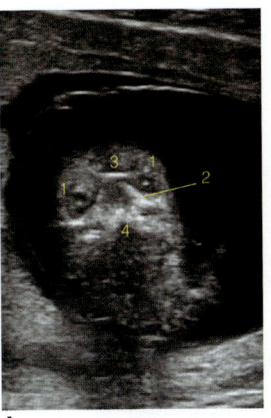 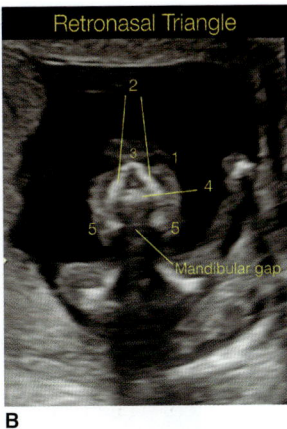

Figure 9-9. Coronal planes in two fetuses (A, B) at 12 weeks of gestation, obtained at the frontal aspects of the bony face. In fetus A, the coronal plane is at the level of the orbits and shows the two eyes (*1*) with orbits and lenses, between the maxillary processes (*2*), the nasal bones (*3*), and the anterior aspect of the maxilla (*4*) with the alveolar ridge. In fetus B, the plane is oblique and demonstrates the retronasal triangle which is formed by the nasal bones superiorly (*3*), the frontal processes of the maxilla laterally (*2*), and the alveolar ridge (primary palate) inferiorly (*4*). This coronal section (B) is posterior to the tip of the mandible, and therefore the two lateral bodies of the mandible are seen (*5*) with a normal gap between, called the mandibular gap.
(Reprinted with permission from Abuhamad A, Chaoui R. *First Trimester Ultrasound Diagnosis of Fetal Abnormalities.* Wolters Kluwer; 2018. Figure 9.7.)

- The tongue can be evaluated in the sagittal plane.
  - Macroglossia is an enlarged tongue and can be associated with Beckwith–Wiedemann syndrome or Down syndrome.
- Ear position and size
  - Low-set ears can be associated with chromosomal abnormalities **(Fig. 9-10)**.
- Orbits **(Fig. 9-11)**
  - Hypotelorism is close-set eyes.
    - A common cause is holoprosencephaly.
  - Hypertelorism is wide-spaced eyes.
    - A common cause is the anterior cephalocele.
- Situs **(Fig. 9-12)**
  - The stomach and heart should be determined to be within the left side of the fetus.

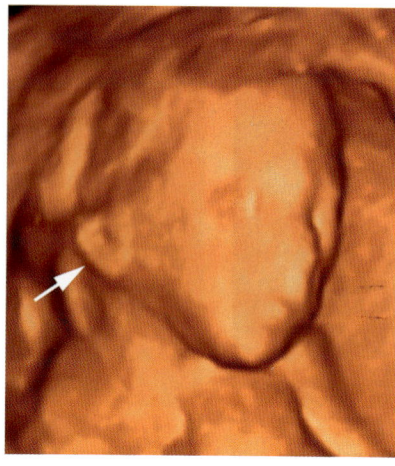

Figure 9-10. Low-set ear. Low-set ear with trisomy 21. 3D sonogram of fetal head and face showing abnormal low positioning of the ear (*arrow*). (Reprinted with permission from Doubilet PM, Benson CB, Benacerraf BR. *Atlas of Ultrasound in Obstetrics and Gynecology: A Multimedia Reference.* 3rd ed. Wolters Kluwer; 2019. Figure 8.8.4.)

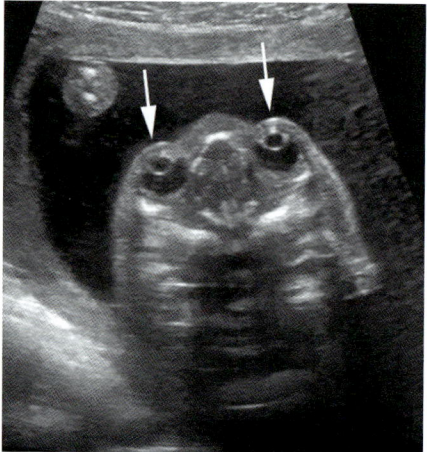

Figure 9-11. Fetal orbits. Both orbits are demonstrated in this image as well as the lenses of the eyes (*arrows*) which appear as small circular structures within the globes. (Reprinted with permission from Doubilet PM, Benson CB, Benacerraf BR. *Atlas of Ultrasound in Obstetrics and Gynecology: A Multimedia Reference.* 3rd ed. Wolters Kluwer; 2019. Figure 2.2.1.)

Chapter 9. Detailed Second- or Third-Trimester Sonography

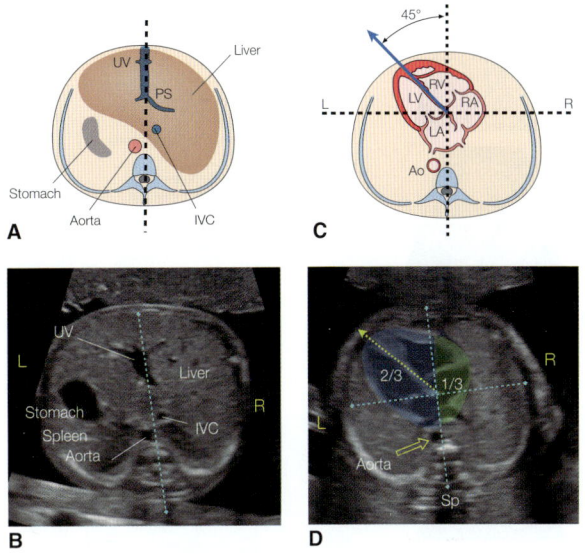

Figure 9-12. Correct situs. Axial view of the upper abdomen shown in a schematic drawing (A) and corresponding sonogram (B) of a fetus with normal situs (situs solitus). The vertical line (A, B) divides the abdomen into right and left sides. The right-sided structures include the gallbladder (not shown), the portal sinus (*PS*), a large part of the liver, and inferior vena cava (*IVC*). The left-sided structures include the descending aorta (*Ao*), the stomach, and the spleen. Axial view of the chest, at the four-chamber view, shown in a schematic drawing (C) and corresponding sonographic image (D) of a fetus with normal situs. The chest is divided into four equal quadrants by a vertical and horizontal line. Note the position of the heart and the descending Ao in the left chest with a normal cardiac axis of 45 degrees. **L,** left; **LA,** left atrium; **LV,** left ventricle; **R,** right; **RA,** right atrium; **RV,** right ventricle; **UV,** umbilical vein. (Reprinted with permission from Abuhamad A, Chaoui R. *A Practical Guide to Fetal Echocardiography: Normal and Abnormal Hearts.* 4th ed. Wolters Kluwer; 2022. Figure 40.1.)

- Heart (**Figs. 9-13** and **9-14**)
  - Aortic arch
  - Superior or inferior venae cavae
  - Ductal arch (see Fig. 9-13)
  - Interventricular septum
  - Three-vessel view (see Fig. 9-14)
  - Three-vessel and trachea view (**Fig. 9-15**)

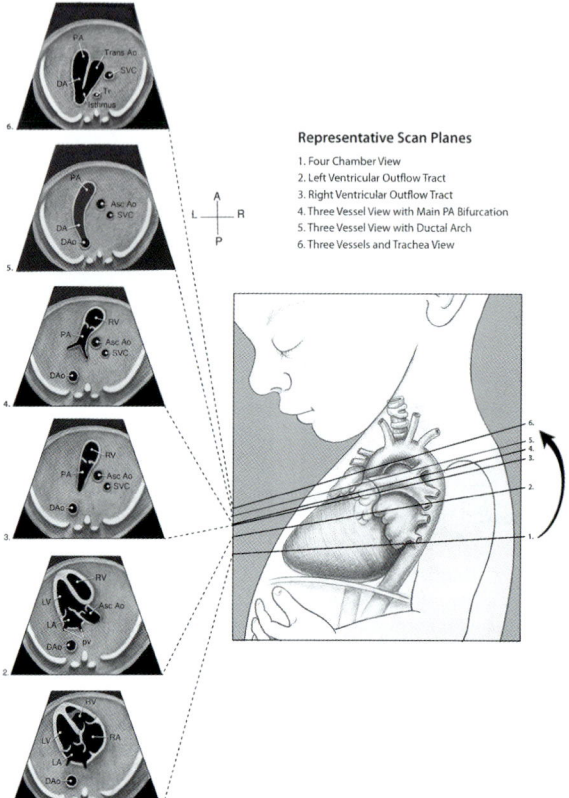

Figure 9-13. Representative scan planes for fetal echocardiography include an evaluation of the four-chamber view (1), left and right arterial outflow tracts (2 and 3, respectively), two variants of the three-vessel view, one demonstrating the main pulmonary artery bifurcation (4) with another more superior plane that demonstrates the ductal arch (5), and the three-vessel and trachea view (6). Not all views may be seen from a single cephalic transducer sweep without some minor adjustments in the position and orientation of the transducer owing to anatomic variations and the fetal lie. Asc Ao, ascending aorta; DAo, descending aorta; LA, left atrium; LV, left ventricle; PA, pulmonary artery; RA, right atrium; RV, right ventricle; Tr, trachea. (From American Institute of Ultrasound in Medicine. AIUM practice parameter for the performance of fetal echocardiography. *J Ultrasound Med.* 2020;39(1):E5–E16. Copyright © 2019 by the American Institute of Ultrasound in Medicine. Reprinted by permission of John Wiley & Sons, Inc.)

Chapter 9. Detailed Second- or Third-Trimester Sonography

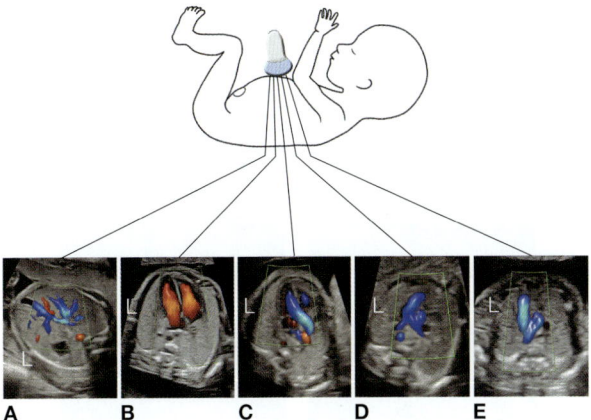

Figure 9-14. Axial planes in color Doppler of the fetal abdomen (A) and chest (B–E) as part of the performance of the fetal echocardiography examination. These axial planes are obtained at the level of the abdominal circumference (A), the four-chamber view (B), the five-chamber view (C), the three-vessel view (D), and the three-vessel trachea view (E). (Reprinted with permission from Abuhamad A, Chaoui R. *A Practical Guide to Fetal Echocardiography: Normal and Abnormal Hearts*. 4th ed. Wolters Kluwer; 2022. Figure 13.15.)

- Lungs
  - Masses can be located within or adjacent to the lungs, including pulmonary sequestration and congenital cystic adenomatoid malformation (congenital pulmonary airway malformation).
  - Fluid around the lung is referred to as a pleural effusion.
    - Pleural effusions may be bilateral.
- Integrity of diaphragm **(Fig. 9-16)**
  - A sagittal or coronal image of the diaphragm can be helpful in evaluating the fetus for signs of a diaphragmatic hernia.
  - The stomach should be noted below the diaphragm on the left side of the fetus.
- Ribs
- Small and large bowel
  - The echogenicity of the bowel should be compared to the fetal bones.
  - Bowel echogenicity may be evaluated with and without harmonics.

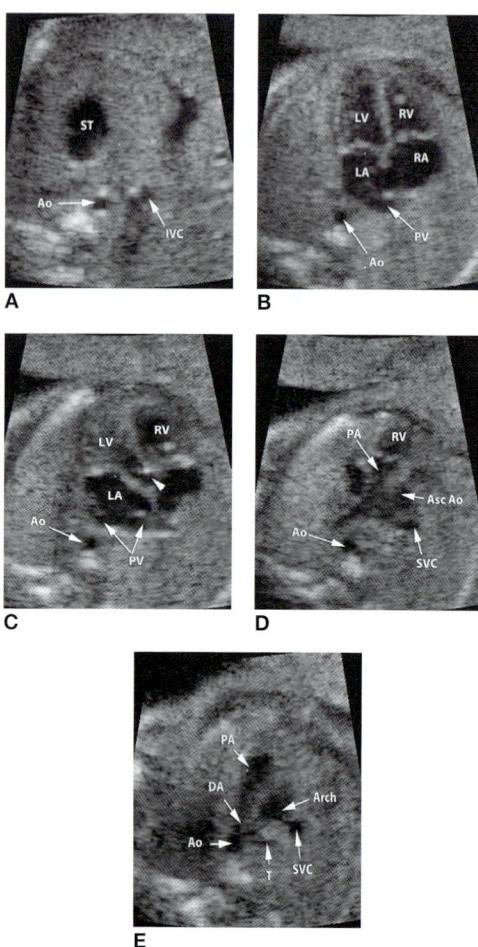

Figure 9-15. Fetal heart and upper abdomen. A. Transverse view of the fetal abdomen. B. Four-chamber view. C. Five-chamber view. D. Three-vessel view. E. Three-vessel and trachea view. Ao, descending aorta; Asc Ao, ascending aorta; DA, ductus arteriosus; IVC, inferior vena cava; LA, left atrium; LV, left ventricle; PA, pulmonary artery; PV, pulmonary veins; RA, right atrium; RV, right ventricle; Short arrow, aortic root; ST, stomach; SVC, superior vena cava; T, trachea. (Reprinted with permission from Gonçalves LF. Three-dimensional ultrasonography. In: Kline-Fath BM, Bulas DI, Lee W, eds. *Fundamental and Advanced Fetal Imaging: Ultrasound and MRI.* 2nd ed. Wolters Kluwer; 2021. Figure 7.33.)

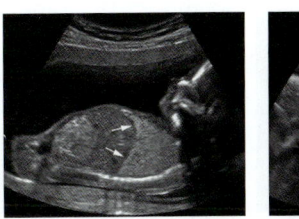
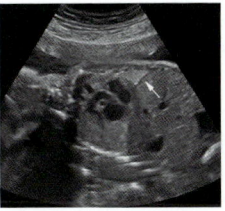

Figure 9-16. Diaphragm. A. Sagittal view of chest and abdomen of an 18-week fetus demonstrating the dome-shaped diaphragm (*arrows*) separating the liver from more echogenic lung tissue. **B.** In the third trimester, the muscles of the diaphragm may be thick enough to be visible as a hypoechoic band (*arrow*). (Reprinted with permission from Doubilet PM, Benson CB, Benacerraf BR. *Atlas of Ultrasound in Obstetrics and Gynecology: A Multimedia Reference.* 3rd ed. Wolters Kluwer; 2019. Figure 2.4.4.)

- The bowel echogenicity should not be the same as or brighter than fetal bone.
- Adrenal glands
  - Normal fetal adrenal glands are readily identifiable.
- Gallbladder
  - Fetal gallstones may be noted.
  - To confirm the gallbladder, utilize color Doppler. The gallbladder will not fill with color.
- Liver
  - Hepatomegaly may be noted in utero.
  - Hepatosplenomegaly can be associated with various fetal anomalies and chromosomal abnormalities, as well as RH sensitization.
  - Always assess the fetus for signs of hydrops.
    - Fluid can be located under the skin (subcutaneous edema), chest (pleural effusion), abdomen (ascites), scrotum (hydrocele), and other locations.
    - The diagnosis of hydrops requires that fluid be located in at least two cavities.
- Renal arteries **(Fig. 9-17)**
  - Renal arteries can be demonstrated in the coronal plane to the fetus using color Doppler.
  - Absence of a renal artery is associated with ipsilateral renal agenesis.
- Spleen
  - Splenomegaly may be noted in utero.

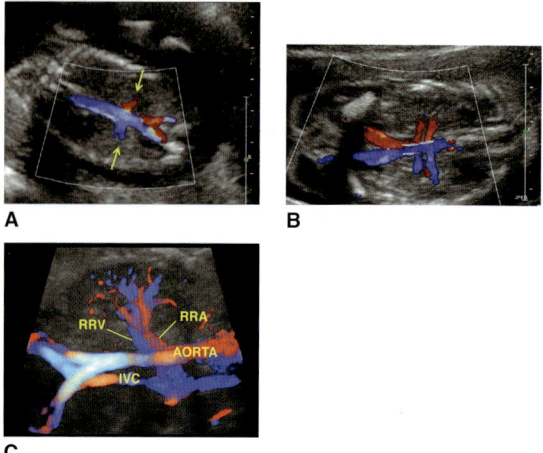

Figure 9-17. Renal arteries. Doppler and three-dimensional (3D) image of the renal vasculature. **A.** Coronal view of the kidneys, using color Doppler to show the renal arteries (*arrows*) arising from the aorta, just above the iliac arteries. **B.** Coronal image of a fetus with two renal arteries bilaterally. **C.** 3D volume data set of the fetal vasculature (aorta, inferior vena cava [*IVC*], right renal artery [*RRA*], and right renal vein [*RRV*]) demonstrated using a transparency render method to allow all vessels to be displayed simultaneously. (Reprinted with permission from Amarillas L. Sonographic assessment of the fetal genitourinary system and fetal pelvis. In: Stephenson SR, Dmitrieva J, eds. *Diagnostic Medical Sonography: Obstetrics & Gynecology.* 4th ed. Wolters Kluwer; 2018. Figure 26-4.)

- Hepatosplenomegaly can be associated with various fetal anomalies and chromosomal abnormalities, as well as RH sensitization.
- Always assess the fetus for signs of hydrops.
- Integrity of abdominal wall
  - Evaluate the abdominal wall for signs of anterior abdominal wall defects such as omphalocele and gastroschisis.
- Integrity of spine and overlying soft tissue
  - The gain should be adjusted to allow the visualization of the overlying soft tissue of the spine.
  - An interruption of the overlying soft tissue may be seen with open spina bifida.
- Shape, curvature, conus medullaris (spine)
  - The distal portion of the spine can reveal where the conus medullaris (distal spinal cord) ends.

- Sagittal and coronal images of the spine can reveal absent spinal elements or fusion, as well as abnormal curvatures including kyphosis and lordosis.
- Coronal images can be used to demonstrate scoliosis.
- Number, architecture, and position of extremities
  - Each extremity should be evaluated closely.
  - Shortening of an extremity or absence of all or part of an extremity may occur.
- Number and position of digits of hands and feet
  - Oligodactyly is a decreased number of digits.
    - Evaluate the fetus closely for signs of other possible amputations that may be associated with amniotic band syndrome.
  - Polydactyly is an increased number of digits.
- External genitalia
  - The external genitalia should be closely evaluated especially when sex-linked abnormalities are suspected.
  - Any dilation of the urinary tract should initiate a more thorough evaluation of the external genitalia.
    - For example, posterior urethral valves are unique to the male fetus and can lead to an enlarged urinary bladder and dilation of the upper urinary tract as well.
  - Hypospadias or epispadias is when the male urethra exits somewhere within the shaft of the penis, instead of the distal penis.
    - An abnormal curvature of the penis will be noted.
  - A hydrocele is the abnormal accumulation of fluid within the scrotum surrounding the testis.
- Assess the placental implantation site (with assessment for abnormal adherence), and for evidence of masses, accessory lobes, abnormal vasculature, and position in relation to the internal cervical os.
- Measurements of the following:
  - Cerebellum **(Fig. 9-18)**
    - Also evaluate the cerebellar hemispheres for signs of asymmetry
  - Inner and outer orbital diameters **(Fig. 9-19)**
    - A small orbit can be measured as well using the ocular diameter **(Fig. 9-20)**
  - Nuchal fold thickness (between 16 and 20 weeks) **(Fig. 9-21)**
  - Humerus **(Fig. 9-22)**

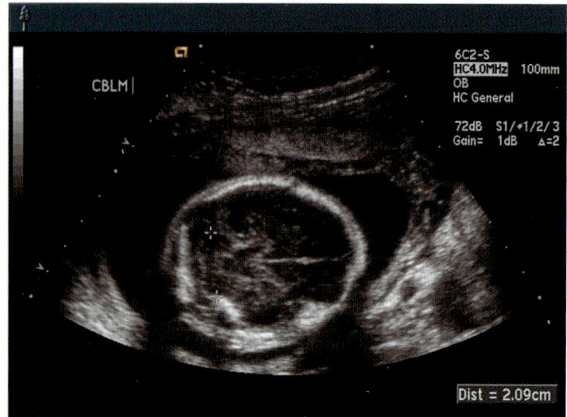

Figure 9-18. Transcerebellar diameter. Measurement of the fetal cerebellum. (Reprinted with permission from Kominiarek M. Intrauterine growth restriction (IUGR). In: Stephenson SR, ed. *Diagnostic Medical Sonography: Obstetrics & Gynecology*. 3rd ed. Wolters Kluwer Health/Lippincott Williams & Wilkins; 2012. Figure 27-3.)

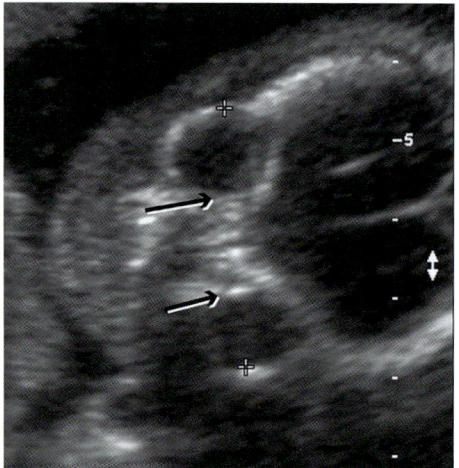

Figure 9-19. Measurement of the inner and outer diameter of the orbits. Transorbital view of the fetal face shows the measurement of the binocular diameter with the calipers on the malar margins of the orbit. The interocular diameter is measured between the two ethmoidal margins (*arrows*). (Reprinted with permission from Robinson AJ. Orbit. In: Kline-Fath BM, Bulas DI, Bahado-Singh R, eds. *Fundamental and Advanced Fetal Imaging: Ultrasound and MRI*. Wolters Kluwer; 2015. Figure 13.1-1.)

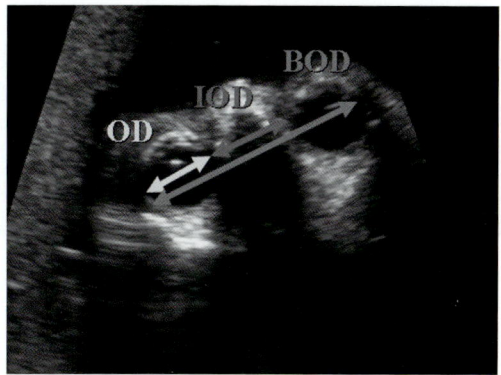

Figure 9-20. Orbital measurements. Transverse view of the face showing normal orbits. Normal orbital measurements of the ocular diameter (*OD*), interocular diameter (*IOD*), and binocular diameter (*BOD*) is demonstrated. (Reprinted with permission from Nyberg DA, McGahan JP, Pretorius DH, Pilu G. *Diagnostic Imaging of Fetal Anomalies*. Lippincott Williams & Wilkins; 2003:339.)

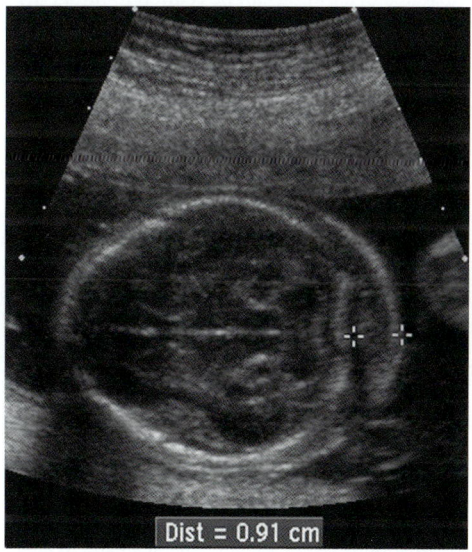

Figure 9-21. Nuchal fold thickness measurement. Abnormal nuchal fold. Image demonstrating a thickened nuchal fold (between *calipers*) measuring 9.1 mm. (Reprinted with permission from Doubilet PM, Benson CB. *Atlas of Ultrasound in Obstetrics and Gynecology: A Multimedia Reference*. 2nd ed. Wolters Kluwer Health/Lippincott Williams & Wilkins; 2012. Figure 7.2.1.)

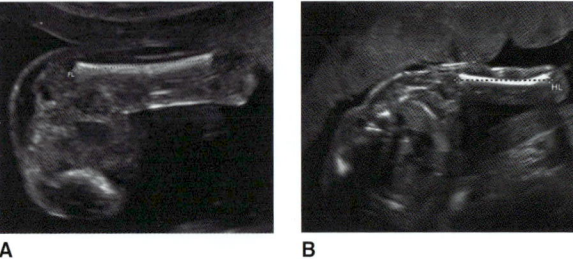

Figure 9-22. Fetal femur and humerus. Longitudinal views of femur (*FL* in A) and humerus (*HL* in B). *Calipers* denote their measurements. (Reprinted with permission from Sonek JD, Retzke JD, Hyett J. Normal fetal ultrasound survey. In: Kline-Fath BM, Bulas DI, Bahado-Singh R, eds. *Fundamental and Advanced Fetal Imaging: Ultrasound and MRI.* Wolters Kluwer; 2015. Figure 1.124.)

- ○ Short or abnormally shaped humeri are associated with dwarfism and skeletal dysplasia
- Measurement of the ulna and radius can be performed (Fig. 9-23)
  - ○ Absence of a radius can be related to radial ray anomaly
  - ○ Short or abnormally shaped ulnae and radiuses are associated with dwarfism and skeletal dysplasia
- Measurement of the tibia and fibula can be performed (Fig. 9-24)
  - ○ Short or abnormally shaped tibias and fibulas are associated with dwarfism and skeletal dysplasia

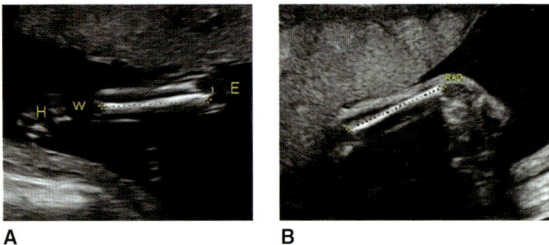

Figure 9-23. Measurements of the fetal forearm bones. A. The ulna (measured) extends further into the elbow (*E*) than the radius (lateral), both bones end at approximately the same level at the wrist (*w*). Lack of wrist bone ossification results in a hypo to anechoic area between the forearm and hand (*H*). B. Fetal radius. Note longer ulna is seen medial. (Reprinted with permission from Johnston S. Assessment of fetal age and size in the second and third trimester. In: Stephenson SR, ed. *Diagnostic Medical Sonography: Obstetrics & Gynecology.* 3rd ed. Wolters Kluwer Health/Lippincott Williams & Wilkins; 2012. Figure 16-12.)

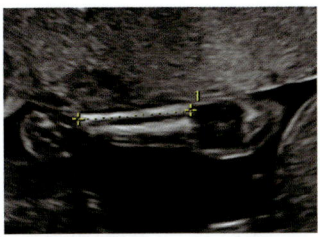 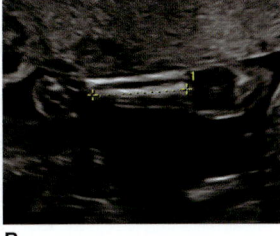

A **B**

Figure 9-24. Fetal lower leg. Long-axis view of the leg demonstrates the ossified portions of the fibula (measured in A) and fibula (measured in B). (Reprinted with permission from Johnston S. Assessment of fetal age and size in the second and third trimester. In: Stephenson SR, ed. *Diagnostic Medical Sonography: Obstetrics & Gynecology.* 3rd ed. Wolters Kluwer Health/Lippincott Williams & Wilkins; 2012. Figure 16-13.)

MULTIPLE GESTATIONS (TWINS)[2,3]

- Important points to remember:
  - The number of fetuses, yolk sacs (if present), and placentas should be documented.
  - The calculation package should be programmed to create a separate worksheet for each twin so that any size discrepancy can be established.
  - Twin A will always be the twin closest to the internal os of the cervix.
  - A complete sonogram should be performed for each fetus present.
  - Amnionicity (number of amniotic sacs) and chorionicity (number of placentas) should be documented when multiple gestations are discovered.
    - There are four types of chorionicity in twin pregnancies **(Fig. 9-25)**:
      - Diamniotic dichorionic (most common)
      - Diamnitoic dichorionic with fused placenta
      - Diamniotic monochorionic
      - Monoamniotic monochorionic
  - The comparison of fetal sizes, the evaluation and documentation of amniotic fluid volume in each gestational sac, and fetal genitalia (if possible) should be provided.
- Clinical findings with multiple gestations
  - A prior history of multiple gestations would increase the likelihood of twins.

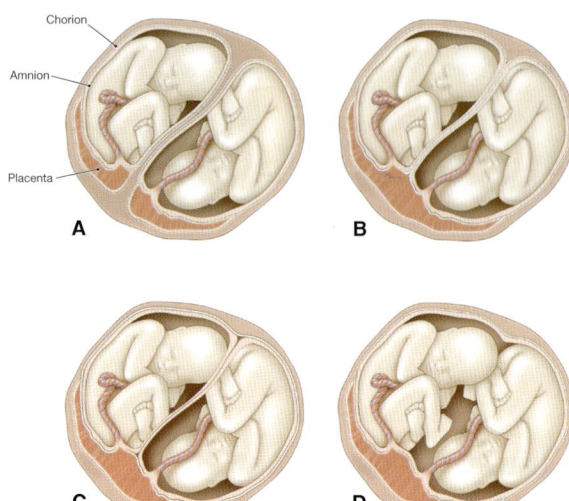

Figure 9-25. Chorionicity in twin pregnancies. A. Two placentas, two amnions, two chorions: diamniotic/dichorionic. B. One placenta, two amnions, two chorions: diamniotic/dichorionic. C. One placenta, two amnions, one chorion: diamniotic/monochorionic. D. One placenta, one amnion, one chorion: monoamniotic/monochorionic. (Reprinted with permission from Casanova R, Goepfert AR, Hueppchen NA, Weiss PM, Connolly A; American College of Obstetricians and Gynecologists. *Beckmann and Ling's Obstetrics and Gynecology*. 9th ed. Wolters Kluwer; 2024. Figure 13.1.)

- Assisted reproductive therapy, including in vitro fertilization and the use of fertility drugs, increases the likelihood of multiple gestations and ectopic pregnancy.
- Family history of twins can increase the risk.
- Elevated human chorionic gonadotropin and other maternal serum screening labs will be evident.
- Twins in the first trimester
  - Two separate gestational sacs will be noted.
  - The thickness of the membrane can be analyzed **(Fig. 9-26)**.
    - A thick membrane denotes dichorionic twinning.
    - A thin membrane denotes monochorionic twinning.
  - Evidence of the twin peak sign and the number of yolk sacs can be used.
    - Twin peak sign is a thick dividing membrane at the placental insertion of the membranes that occurs with dichorionic pregnancies **(Fig. 9-27)**.

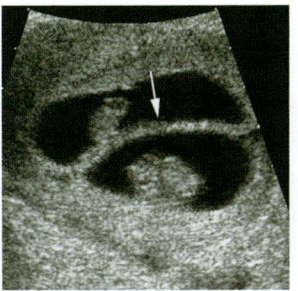 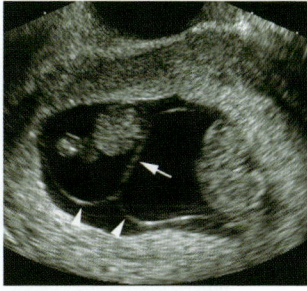

A   **B**

Figure 9-26. Determination of chorionicity based on membrane thickness in the first trimester. A. Dichorionic twins—Sonogram demonstrates a twin gestation in which the two fetuses are separated by a thick membrane (*arrow*), indicating that the twins are dichorionic. **B. Monochorionic twins**—Sonogram demonstrates a twin gestation with two amniotic membranes (*arrowheads*), which meet to form a thin membrane (*arrow*) between the two fetuses. (Reprinted with permission from Doubilet PM, Benson CB. *Atlas of Ultrasound in Obstetrics and Gynecology: A Multimedia Reference*. 2nd ed. Wolters Kluwer Health/Lippincott Williams & Wilkins; 2012. Figure 20.2.1.)

- Two yolk sacs suggest diamniotic pregnancy (see Fig. 9-27).
- Twins in the second or third trimester
  - Always try to obtain any previous sonogram reports, as those measurements, especially if obtained in the first trimester, will be more accurate dating than a sonogram performed in the second or third trimester.
  - Useful sonographic findings:
    - The twin peak sign will be better delineated, which is a sign of dichorionic twinning.
    - The "T" sign denotes monochorionic diamniotic twinning **(Fig. 9-28)**.
    - The thickness of the membrane can be helpful **(Fig. 9-29)**.
      - A thick membrane typically indicates dichorionic twins.
      - A thin membrane typically indicates monochorionic twins.
    - Two placentas with two locations (e.g., anterior and posterior) are helpful to denote a dichorionic pregnancy **(Fig. 9-30)**
    - Two different genders indicate dichorionic twinning **(Fig. 9-31)**.

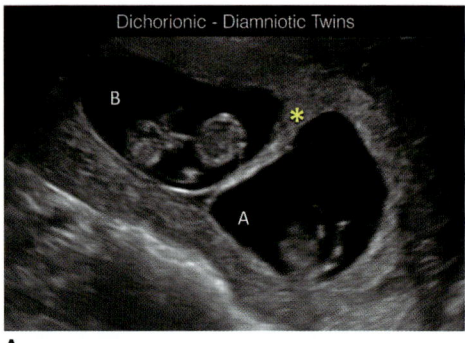

A

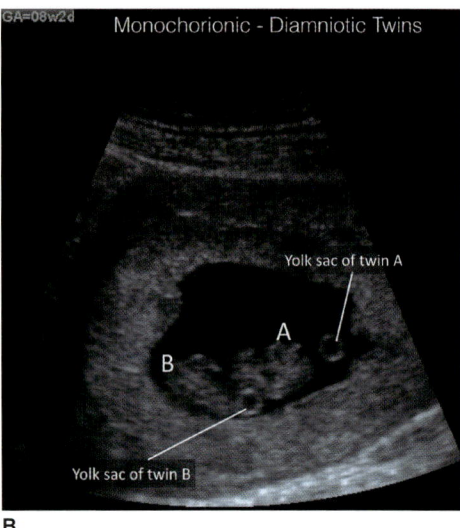

B

Figure 9-27. Twin peak and number of yolk sacs. A. Dichorionic-diamniotic twins (A and B) at 11 weeks of gestation. Note the thick dividing membrane with a twin-peak sign (*asterisk*) at the placental insertion of the membranes. B. Monochorionic–diamniotic twins (A and B) at 8 weeks of gestation. Note the presence of two yolk sacs. A thin separating membrane is not visible in this image. The presence of two yolk sacs at this gestation suggests monochorionic–diamniotic pregnancy but does not confirm it. The presence of a dividing membrane on follow-up sonogram with high-resolution transducers, confirmed this diagnosis. (Reprinted with permission from Abuhamad A, Chaoui R. *First Trimester Ultrasound Diagnosis of Fetal Abnormalities.* Wolters Kluwer; 2018. Figures 7.3 and 7.7.)

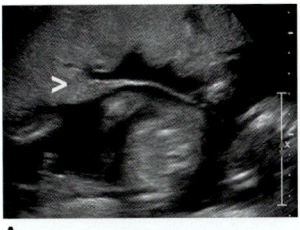 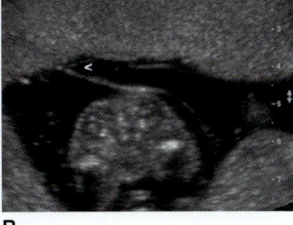

A   **B**

Figure 9-28. Second-trimester twin peak sign verses T-sign. Twin peak sign in a second-trimester DC/DA twin gestation (A). T-sign in a second-trimester MC/DA twin gestation (B). (Reprinted with permission from Drose JA. Multiple gestations. In: Stephenson SR, ed. *Diagnostic Medical Sonography: Obstetrics & Gynecology.* 3rd ed. Wolters Kluwer Health/Lippincott Williams & Wilkins; 2012. Figure 26-8.)

- Twin pathology
  - Conjoined twins
    - Results from monochorionic monoamniotic twinning
    - Many variants exist including omphalopagus (abdominal connection), craniopagus (cranial connection), and pyopagus (sacral connection) **(Fig. 9-32).**
  - Twin–twin transfusion syndrome **(Fig. 9-33)**
    - Often a fatal syndrome is characterized initially by monochorionicity with subsequent discordant fetal growth **(Fig. 9-34).**

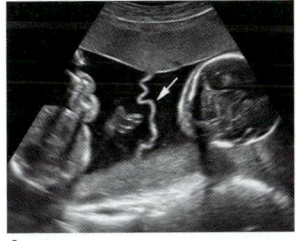 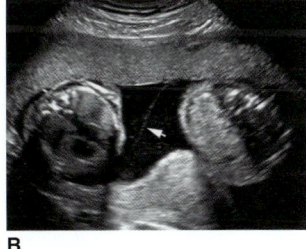

A   **B**

Figure 9-29. The thickness of the membrane. These two images demonstrate (A) a thick membrane (*arrow*) separating dichorionic twins and (B) a thin membrane (*arrow*) separating monochorionic twins. The difference in membrane thickness between monochorionic and dichorionic twins is less pronounced at this stage of pregnancy than in the first trimester. (Reprinted with permission from Doubilet PM, Benson CB, Benacerraf BR. *Atlas of Ultrasound in Obstetrics and Gynecology: A Multimedia Reference.* 3rd ed. Wolters Kluwer; 2019. Figure 23.2.4.)

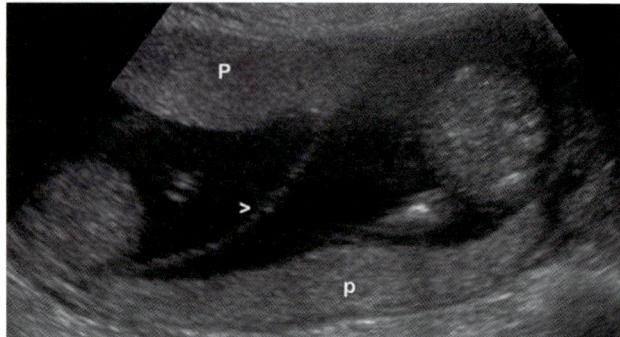

Figure 9-30. The number of placentas. Second-trimester dichorionic/diamniotic twin pregnancy in which two separate placentas (*P* is anterior, *p* is posterior) are visualized, along with an intertwin membrane (***arrowhead***). (Reprinted with permission from Matuzak A. Multiple gestations. In: Stephenson SR, Dmitrieva J, eds. *Diagnostic Medical Sonography: Obstetrics & Gynecology*. 4th ed. Wolters Kluwer; 2018. Figure 29-8.)

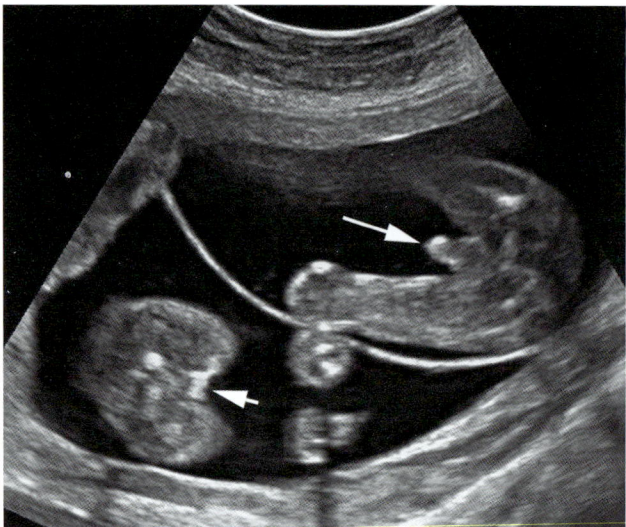

Figure 9-31. Dichorionicity based on different genders. Sonography of the genitalia in the twin gestation reveals a male (***long arrow***) and female (***short arrow***), thus confirming dichorionicity. (Reprinted with permission from Penny SM. *Examination Review for Ultrasound: Abdomen & Obstetrics and Gynecology*. 3rd ed. Wolters Kluwer; 2023. Figure 31-10.)

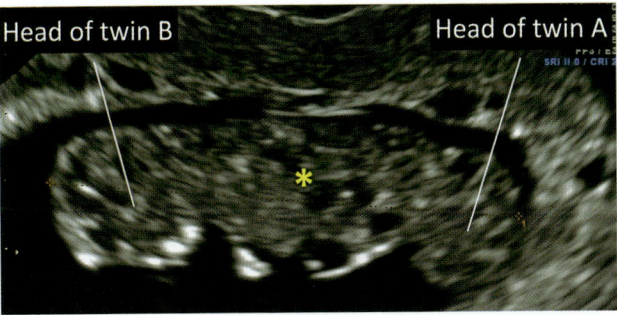

A

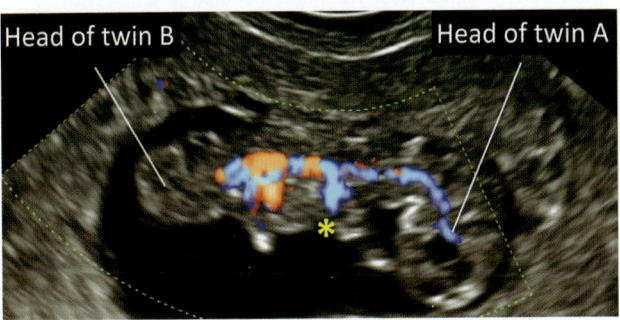

B

Figure 9-32. Conjoined twins. Conjoined twins noted on two-dimensional grayscale ultrasound at 9 weeks of gestation (A). Note the fusion of twins in the pelvic area (*asterisk*). Cephalic regions of twins are labeled. B. The conjoined twins with color Doppler sonogram confirming vascular connectivity between the two embryos (*asterisk*). (Reprinted with permission from Abuhamad A, Chaoui R. *First Trimester Ultrasound Diagnosis of Fetal Abnormalities*. Wolters Kluwer; 2018. Figure 7.16.)

- Associated with monochorionic twinning only.
- Both fetuses suffer:
  - Donor twin
    - Smaller twin
    - Oligohydramnios
  - Recipient twin
    - Larger twin
    - Polyhydramnios

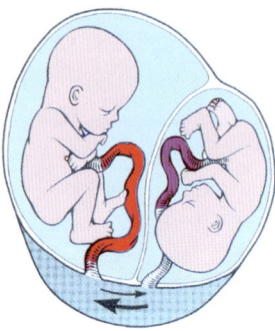

Figure 9-33. Diagram illustrates monochorionic gestation with twin-to-twin transfusion syndrome. The recipient twin is larger and in a polyhydramniotic sac. The donor twin is smaller and in an oligohydramniotic sac. (Reprinted with permission from Habli M. Multiple gestation. In: Kline-Fath BM, Bulas DI, Bahado-Singh R, eds. *Fundamental and Advanced Fetal Imaging: Ultrasound and MRI*. Wolters Kluwer; 2015. Figure 11.20.)

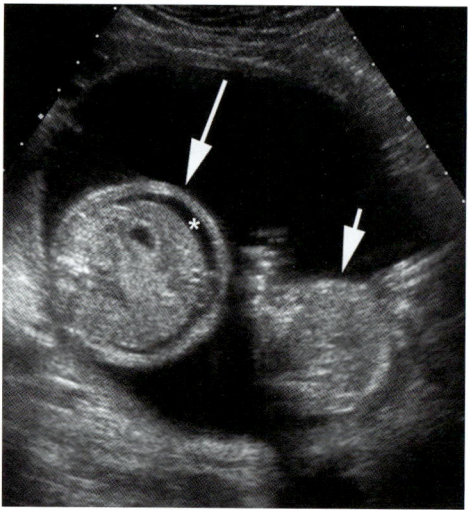

Figure 9-34. The two fetal abdomens differ in size with these twins, with one smaller (*short arrow*) than the other (*long arrow*), indicating discordant growth. Ascites (*asterisk*) in the larger, recipient twin's abdomen indicate possible hydrops. (Reprinted with permission from Doubilet PM, Benson CB, Benacerraf BR. *Atlas of Ultrasound in Obstetrics and Gynecology: A Multimedia Reference*. 3rd ed. Wolters Kluwer; 2019. Figure 24.1.3.)

REFERENCES

1. AIUM. Practice parameter for the performance of detailed second- and third-trimester diagnostic obstetric ultrasound examinations. *J Ultrasound Med*. 2019;38:3093–3100.
2. Kline-Fath BM, Bulas DI, Lee W. *Fundamental and Advanced Fetal Imaging: Ultrasound and MRI*. 2nd ed. Wolters Kluwer; 2020:1–156.
3. Penny SM. *Examination Review for Ultrasound: Abdomen & Obstetrics and Gynecology*. 3rd ed. Wolters Kluwer; 2022:11–19 & Section III.

CHAPTER 10

Chromosomal Abnormalities and Neural Tube Defects

INTRODUCTION

This chapter will provide the sonographic findings and clinical findings of the most common chromosomal abnormalities, including trisomy 13, 18, and 21, triploidy, and monosomy X. Also, information regarding two common neural tube defects—anencephaly and spina bifida—is provided. A thorough clinical history analysis should be conducted when chromosomal anomalies are suspected. Ultrasound practitioners should be capable of detecting many of these findings while performing the routine protocols mentioned in Chapters 6 and 8 of this text. This chapter concludes with a section that contains additional images of these abnormalities.

CHROMOSOMAL ABNORMALITIES[1-3]

- Noninvasive maternal serum screening
  - Triple screen includes:
    - Maternal serum alpha-fetoprotein (MSAFP)
      - A protein produced by the fetus.
    - Human chorionic gonadotropin (hCG)
      - A hormone produced by the placenta.
    - Estriol (UE)
      - A form of estrogen produced by the fetus and placenta.
  - Quadruple screen includes:
  - MSAFP
  - hCG
  - UE
  - Inhibin-A
    - Protein produced by the placenta and ovaries.

- Pregnancy-associated plasma protein-A (PAPP-A)
  - Protein produced by the placenta that can be measured as part of the pregnancy screening blood test.
- Cell-free DNA prenatal test (cfDNA)
  - cfDNA is the straightforward screening of maternal blood.
  - Highly accurate test used for trisomy 21, 18, and 13 screening.
  - May detect sex chromosomal aneuploidies, including monosomy X, and Klinefelter syndrome.
- Trisomy 21 (Fig. 10-1)
  - Facts to note:
    - Trisomy 21 is the most common chromosomal abnormality.
    - The fetus with trisomy 21 has a third chromosome 21.
    - It is associated with Down syndrome, a group of clinical findings.
    - Down syndrome is associated with advanced maternal age (≥ 35).
  - Clinical findings of trisomy 21:
    - Low MSAFP
    - Elevated hCG
    - Elevated Inhibin-A
    - Low UE
    - Low PAPP-A

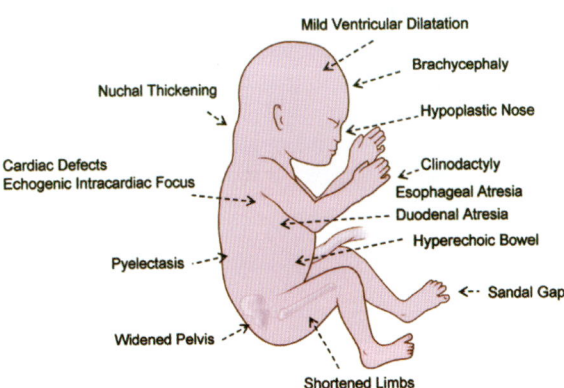

Figure 10-1. Features of trisomy 21. (Reprinted with permission from Rapp C, Mathew D. Patterns of fetal anomalies. In: Stephenson SR, Dmitrieva J, eds. *Diagnostic Medical Sonography: Obstetrics & Gynecology*. 4th ed. Wolters Kluwer; 2018. Figure 31-30.)

- Common sonographic findings of trisomy 21:
  - Thickened nuchal translucency in the first trimester and thickened nuchal fold in the second/third trimester (Fig. 10-1)
  - Absent or hypoplastic nasal bones (Fig. 10-2)
  - Clinodactyly
    - Abnormal bending of the fifth digit toward the fourth digit
  - Duodenal atresia
    - Absence of the proximal portion of the small bowel
    - Seen as an anechoic "double-bubble" in the abdomen at the level of the stomach
  - Echogenic intracardiac focus (EIF) and ventricular septal defect (Fig. 10-3)
    - EIF is typically found within the left ventricle.
  - Macroglossia (Fig. 10-4)
    - Enlarged tongue

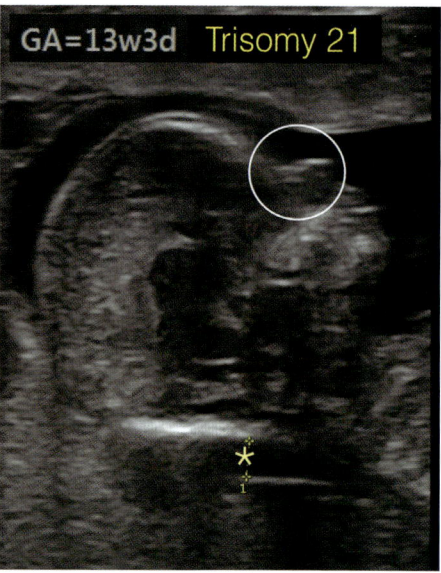

Figure 10-2. Absent nasal bones. Midsagittal plane of the fetal head at 13 weeks of gestation with trisomy 21. Note the presence of thickened nuchal translucency (3.3 mm) (*asterisk*) and absent nasal bone (*circle*). (Reprinted with permission from Doubilet PM, Benson CB, Benacerraf BR. *Atlas of Ultrasound in Obstetrics and Gynecology: A Multimedia Reference.* 3rd ed. Wolters Kluwer; 2019. Figure 12.2.1.)

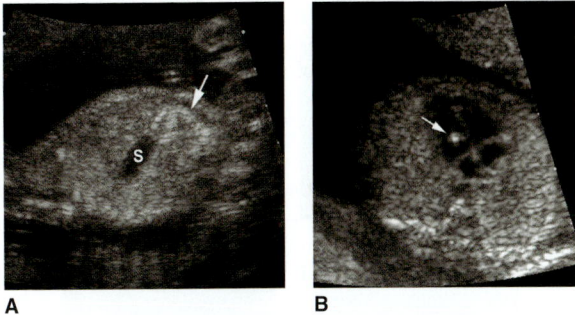

Figure 10-3. Echogenic bowel and echogenic intracardiac focus. A. Longitudinal image of fetus with trisomy 21 demonstrating echogenic bowel (*arrow*) inferior to the stomach (*S*). B. Four-chamber view of the heart in a different fetus with trisomy 21, showing an echogenic intracardiac focus (*arrow*) in the left ventricle. (Reprinted with permission from Doubilet PM, Benson CB. *Atlas of Ultrasound in Obstetrics and Gynecology: A Multimedia Reference*. 2nd ed. Wolters Kluwer Health/Lippincott Williams & Wilkins; 2012. Figure 14.3.4.)

- Pyelectasis (also known as hydronephrosis)
  - Enlarged renal pelvis
  - Hydronephrosis can be graded **(Fig. 10-5)**
- Echogenic bowel (see Fig. 10-3)
- Widened pelvic angles

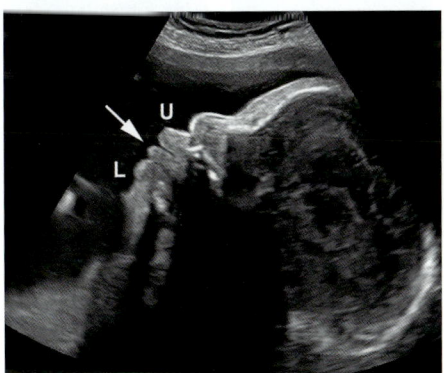

Figure 10-4. Profile image demonstrating macroglossia. Sagittal image of face demonstrating large tongue (*arrow*) protruding anteriorly between upper (*U*) and lower (*L*) lips. (Reprinted with permission from Doubilet PM, Benson CB, Benacerraf BR. *Atlas of Ultrasound in Obstetrics and Gynecology: A Multimedia Reference*. 3rd ed. Wolters Kluwer; 2019. Figure 8.2.1.)

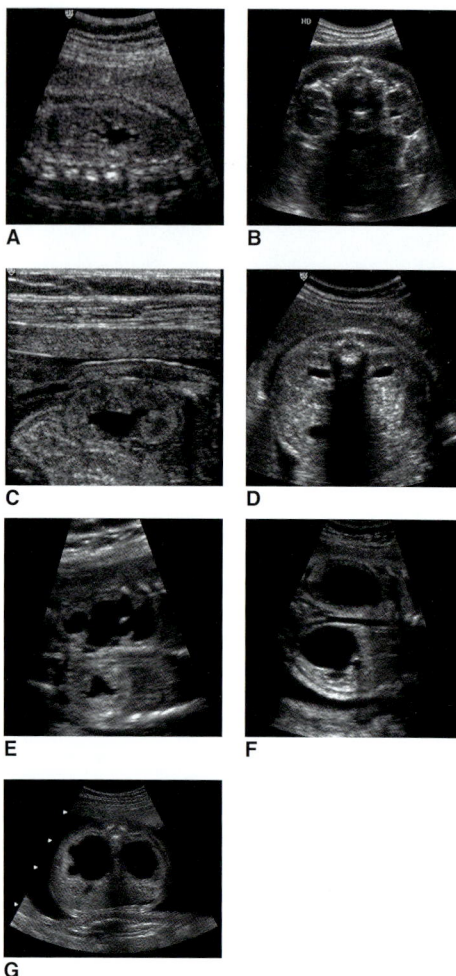

Figure 10-5. Various degrees of fetal hydronephrosis grading. Mild, grade I, on a longitudinal (A) and transverse (B) image. Moderate, grade II, on a longitudinal (C) and transverse (D) image. Increasing hydronephrosis, grade IV, demonstrating dilatation of the calyces (E) on a longitudinal image. A grade V on a coronal (F) and transverse (G) image. (Reprinted with permission from Layton GA. Ultrasound of the abnormal fetal chest, abdomen, and pelvis. In: Stephenson SR, ed. *Diagnostic Medical Sonography: Obstetrics & Gynecology.* 3rd ed. Wolters Kluwer Health/Lippincott Williams & Wilkins; 2012. Figure 21-31.)

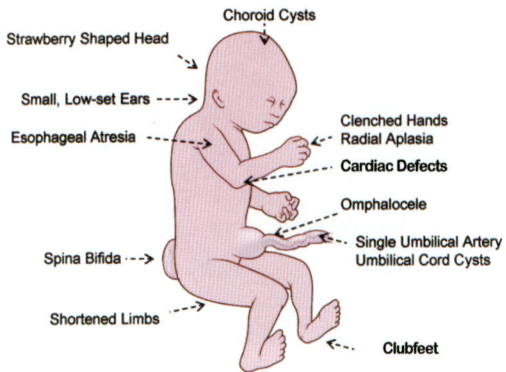

Figure 10-6. Features of trisomy 18. (Reprinted with permission from Rapp C, Mathew D. Patterns of fetal anomalies. In: Stephenson SR, Dmitrieva J, eds. *Diagnostic Medical Sonography: Obstetrics & Gynecology.* 4th ed. Wolters Kluwer; 2018. Figure 31-27.)

- Sandal gap
  - Large space between the first and second toes.
- Trisomy 18 **(Fig. 10-6)**
  - Facts to note:
    - Trisomy 18 is the second most common chromosomal abnormality.
    - The fetus with trisomy 18 has a third chromosome 18.
    - It is associated with Edwards syndrome, a group of clinical abnormalities.
  - Clinical findings of trisomy 18:
    - All labs are typically lower than normal.
  - Sonographic findings of trisomy 18:
    - Agenesis of the corpus callosum
      - Absence of corpus callosum
      - In the profile image, this will produce a "sunburst" appearance of the sulci **(Fig. 10-7)**
      - Elevated and dilated third ventricle
    - Choroid plexus cyst (may be bilateral)
      - Located within the lateral ventricle **(Fig. 10-8)**
    - Hypoplastic cerebellum
    - Enlarged cisterna magna
    - Strawberry-shaped skull **(Fig. 10-9)**
    - Micrognathia
      - Recessed chin is best seen in profile image **(Fig. 10-10)**

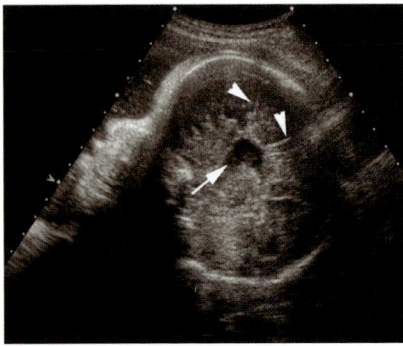

Figure 10-7. Agenesis of the corpus callosum. Apert syndrome with agenesis of the corpus callosum. Sagittal image of a fetus with Apert syndrome revealing agenesis of the corpus callosum with the typical spoke-wheel or sunburst pattern of the sulci (*arrowheads*) and the elevation and dilation of the third ventricle (*arrow*). (Reprinted with permission from Doubilet PM, Benson CB. *Atlas of Ultrasound in Obstetrics and Gynecology: A Multimedia Reference.* 2nd ed. Wolters Kluwer Health/Lippincott Williams & Wilkins; 2012. Figure 4.17.2.)

- Small, low-set ears
- Clenched hands, overlapping index finger, fixed wrist **(Fig. 10-11)**
- Omphalocele

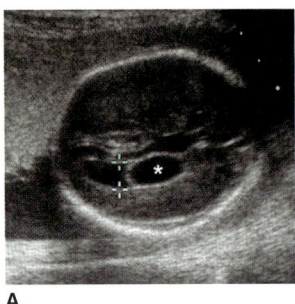
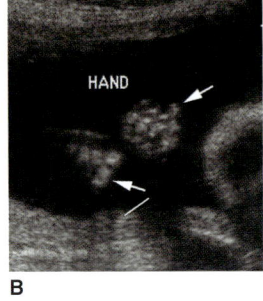

Figure 10-8. Trisomy 18 with choroid plexus cyst and clenched hands with overlapping digits. A. Axial image of head depicting a cyst (*asterisk*) within the choroid plexus of the lateral ventricle (*calipers*). **B.** Image of both hands showing abnormal overlapping of index finger over middle finger bilaterally (*arrows*). (Reprinted with permission from Doubilet PM, Benson CB. *Atlas of Ultrasound in Obstetrics and Gynecology: A Multimedia Reference.* 2nd ed. Wolters Kluwer Health/Lippincott Williams & Wilkins; 2012. Figure 14.2.5.)

Chapter 10. Chromosomal Abnormalities and Neural Tube Defects

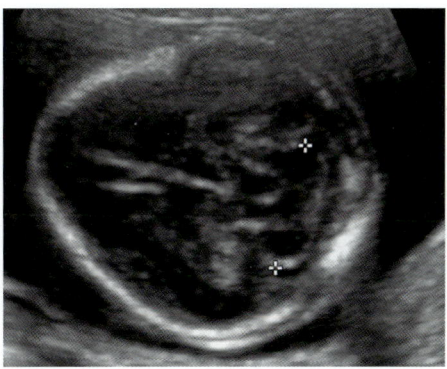

Figure 10-9. Strawberry skull associated with trisomy 18. A strawberry-shaped calvarium in this 19-week fetus with trisomy 18. The calipers are measuring the cerebellum. (Reprinted with permission from Chapman T, Santoro SL, Hopkin RJ. Genetic abnormalities and syndromes. In: Kline-Fath BM, Bulas DI, Bahado-Singh R, eds. *Fundamental and Advanced Fetal Imaging: Ultrasound and MRI*. Wolters Kluwer; 2015. Figure 20.7A.)

- ○ Mass located at the level of the umbilicus that often contains abdominal organs **(Fig. 10-12)**
- ● Heart defects
  - ○ Ventriculoseptal defects

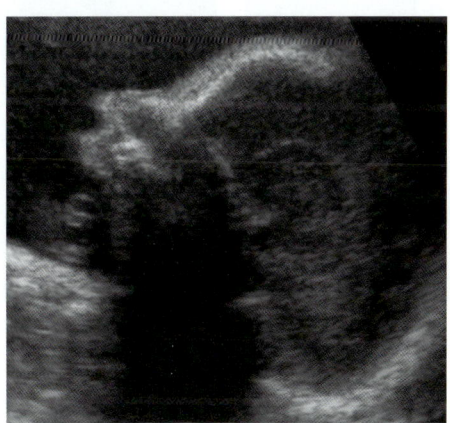

Figure 10-10. Micrognathia. Micrognathia (recessed chin) is noted on this sagittal view of the facial profile. (Reprinted with permission from Chapman T, Santoro SL, Hopkin RJ. Genetic abnormalities and syndromes. In: Kline-Fath BM, Bulas DI, Bahado-Singh R, eds. *Fundamental and Advanced Fetal Imaging: Ultrasound and MRI*. Wolters Kluwer; 2015. Figure 20.37B.)

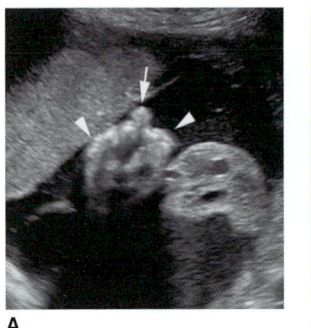
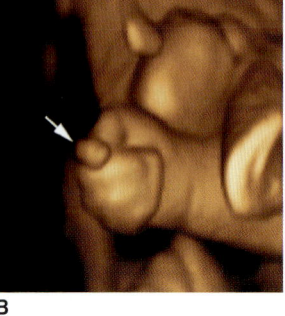

Figure 10-11. Overlapping fingers. A. Image of hand in fetus with trisomy 18 demonstrating a finger (*arrow*) protruding abnormally above the clenched fist (*arrowheads*). **B.** 3D image of same hand demonstrating abnormal overlapping of index finger (*arrow*) in the persistently clenched fist. (Reprinted with permission from Doubilet PM, Benson CB, Benacerraf BR. *Atlas of Ultrasound in Obstetrics and Gynecology: A Multimedia Reference*. 3rd ed. Wolters Kluwer; 2019. Figure 16.6.1A-B.)

- Tetralogy of Fallot **(Fig. 10-13)**
  - Overriding aortic root
  - Subaortic ventricular septal defect

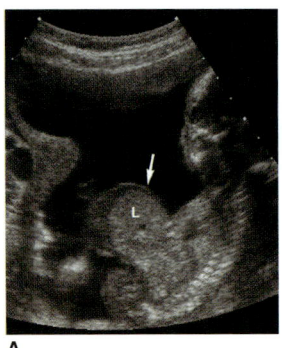
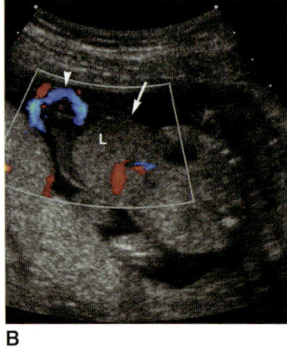

Figure 10-12. Omphalocele containing liver. A. Sagittal image of fetus demonstrating large omphalocele (*arrow*) containing a region of homogeneous tissue representing liver (*L*). **B.** Color Doppler image of large omphalocele (*arrow*) showing vessels in the herniated portion of the liver (*L*). Umbilical vessels (*arrowhead*) are seen inserting into the omphalocele sac. (Reprinted with permission from Doubilet PM, Benson CB. *Atlas of Ultrasound in Obstetrics and Gynecology: A Multimedia Reference*. 2nd ed. Wolters Kluwer Health/Lippincott Williams & Wilkins; 2012. Figure 11.1.2.)

Chapter 10. Chromosomal Abnormalities and Neural Tube Defects

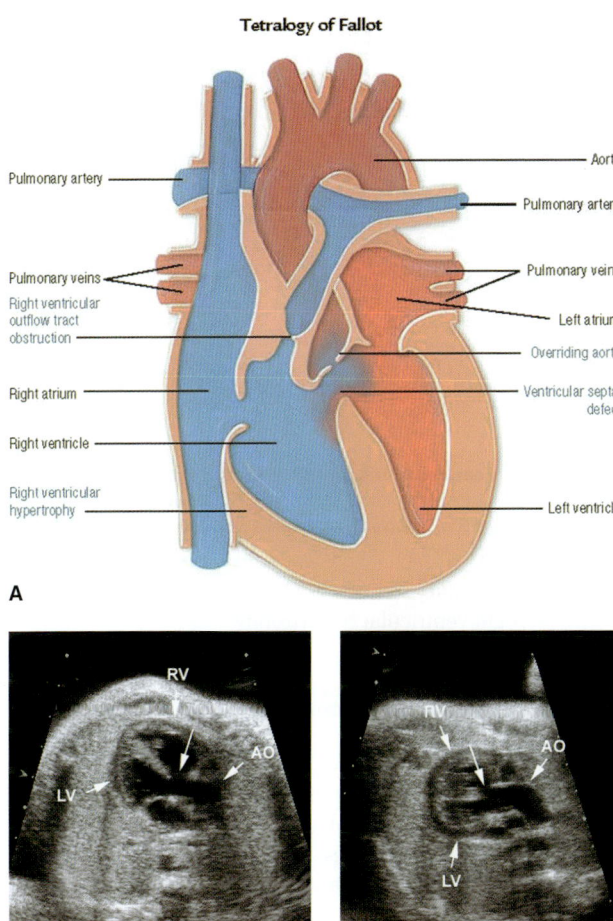

Figure 10-13. Tetralogy of Fallot sonographic findings. **A.** Drawing of findings of tetralogy of Fallot. **B.** Ventricular septal defect with tetralogy of Fallot (long *arrow* in both B and C). **C.** Oblique view of the left ventricular outflow tract demonstrating overriding aorta (AO *arrow*). LV arrow, left ventricle; RV arrow, right ventricle. (A. Reprinted with permission from Kline-Tilford AM, Haut C. Lippincott Certification Review: Pediatric Acute Care Nurse Practitioner. Wolters Kluwer; 2016. Figure 5-8. **B, C.** Reprinted with permission from Doubilet PM, Benson CB. *Atlas of Ultrasound in Obstetrics and Gynecology: A Multimedia Reference.* 2nd ed. Wolters Kluwer Health/Lippincott Williams & Wilkins; 2012. Figure 9.7.1.)

330   Chapter 10. Chromosomal Abnormalities and Neural Tube Defects

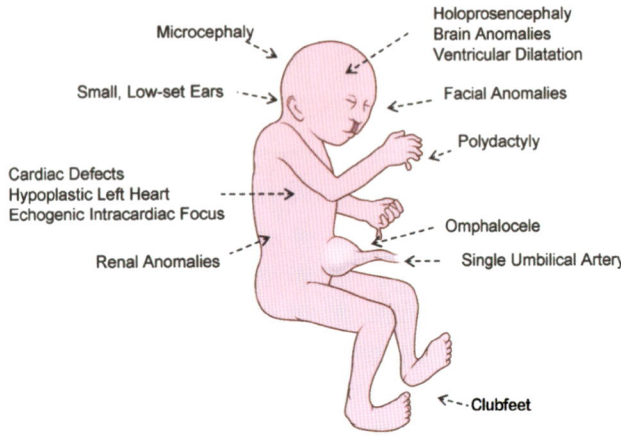

Figure 10-14. Features of trisomy 13. (Reprinted with permission from Rapp C, Mathew D. Patterns of fetal anomalies. In: Stephenson SR, Dmitrieva J, eds. *Diagnostic Medical Sonography: Obstetrics & Gynecology*. 4th ed. Wolters Kluwer; 2018. Figure 31-25.)

- Pulmonary stenosis
- Right ventricular hypertrophy
- Renal anomalies
- Single umbilical cord
- Clubfeet or rocker-bottom feet
- Trisomy 13 **(Fig. 10-14)**
  - Facts to note:
    - The fetus with trisomy 13 has a third chromosome 13.
    - Trisomy 13 is associated with Patau syndrome, which is a group of clinical findings.
    - There is a strong association between trisomy 13 and holoprosencephaly.
  - Clinical findings of trisomy 13:
    - Simple blood tests like the triple screen may not be helpful.
    - Cell-free DNA is most useful.
  - Sonographic findings of trisomy 13:
    - Microcephaly
    - Holoprosencephaly **(Fig. 10-15)**
    - Ventriculomegaly
    - Polydactyly
    - Facial anomalies
      - Cleft lip

Chapter 10. Chromosomal Abnormalities and Neural Tube Defects   **331**

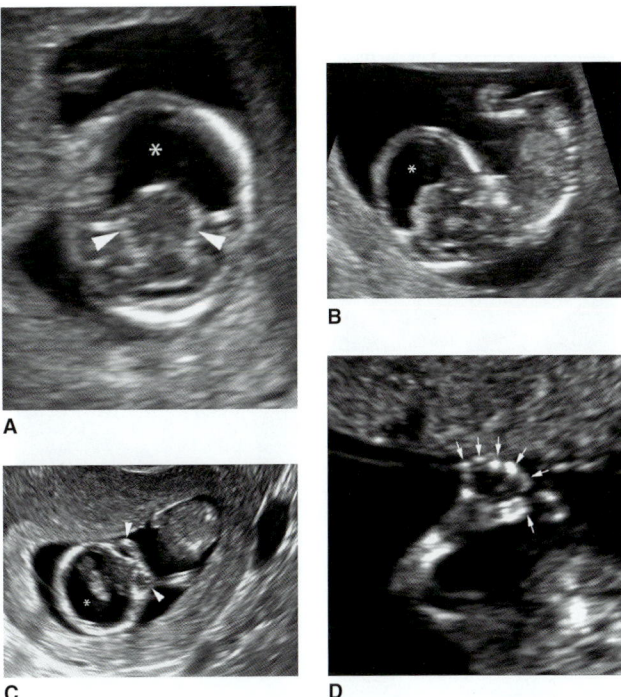

Figure 10-15. Holoprosencephaly. A. Coronal view through the fetal head showing a single fused ventricle (*asterisk*), fused thalami (*arrowheads*), and absence of the falx, typical of alobar holoprosencephaly. **B.** Sagittal view showing the large monoventricle (*asterisk*) distending the head. **C.** Frontal view of head showing the large single ventricle (*asterisk*) and hypotelorism, where the orbits (*arrowheads*) are abnormally close together. **D.** View of the hand showing six digits (*arrows*), a common finding **with trisomy 13.** (Reprinted with permission from Doubilet PM, Benson CB, Benacerraf BR. *Atlas of Ultrasound in Obstetrics and Gynecology: A Multimedia Reference.* 3rd ed. Wolters Kluwer; 2019. Figure 4.2.5.)

- ○ Cleft palate
- ○ Micropthalmia
  - Small orbit
- ○ Hypotelorism (see Fig. 10-15)
  - Close-spaced eyes
- Cardiac defects
  - ○ Hypoplastic left heart

Echogenic intracardiac focus

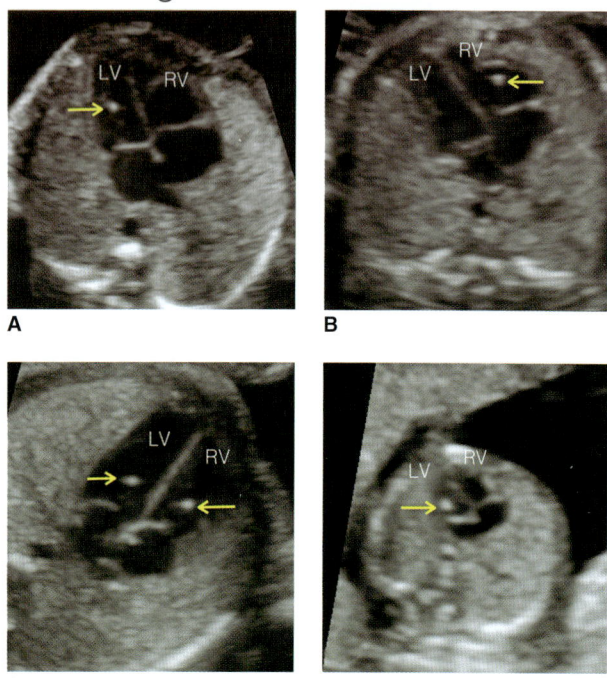

Figure 10-16. Apical four-chamber views in four fetuses (A–D) with echogenic intracardiac foci (*arrows*). The echogenic intracardiac focus (EIF) is typically located in the papillary muscle, most commonly in the left ventricle (*LV*) (A). Occasionally, it can be located in the right ventricle (*RV*) (B) or in both the LV and RV (C). EIF can also be present at 11 to 13 weeks' scan as shown in D. (Reprinted with permission from Abuhamad A, Chaoui R. *A Practical Guide to Fetal Echocardiography: Normal and Abnormal Hearts.* 3rd ed. Wolters Kluwer; 2016. Figure 7.10.)

- Small left ventricle
- EIF **(Fig. 10-16)**
- Triploidy **(Fig. 10-17)**
  - Facts to note:
    - The fetus with triploidy has an extra chromosome for every chromosome.
    - There is a strong association between triploidy and gestational trophoblastic disease (partial mole).

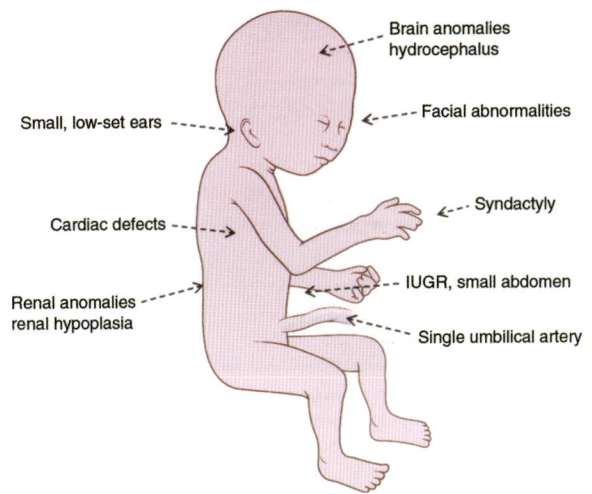

Figure 10-17. Features of triploidy. (Reprinted with permission from Chapman T, Santoro SL, Hopkin RJ. Genetic abnormalities and syndromes. In: Kline-Fath BM, Bulas DI, Bahado-Singh R, eds. *Fundamental and Advanced Fetal Imaging: Ultrasound and MRI.* Wolters Kluwer; 2015. Figure 20.11.)

- Clinical findings of triploidy:
  - Markedly elevated hCG
  - Hyperemesis gravidarum
    - Excessive vomiting during pregnancy
- Sonographic findings of triploidy:
  - First trimester findings of triploidy:
    - Cystic spaces within an enlarged placenta **(Fig. 10-18)**
    - Fetal hydrops or demise
    - Bilateral, enlarged cystic structures on the ovaries (theca lutein cysts)
  - Second-trimester findings of triploidy:
    - Dandy–Walker malformation **(Fig. 10-19)**
      - Enlarged cisterna magna
      - Absent cerebellar vermis
    - Hydrocephalus
    - Facial abnormalities
    - Renal abnormalities
    - Cardiac defects
    - Syndactyly (webbed fingers or toes)
    - Clubfeet **(Fig. 10-20)**

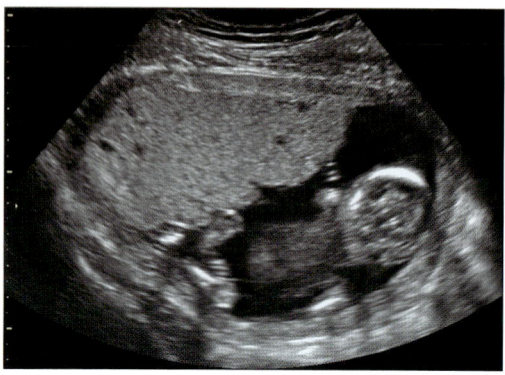

Figure 10-18. Triploidy with a live fetus. A partial mole is noted demonstrating an enlarged placenta with cystic avascular areas, the fetus is very small for gestational age due to the association with fetal triploidy.
(Reprinted with permission from Hernandez-Andrade E, Soto Torres EE, Tirosh D. Ultrasound evaluation of the placenta, amniotic fluid, umbilical cord, and amniotic membranes. In: Kline-Fath BM, Bulas DI, Lee W, eds. *Fundamental and Advanced Fetal Imaging: Ultrasound and MRI*. 2nd ed. Wolters Kluwer; 2021. Figure 13.1-20.)

- Monosomy X **(Fig. 10-21)**
  - The fetus with monosomy X has only one X chromosome.
  - There is a strong association between monosomy X and Turner syndrome, which is a group of clinical findings.

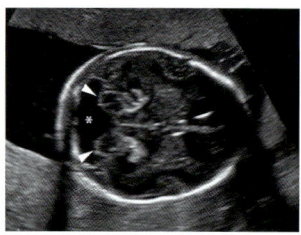
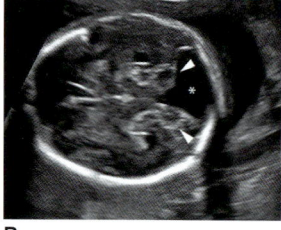

A **B**

Figure 10-19. Dandy–Walker malformation with large posterior fossa cyst and flattened cerebellar hemispheres. **(A)** and **(B)** Axial images of two different fetuses demonstrating an abnormal posterior fossa with absence of the cerebellar vermis, and splaying and flattening of the cerebellar hemispheres (*arrowheads*) by a large fluid-filled space (*asterisk*) connecting the fourth ventricle to the cisterna magna.
(Reprinted with permission from Doubilet PM, Benson CB, Benacerraf BR. *Atlas of Ultrasound in Obstetrics and Gynecology: A Multimedia Reference*. 3rd ed. Wolters Kluwer; 2019. Figure 6.3.1.)

Chapter 10. Chromosomal Abnormalities and Neural Tube Defects 335

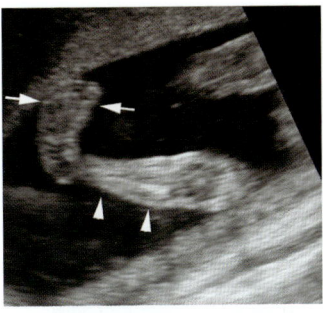

A

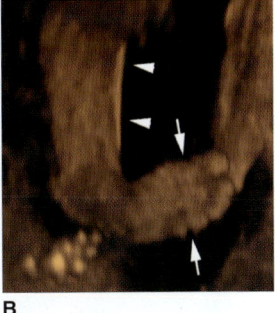

B

Figure 10-20. Clubfoot. Clubfoot in 2D and 3D ultrasound. **A.** 2D sonogram of lower leg and foot showing that the foot (*arrows*) is turned such that its bones lie in the same plane as the bones of the calf (*arrowheads*). **B.** 3D image of same foot (*arrows*) showing abnormal relationship of the foot to the lower leg (*arrowheads*) due to clubfoot deformity. (Reprinted with permission from Doubilet PM, Benson CB. *Atlas of Ultrasound in Obstetrics and Gynecology: A Multimedia Reference.* 2nd ed. Wolters Kluwer Health/Lippincott Williams & Wilkins; 2012. Figure 13.7.2.)

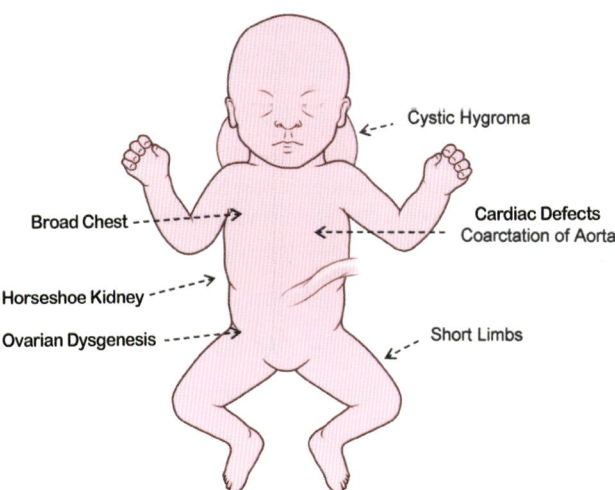

Figure 10-21. Feature of Turner syndrome. (Reprinted with permission from Rapp C, Mathew D. Patterns of fetal anomalies. In: Stephenson SR, Dmitrieva J, eds. *Diagnostic Medical Sonography: Obstetrics & Gynecology.* 4th ed. Wolters Kluwer; 2018. Figure 31-18.)

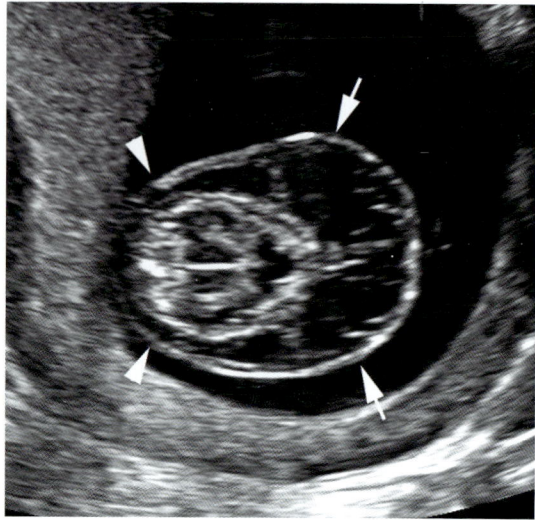

Figure 10-22. Large cystic hygroma. A. Axial image of neck showing large posterior cystic hygroma (*arrows*) with septations. Subcutaneous edema is visible extending around the head laterally and anteriorly (*arrowheads*). (Reprinted with permission from Doubilet PM, Benson CB, Benacerraf BR. *Atlas of Ultrasound in Obstetrics and Gynecology: A Multimedia Reference*. 3rd ed. Wolters Kluwer; 2019. Figure 9.2.5.)

- Clinical findings of monosomy X:
  - All labs will be lower than normal.
- Sonographic findings of monosomy X:
  - Enlarged placenta containing cystic spaces
  - Increased nuchal translucency
  - Cystic hygroma **(Fig. 10-22)**
  - Fetal hydrops
    - Fluid collection within at least two cavities
  - Renal anomalies
  - Cardiac defects

NEURAL TUBE DEFECTS[1-3]

- Anencephaly
  - Facts to note:
    - Absence of the cranial vault.
    - Some cerebral tissue may be present.
    - Fetal heart activity and fetal movement may be present.

Chapter 10. Chromosomal Abnormalities and Neural Tube Defects 337

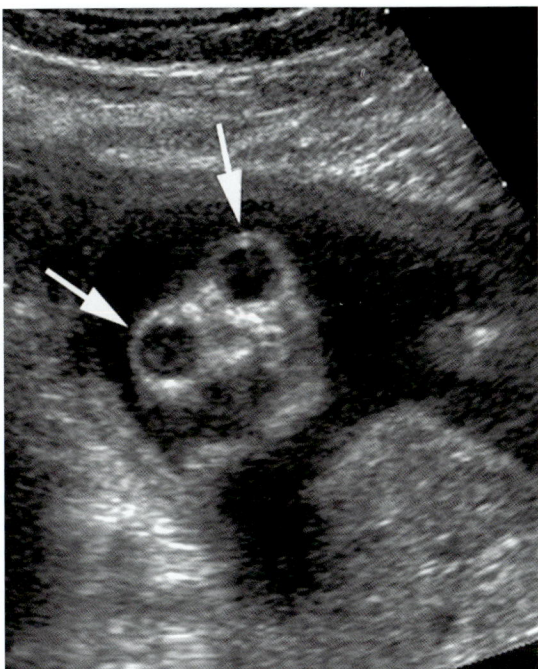

Figure 10-23. Anencephaly. This coronal image of the fetal face demonstrates "froglike" facies and the absence of the forehead and cranium above orbits (*arrows*). (Reprinted with permission from Doubilet PM, Benson CB, Benacerraf BR. *Atlas of Ultrasound in Obstetrics and Gynecology: A Multimedia Reference.* 3rd ed. Wolters Kluwer; 2019. Figure 6.4.1.)

- Clinical findings of anencephaly:
  - Elevated MSAFP
- Sonographic findings of anencephaly:
  - Absent cranial vault
  - Exposed brain tissue
  - "Froglike" facies and bulging eyes **(Fig. 10-23)**
  - Fetal heart activity may be noted
- Spina bifida
  - Facts to note:
    - Open spina bifida is often associated with Arnold–Chiari II malformation, which is a group of cranial abnormalities.
    - Abnormal head shape (lemon-shaped skull) is often an obvious finding.

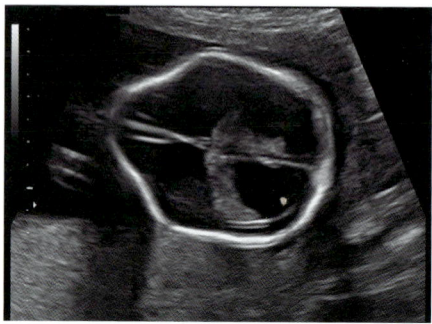

Figure 10-24. Lemon-shaped skull. Lemon-shaped skull associated with open spina bifida. Ventriculomegaly can also be noted in this image. (Reprinted with permission from Provenzale JM, Nelson RC, Vinson EN. *Duke Radiology Case Review: Imaging, Differential Diagnosis, and Discussion.* 2nd ed. Wolters Kluwer Health/Lippincott Williams & Wilkins; 2012. Figure 9-4C.)

- The associated myelomeningocele (spinal mass) is most often located at the level of the distal spine.
- Myelomeningocele may be demonstrated in the transverse or sagittal plane to the fetal spine. Coronal may also be utilized.
- Clinical findings of spina bifida:
  - Elevated MSAFP
- Sonographic findings of spina bifida:
  - Lemon-shaped skull **(Fig. 10-24)**
  - Banana-shaped cerebellum **(Fig. 10-25)**
  - Obliterated cisterna magna
  - Colpocephaly
    - Narrow frontal horns and enlarged occipital horns of lateral ventricles
  - Ventriculomegaly (see Fig. 10-24)
  - Splaying of the spinal laminae at the level of the defect (typically located in the distal spine) **(Fig. 10-26)**
  - Complex mass emanating from the distal spine (myelomeningocele)

ADDITIONAL IMAGES OF COMMON CHROMOSOMAL ABNORMALITIES AND NEURAL TUBE DEFECTS

- Some facial sonographic findings of trisomy 21 are provided in **Figure 10-27**.
- Various sonographic findings of trisomy 18 are seen in **Figure 10-28**.

Chapter 10. Chromosomal Abnormalities and Neural Tube Defects

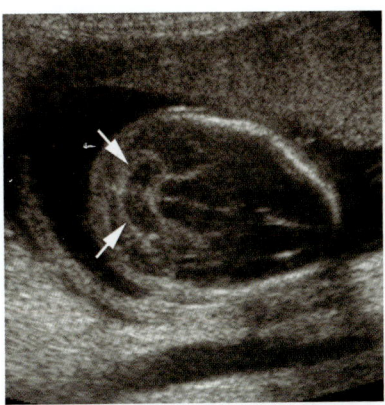

Figure 10-25. Banana-shaped cerebellum. Banana sign associated with meningomyelocele. Axial image of posterior fossa demonstrating banana-shaped cerebellum (*arrows*) in a small posterior fossa with effacement of the cisterna magna, due to the Chiari II malformation. This fetus had a lumbosacral meningomyelocele. (Reprinted with permission from Doubilet PM, Benson CB. *Atlas of Ultrasound in Obstetrics and Gynecology: A Multimedia Reference.* 2nd ed. Wolters Kluwer Health/Lippincott Williams & Wilkins; 2012. Figure 5.1.4.)

- Anencephaly in 2D and 3D can be seen in **Figure 10-29**.
- 3D and surface mode of spina bifida is demonstrated in **Figure 10-30**.

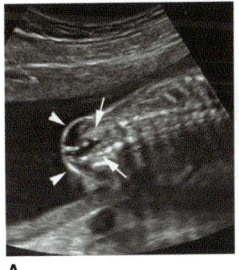 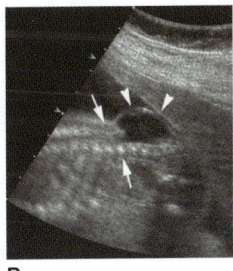 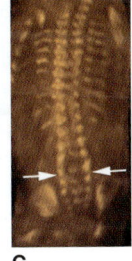

A　　　　　　　　　B　　　　　　　　C

Figure 10-26. Myelomeningocele. A. Coronal image of the distal spine (*arrows*) revealing herniation of the spinal cord (*arrowheads*). **B.** A large myelomeningocele (*arrowheads*) is noted protruding from the distal spine (*arrows*) in this image. **C.** Three-dimensional image of the fetal spine demonstrating widening of the distal spine in the area of the defect (*between arrows*). (Reprinted with permission from Doubilet PM, Benson CB. *Atlas of Ultrasound in Obstetrics and Gynecology: A Multimedia Reference.* 2nd ed. Wolters Kluwer Health/Lippincott Williams & Wilkins; 2012. Figure 5.1.1.)

Trisomy 21: Cranial and Facial Markers

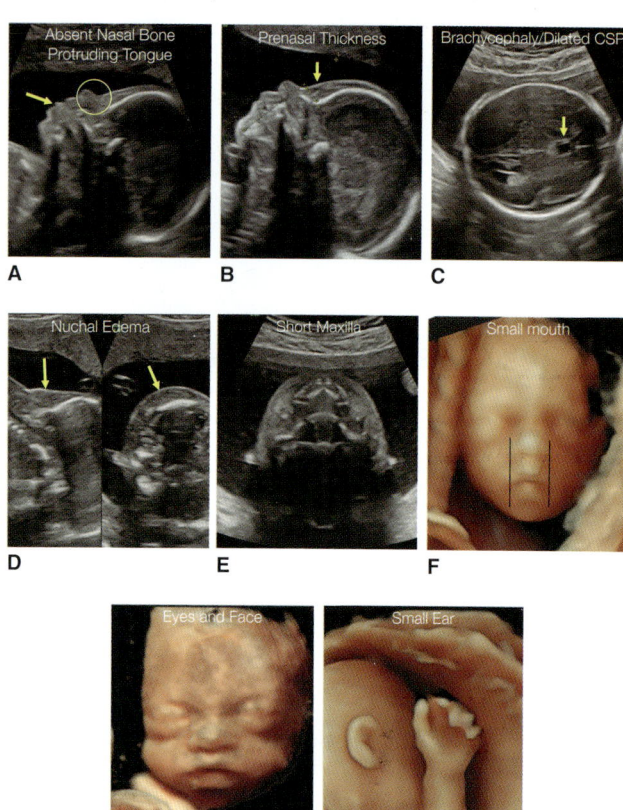

Figure 10-27. Trisomy 21 cranial and facial findings. Cranial and facial markers in trisomy 21 fetuses including absent nasal bone (A-*circle*), protruding tongue with an open mouth (A, *arrow*), prenasal thickness (B, *arrow*), brachycephaly (C), dilated cavum septi pellucidi (CSP) (C, *arrow*), nuchal edema (D, *arrows*), as seen in sagittal (D-left) or axial (D-right) view. The midfacial hypoplasia in trisomy 21 is associated with a short maxilla (E) and small mouth, as microstoma (F). Facial features of trisomy 21 can be recognized on three-dimensional sonography and are shown in panel (G). A small ear (H) can also be found but is not very specific. (Reprinted with permission from Abuhamad A, Chaoui R. *A Practical Guide to Fetal Echocardiography: Normal and Abnormal Hearts.* 4th ed. Wolters Kluwer; 2022. Figure 2.4.)

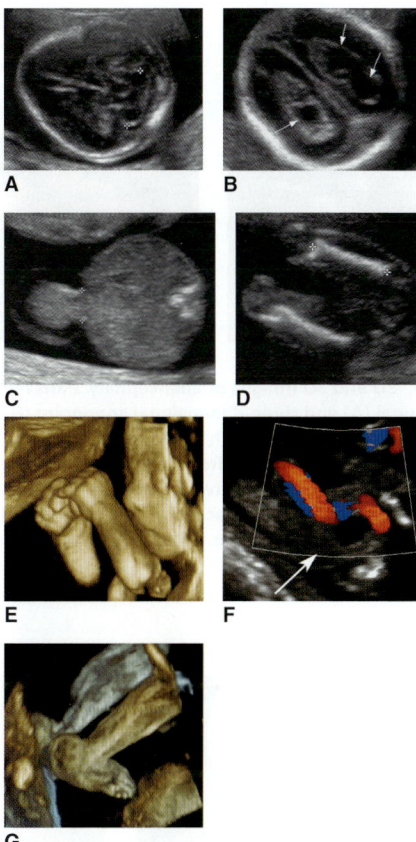

Figure 10-28. Trisomy 18. A. A strawberry-shaped calvarium. B. Choroid plexus cysts are noted as well-demarcated anechoic spaces within the bulk (*arrows*) of the echogenic choroid. C. Small omphaloceles are additional features of this disorder. D. Bilateral femurs and remaining long bones are abnormally short. E. Clenched hands may be observed by two-dimensional US and easily seen with three-dimensional images. F. A single umbilical artery with other malformations contributes to the likelihood of a chromosomal anomaly. The arrow indicates the expected location of a non-visualized umbilical artery. G. Foot abnormalities include rocker-bottom foot, as seen in a different 23-week fetus on the three-dimensional image. (Reprinted with permission from Santoro SL, Hopkin RJ, Chapman T, Kline-Fath BM. Chromosomal and genetic syndromes. In: Kline-Fath BM, Bulas DI, Lee W, eds. *Fundamental and Advanced Fetal Imaging: Ultrasound and MRI.* 2nd ed. Wolters Kluwer; 2021. Figure 30.7A-B.)

342   **Chapter 10.** Chromosomal Abnormalities and Neural Tube Defects

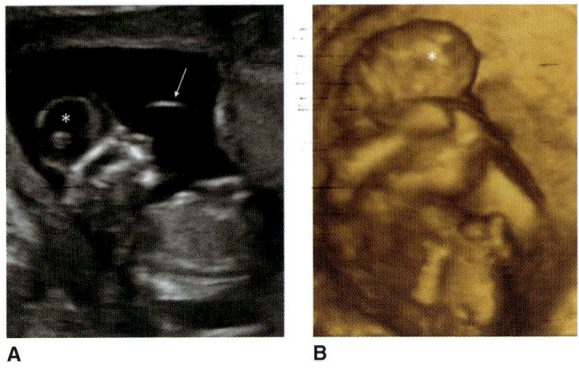

Figure 10-29. 2D and 3D images of anencephaly. Transvaginal two-dimensional (A) and three-dimensional sonogram (B) of a fetus at 13 weeks of gestation with severe brain malformation (anencephaly—*asterisk*) resulting from amniotic band syndrome. Note the presence in A of a reflective membrane within the amniotic cavity (*arrow*) that is attached to the fetal head. This reflective membrane represents an amniotic band. (Reprinted with permission from Abuhamad A, Chaoui R. *First Trimester Ultrasound Diagnosis of Fetal Abnormalities.* Wolters Kluwer; 2018. Figure 15.24.)

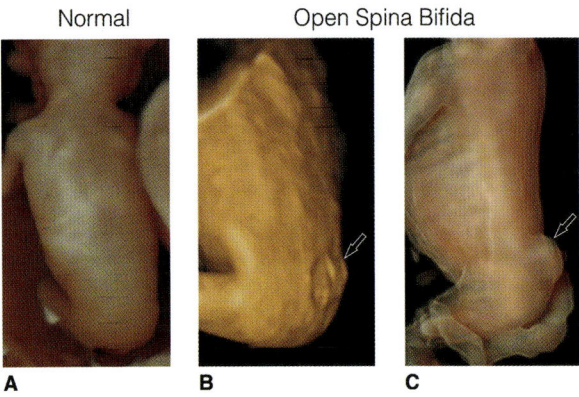

Figure 10-30. Three-dimensional sonogram in surface mode of a normal fetus (A) and two fetuses with open spina bifida as myelomeningocele (B and C) at 13 weeks of gestation. Note in B and C the direct visualization of the spina bifida in the lower lumbosacral spine (*arrows*). (Reprinted with permission from Abuhamad A, Chaoui R. *First Trimester Ultrasound Diagnosis of Fetal Abnormalities.* Wolters Kluwer; 2018. Figure 8.45.)

REFERENCES

1. Norton ME, Scoutt LM, Feldstein VA. *Callen's Ultrasonography in Obstetrics and Gynecology.* 6th ed. Elsevier; 2017:805-882.
2. Kline-Fath BM, Bulus DI, Lee W. *Fundamental and Advanced Fetal Imaging.* 2nd ed. Wolters Kluwer; 2021:902-947.
3. Penny SM. *Examination Review for Ultrasound: Abdomen & Obstetrics and Gynecology.* 3rd ed. Wolters Kluwer; 2022:Chapter 30:729-749.

INDEX

Note: Page numbers followed by f indicate figures; those followed by t indicate tables.

A

Abdomen, fetal, 166-168, 223-227, 223f-228f
Abortion, 130t, 198-199
Acoustic shadowing, 7t, 8f, 133, 134f
Acrania, in first trimester, 180, 182f, 237, 241f
Adnexa, 79
  AIUM recommendations for sonography of, 32-33
  anatomy, 40, 41f
Adult female pelvic sonography, 30-75
  AIUM indications for, 1-2
  AIUM recommendations for, 30-33
    adnexa, 32-33
    ALARA (As Low as Reasonably Achievable) principle, 33
    cul-de-sac, 33
    Doppler sonography, 33
    ovaries, 32
    uterus, 30-32
  clinical investigation for, 44
  equipment for, 43-44
  image orientation, 45-48
    transabdominal, 45-47, 45f-47f
    transvaginal, 47-48, 47f, 49f-50f
  normal measurements, 59-60
    ovaries size, 60
    uterine size, 59-60
  normal sonographic description, 44
    ovaries, 44
    uterus, 44
  patient positioning
    for transabdominal female pelvic sonogram, 21, 22f
    for transvaginal sonography, 22, 23f
  patient preparation
    for transabdominal pelvic sonography, 20-21, 20f, 21f
    for transvaginal female pelvic examination, 21
  protocol for, 48, 51, 52f, 53-54, 54f-59f, 56
  scanning tips, 56-59
AFI. *See* Amniotic fluid index
Agenesis of corpus callosum, 325, 326f
AIUM. *See* American Institute of Ultrasound in Medicine
ALARA (as low as reasonably achievable) principle, 6, 33, 79
  obstetric sonography, 127
Ambiguous genitalia, 95-96

Amenorrhea, 41t, 130t
American Institute of Ultrasound in Medicine (AIUM), 1
  equipment selection and quality control, 2-6
  female pelvis sonography
    indications for, 1-2
    recommendations for, 30-33
  Guidelines for Nuchal Translucency Measurements between 11 and 14 weeks, 180, 182-183, 182f-183f
  HyCoSy
    indications for, 2
    procedure recommendations for, 108
    protocol images for, 110
    recommendations for performance of, 105, 107f
  recommendations for standard second-/third-trimester sonography, 245-267
  SIS
    indications for, 2
    procedure recommendations for, 108
    protocol images for, 108-110, 110f, 111f
    recommendations for performance of, 105, 106f
  standard first-trimester sonography, recommendations for, 158-159
  standard second-/third-trimester sonography, recommendations for, 245-267
Amnion, 160
Amnionicity (number of amniotic sacs), 311
Amniotic fluid index (AFI), 247, 247f
Amniotic fluid volume, 247, 247f
Anatomy and physiology of first trimester, 159-169
  abdomen and pelvis, 166-168
  chest, 166, 167f-168f
  conception, 159-160
  early gestational structures, development of, 160, 162, 162f
  extremities, 169
  fetus, development of, 162, 163f
  genitalia, 168
  gestational sac, 160, 161f
  heart activity, 162-163, 164f
  kidneys, 167

Anatomy and physiology of first trimester (*Continued*)
  skull, 163, 165f, 166
  spine, 166, 166f
  stomach, 166–167
  umbilical cord insertion, 167, 169f
Anembryonic gestation, 196
Anencephaly, 336–337, 337f
  clinical findings of, 337
  in 2D and 3D, 339, 342f
  facts, 336
  in first trimester, 237, 241f
  sonographic findings of, 337, 337f
Aneuploidy, 130t, 138, 139t, 140
Appendicitis, 71, 72f, 100, 101f, 103f
Appendix, 274, 275f
Arnold–Chiari malformation, 237, 241, 242f
Asherman syndrome, SIS of, 116, 117f
Assisted reproductive therapy, 130t

B
Benign ovarian teratoma, 103f
Beta-human chorionic gonadotropin (β-hCG), 138, 160
Bicornuate pregnancy, 235f
Bicornuate uterus, 37, 38f
Birth control pills, 18
Bladder diverticulum, 70, 72f
Blighted ovum, 130t
Blood (serum) testing, 138, 139t
Brain stemoccipital bone ratio (BS/BSOB), 237, 241, 242f

C
Cell-free DNA testing (cfDNA), 140, 235, 321, 321f
Cervical incompetence, 148–149, 150f–154f, 151–152
Cervix, 32, 34
CfDNA. *See* Cell-free DNA testing
Chest, fetal, 166, 167f–168f
Chorioangioma, 280, 280f
Chorion, 160
Chorionicity (number of placentas), 311, 312f
Choroid plexus cyst, 325, 326f
Chromosomal abnormalities, 320–336
  monosomy X, 334, 335f, 336
    clinical findings of, 336
    sonographic findings of, 336
  noninvasive maternal serum screening, 320–325
    cfDNA, 321, 321f
    monosomy X, 334, 335f, 336
    PAPP-A, 321
    quadruple screen, 320
    triple screen, 320
    triploidy, 332–333
    trisomy 13, 330–332
    trisomy 18, 325–330
    trisomy 21, 321–323
  triploidy, 332–333
    clinical findings of, 333
    facts, 332
    sonographic findings of, 333, 334f–335f
  trisomy 13, 330–332
    clinical findings of, 330
    facts, 330, 330f
    sonographic findings of, 330–332, 331f–332f
  trisomy 18, 325–330
    agenesis of corpus callosum, 325, 326f
    choroid plexus cyst, 325, 326f
    clenched hands, 326, 328f
    clinical findings of, 325
    clubfeet/rocker-bottom feet, 330
    enlarged cisterna magna, 325
    facts, 325
    heart defects, 327–328, 329f, 330
    hypoplastic cerebellum, 325
    micrognathia, 325, 327f
    omphalocele, 326–327, 328f
    renal anomalies, 330
    single umbilical cord, 330
    small, low-set ears, 326
    sonographic findings of, 325–330, 338, 341f
    strawberry-shaped skull, 325, 327f
  trisomy 21, 321–323, 321f–324f
    absent/hypoplastic nasal bones, 321f, 322
    clinical findings of, 321
    clinodactyly, 322
    common sonographic findings of, 321f–324f, 322–323
    duodenal atresia, 322, 322f
    echogenic bowel, 323, 323f
    echogenic intracardiac focus (EIF), 322, 323f
    facial sonographic findings of, 338, 340f
    features of, 321, 321f
    macroglossia, 322, 323f
    pyelectasis, 323, 324f
    sandal gap, 325
    thickened nuchal translucency, 321f, 322
    ventricular septal defect, 322, 323f
    widened pelvic angles, 323
Cisterna magna, 283
Clubfoot, 335f
Color Doppler (CD) sonography, 10, 13, 13f, 133, 135, 136f
Comet tail artifact, 7t, 8f, 133, 134f
Common artifacts, ultrasound, 6, 7t, 8f–10f
  acoustic shadowing, 7t, 8f

comet tail artifact, ultrasound, 7t, 8f
dirty shadowing artifact, 7t, 9f
edge shadowing artifact, 7t, 9f
mirror image artifact, 7t, 10f
posterior acoustic enhancement (through transmission) artifact, 7t, 10f
refraction artifact, 7t, 11f
reverberation artifact, 7t, 12f
ring-down artifact, 7t, 12f
Common artifacts in obstetric sonography, 133, 133t
Common clinical obstetric terms, 130, 130t–133t
Complex fluid, 184
Conception, 159–160
Conjoined twins, 315, 317f
Continuous-wave (CW) Doppler sonography, 15
Cornua (uterine horns), 34
Coronal uterine anatomy, 35f
Corpus luteum, 40, 160, 161f
 of pregnancy, 183, 187f
CRL. *See* Crown-rump length
Crown-rump length (CRL), 159
Cul-de-sacs
 AIUM recommendations for sonography of, 33
 fluid during pregnancy, 183–184, 188f
Cystic hygroma (large), 336f
Cystic teratoma, 65–66, 67f, 157
Cystitis, 70, 70f

D

Dandy-Walker malformation, 334f
Detailed first-trimester sonography, 201–244
 common fetal anomalies, 237, 241–244
 fetal anomalies identifiable in, 237, 241–244
  acrania, 237, 241f
  anencephaly, 237, 241f
  Arnold–Chiari malformation, 237, 241, 242f
  exencephaly, 237, 241f
  gastroschisis, 244, 244f
  omphalocele, 241, 243f, 244
  spina bifida, 237, 241, 242f
 genitalia in first trimester, 235, 236f
 protocol for, 237
 scanning planes and structures required for, 201–235
  extremities, 227–228, 229f–230f
  facial structures, 207–215, 208f–216f
  fetal abdomen, 223–227, 223f–228f
  fetal biometry, 202–205, 203f–206f
  fetal head, 205–207, 207f
  fetal thorax, 216–222, 217f–222f
  general assessment, 201–202
  neck, 216
  placenta, 230–231, 233f–234f, 234
  spine, 228, 230, 231f–232f
  uterus, adnexa, cul-de-sac, 234–235, 235f
 specifications of, 201
 trisomy sonographic detection, 237, 238f–240f
Detailed second-/third-trimester sonography, 292–318
 abdominal wall, integrity of, 306
 adrenal glands, 305
 brain parenchyma, 295
 cerebellar lobes, 294
 cerebellum, 307, 308f
 components of, 292–310
 coronal face (nose/lips, lens), 296, 297f–298f, 298
 corpus callosum, 294–295, 294f
 cranial vault, 295, 295f–296f
 description, 292
 diaphragm, integrity of, 303, 305f
 ear position and size, 299, 300f
 external genitalia, 307
 extremities, 307
 fibula, 310, 311f
 fourth ventricle, 293, 293f
 gallbladder, 305
 hands and feet, 307
 heart, 301, 302f–304f
 humerus, 307, 310, 310f
 hypertelorism, 299, 300f
 hypotelorism, 299, 300f
 inner and outer orbital diameters, 307, 308f–309f
 lateral ventricular, 294
 liver, 305
 lungs, 303
 mandible, 298, 299f
 maxilla, 298, 299f
 multiple gestations (twins), 311–318
  amnionicity (number of amniotic sacs), 311
  chorionicity (number of placentas), 311, 312f
  clinical findings with, 311–312
  conjoined, 315, 317f
  in first trimester, 312–313, 313f–314f
  important points to remember, 311, 312f
  pathology, 315, 317, 318f
  in second/third trimester, 313, 315f–316f
  twin–twin transfusion syndrome, 315, 317, 318f

Detailed second-/third-trimester sonography (*Continued*)
  neck, 295–296
  nuchal fold, 307, 309f
  orbits, 299, 300f
  palate, 298
  placental implantation site, 307
  profile, 296
  renal arteries, 305, 306f
  ribs, 303
  shape, curvature, conus medullaris (spine), 306–307
  situs, 299, 301f
  small and large bowel, 303, 305
  spine and overlying soft tissue, 306
  spleen, 305–306
  third ventricle, 292, 293f
  tibia, 310, 311f
  tongue, 299
  ulna, 310, 310f
DIA. *See* Dimeric inhibin A
Diaphragmatic hernia, 287f
Didelphys, uterus, 37, 38f
Dimeric inhibin A (DIA), 140
Dirty shadowing artifact, ultrasound, 7t, 9f
Discriminatory zone, 130t, 160
Doppler sonography in gynecologic sonography, 10–16
  color, 10, 13, 13f
  continuous-wave, 15
  of female pelvis, 60
  motion mode (M-mode), 15
  power, 13, 14f
  pulsed-wave, 13–14, 15f, 16f
Down syndrome, 321
Dyschezia, 130t
Dysmenorrhea, 41t, 130t
Dyspareunia, 131t

E

Early gestational structures, development of, 160, 162, 162f
Eclampsia, 131t, 148
Ectopic pregnancy, 131t, 196, 197f
Edge shadowing artifact, ultrasound, 7t, 9f
Embryonic (fetal) demise, 131t, 198
Endocavity transducer, 3
  for transabdominal pelvic imaging, 4f
  for transvaginal pelvic imaging, 5f
Endometrial carcinoma, 62, 63f
Endometrial hyperplasia, 118, 120f
Endometrioma, 64–65, 66f, 157
Endometrium, 31–32, 35–36
Epispadias, 307
Equipment selection and quality control, 2–6
Ergonomics, 25–27
  obstetric sonography, 145

Estimated date of confinement, 131t
Estriol (UE), 138, 320
Estrogen, 39
Exencephaly, in first trimester, 237, 241f
Extremities, fetal, 169

F

Fallopian tube anatomy, 41f
Female pelvic
  adult, sonography of, 30–75
  anatomy, 34f
    computed tomography (CT), 27, 27f
    magnetic resonance imaging (MRI), 27, 28f
  pathology, 60–70
    bladder diverticulum, 70, 72f
    cystic teratoma, 65–66, 67f
    cystitis, 70, 70f
    endometrial carcinoma, 62, 63f
    endometrioma, 64–65, 66f
    follicular cyst, 63–64, 64f–65f
    inflamed appendix, 71, 72f
    ovarian carcinoma, 68, 69f, 70
    ovarian torsion, 62–63, 64f
    pelvic inflammatory disease (PID), 67–68, 69f
    polycystic ovary syndrome (PCOS), 66, 68f
    transitional cell carcinoma of bladder, 70, 71f
    uterine leiomyoma (fibroid uterus), 60–61, 61f–62f
Fertility drugs, 18
Fetal biometry, 248–251, 250f
Fetal heart and circulation, 166, 167f–168f
Fetal karyotyping, 131t
Fetal lie, 131t
Fetal pole, 188
Fetal presentation, 131t
Fetal skull anatomy, 163, 165f, 166
Fetal stomach, 183, 184f–185f
Fetus, development of, 162, 163f
Fetuses with trisomy 13, 240f
Fetuses with trisomy 18 (Edwards syndrome), 239f
First-trimester trisomy 21, 238f
Follicles, 40
Follicular cyst, 63–64, 64f–65f
Fundal height, 127, 128f, 129–130, 129f

G

Gastroschisis, 244, 244f
General clinical history queries, 16–19
Genitalia, fetal, 168
Genital tubercle
  of female fetus, 236f
  of male fetus, 236f
Gestational diabetes, 131t

Index **349**

Gestational/menstrual age, 131t
Gestational sac, 160, 161f
Gestational trophoblastic disease (GTD), 131t
Graffian follicle, 40
Gravida (gravidity), 131t
Gravidity, 17
GTD. *See* Gestational trophoblastic disease
Gynecologic imaging. *See* Endocavity transducer

H
HCG. *See* Human chorionic gonadotropin
Heart activity, 162-163, 164f
Hemorrhagic ovarian cysts, 154
Hirsutism, 132t
Holoprosencephaly, 330-332, 331f
Human chorionic gonadotropin (hCG), 160, 320
HyCoSy. *See* Hysterosalpingo-contrast sonography
Hydrocele, 307
Hydronephrosis, 153, 155f-156f
Hyperemesis gravidarum, 132t
Hypospadias, 307
Hysterosalpingo-contrast sonography (HyCoSy)
  AIUM
    indications, 2
    procedure recommendations, 108, 109f
    protocol images, 110
    recommendations for performance, 105, 107f
  contraindications of, 105
  patient preparation for, 108
  primary focus of, 105
Hysterosonography. *See* Sonohysterography

I
Image correlation, 73, 74f-75f
Infertility, 132t
Inflamed appendix, 71, 72f
Inhibin-A, 320
Intrauterine device (IUD), 132t
Intrauterine growth restriction (IUGR), 132t
Intussusception, 100, 101f, 102
IUD. *See* Intrauterine device
IUGR. *See* Intrauterine growth restriction

K
Kidneys, fetal, 167, 258, 259f-260f

L
Laboratory findings, 19t

Leiomyoma/fibroids, 154, 273, 273f
Linear transducer, 5, 5f

M
Macrosomia, 132t, 148, 148f
Maternal and gestational diabetes, 148, 148f
Maternal hydronephrosis, 153, 155f-156f
Maternal serum alpha-fetoprotein (MSAFP), 138, 320
Mean sac diameter (MSD), 159
Menarche, 40, 41t
Menometrorrhagia, 41t
Menorrhagia, 41t
Menstrual cycle, 16-17, 40-43
  begins, 40
  common terms, 41, 41t
  diagram of, 42f
  first, 40
  lasts, 41
  phases of, 41, 43
    endometrial cycle, 43
    follicular phase (days 1 to 14), 41, 43
    luteal phase (days 15 to 28), 43
    ovarian cycle, 41, 43
    ovulation (day 14), 43
    proliferative phase (days 1 to 14), 43
    secretory phase (days 15 to 28), 43
Metrorrhagia, 41t, 132t
Mirror image artifact, ultrasound, 7t, 10f
Miscarriage. *See* Abortion
Mittelschmerz, 41t
Molar pregnancy, 196-198, 198f
Motion mode (M-mode) Doppler sonography, 15, 138, 139f
MSAFP. *See* Maternal serum alpha-fetoprotein
MSD. *See* Mean sac diameter
Mullerian duct anomalies, 111, 112f
Multigravida, 132t
Myometrial contraction *(MyC)*, 273, 274f
Myometrium, 31, 35

N
Neural tube defects, 132t, 336-338
  anencephaly, 336-337, 337f
  spina bifida, 337-338, 338f-339f
Nuchal fold, 283, 284f
Nulligravida, 132t

O
Obstetric sonography, 123-157
  AIUM
    first-trimester detailed ultrasound indications, 124

Obstetric sonography (*Continued*)
first-trimester ultrasound indications, 123–124
second- and third-trimester detailed ultrasound indications, 125–126
second- and third-trimester ultrasound indications, 124–125
ALARA principle, 127
cervical incompetence and, 148–149, 150f–156f, 151–152
common artifacts in, 133, 133t
common clinical obstetric terms, 130, 130t–133t
Doppler in, 133
 color, 133, 135, 136f
 M-mode, 138, 139f
 power, 135, 137f
 pulsed-wave, 136–137, 138f
eclampsia and, 148
ectopic pregnancy emergency situations during, 145, 146f, 147
equipments
 maintenance, 144
 selection and quality control, 126–127
ergonomics, 145
general clinical history queries, 140–142
infection control, 143–144
labeling of examinations, 143
maternal and gestational diabetes and, 148, 148f
maternal hydronephrosis and, 153, 155f–156f
maternal serum screening for aneuploidy, 138, 139t, 140
patient positioning for, 143
patient preparation for, 142–143
pelvic masses associated with pregnancy, 154, 156f, 157
preeclampsia and, 148, 149f
Rh sensitization and, 152–153, 154f
supine hypotensive syndrome and, 147, 147f
trimesters and fundal height, 127, 128f, 129–130, 129f
Oligodactyly, 307
Omphalocele, 241, 243f, 244
Ovarian-adnexal reporting and data system (O-RADS), 71–73, 73f
Ovarian carcinoma, 68, 69f, 70
Ovarian fossa, 38–39
Ovarian torsion, 62–63, 64f, 98, 102f
Ovaries, 44
abnormalities, 32
AIUM recommendations for sonography of, 32
anatomy, 37–40, 39f

blood supply in, 40
corpus luteum, 40
estrogen and, 39
follicles, 40
inner medulla, 40
orthogonal planes, 32
outer cortex, 40
ovarian fossa, 38–39
positions of, 39f
progesterone and, 39
size, 32
vein, 40

P

Pain, 17, 18f
PAPP-A. *See* Pregnancy-associated plasma protein-A; Pregnancy-associated plasma protein A
Para (parity), 132t
Parity score, 17
PAS. *See* Placenta accreta spectrum
Patient positioning
for pediatric female pelvic sonography, 89
for standard first-trimester sonography, 171
for standard second-/third-trimester sonography, 268–269
for transabdominal female pelvic sonogram, 21, 22f
for transabdominal obstetric sonogram, 21
for transvaginal female pelvic sonogram, 22, 23f
for transvaginal obstetric sonogram, 143
Patient preparation
for first-trimester pelvic sonogram, 142
for pediatric female pelvic sonography, 87–89
for standard first-trimester sonography, 169–170
for standard second-/third-trimester sonography, 268
for transabdominal female pelvic sonogram, 20–21, 20f, 21f
for transvaginal female pelvic examination, 21
for transvaginal first-trimester pelvic examination, 142–143
PCOS. *See* Polycystic ovary syndrome
Pediatric female pelvic
anatomy of, 79–85
 ovaries, 82, 84–85, 85f–86f
 uterus, 79–80, 80f–84f, 82
pathology of, 95–100
 ambiguous genitalia, 95–96
 appendicitis, 100, 101f, 103f
 congenital anomalies of uterus, 102

free fluid within pelvis, 100
intussusception, 100, 101f, 102
ovarian masses, 100
ovarian torsion, 98, 102f
pediatric ovarian masses, 99–100, 100f
precocious puberty, 97
pseudoprecocious puberty, 97–98
right lower quadrant pain, 100
urinary bladder, 102
vaginal obstructions, 95, 95t
physiology of, 79–85
Pediatric female pelvic sonography, 76–103
clinical investigation for, 87, 89–90
Doppler of, 94
equipment and quality control for, 85–87
image correlation for, 102, 102f–103f
normal measurements, 93–94
patient positioning for, 89
transabdominal, 89
transvaginal, 89
patient preparation for, 87–89
transabdominal sonography, 87–88
transvaginal sonography, 88–89
protocol for, 90–92
recommendations for, 76–79
adnexa, 79
ALARA (As Low As Reasonably Achievable) principle, 79
cervix, 78
cul-de-sac, 79
Doppler sonography, 79
ovaries, 78
three-dimensional sonography, 78
uterus, 76–78
vagina, 78
scanning tips, 92–93
Pediatric ovarian masses, 99–100, 100f
Pelvic inflammatory disease (PID), 67–68, 69f
Pelvic masses associated with pregnancy, 154, 156f, 157
Pelvic pain, 17, 18f
Pelvic pathologies findings, 19t
Pelvis, fetal, 166–168
PID. *See* Pelvic inflammatory disease
Placenta, 162
accreta in first trimester, 230–231, 233f–234f, 234
in first trimester, 183, 186f
Placenta accreta, 277
Placenta accreta spectrum (PAS), 276, 278f
Placenta increta, 277
Placental abruption, 277, 279, 279f
Placental grading, 276, 277f

Placenta percreta, 277
Placenta previa, 274, 276f
Polycystic ovary syndrome (PCOS), 66, 68f
Polydactyly, 307
Posterior acoustic enhancement (through transmission) artifact, ultrasound, 7t, 10f, 133, 135f
Power Doppler (PD) sonography, 13, 14f, 135, 137f
Precocious puberty, 97
Preeclampsia, 148, 149f
Preeclampsia, 132t
Pregnancy-associated plasma protein-A (PAPP-A), 140, 321
Premature rupture of membranes (PROM), 132t
Primigravida, 132t
Progesterone, 39
PROM. *See* Premature rupture of membranes
Pseudoprecocious puberty, 97–98
Pulsed-wave (PW) Doppler sonography, 13–14, 15f, 16f, 136–137, 138f

R

Refraction, 133
Refraction artifact, ultrasound, 7t, 11f
Retained products of conception (RPOC), 153
Reverberation artifact, ultrasound, 7t, 12f, 133
Rhombencephalon, 163
Rh sensitization, 152–153, 154f
Ring-down artifact, ultrasound, 7t, 12f, 133
RPOC. *See* Retained products of conception

S

Saline infusion sonography (SIS), 105, 106f
AIUM
indications, 2
procedure recommendations, 108
protocol images, 108–110, 110f, 111f
recommendations for performance, 105, 106f
of Asherman syndrome, 116, 117f
color Doppler, 111f
contraindications of, 105
3D imaging, 111f
for examination of uterus, 32
pathology noted on, 116–120
Asherman syndrome, 116, 117f
endometrial hyperplasia, 118, 120f
uterine adhesions, 116

352 Index

Saline infusion sonography (*Continued*)
    uterine myoma (fibroid), 116, 118, 119f
    uterine polyps, 116, 118f
  patient preparation for, 108
  primary focus of, 105
  and uterine myoma, 119f
Scaphocephaly, 295, 295f
Septate uterus, 37, 38f
SIS. *See* Saline infusion sonography
Sonography, gynecologic
  adult female pelvic, 30–75
  AIUM indications for, 1–2
  AIUM recommendations for female pelvis, 30–33
  common artifacts, ultrasound, 6, 7t, 8f–10f
  detailed first-trimester, 201–244
  detailed second-/third-trimester, 292–318
  Doppler sonography in, 10–16
  equipment maintenance, 24–25
  hysterosalpingo-contrast-sonography, 2
  infection control, 23–24
  labeling of examinations, 22–23, 23f
  laboratory findings, 19t
  overview, 1
  patient positioning for, 21–22, 22f
  patient preparation for, 20–21
  pediatric female pelvic, 76–103
  pelvic pathologies findings, 19t
  standard first-trimester, 158–199
  terminology, 6, 7t
Sonohysterography
  AIUM
    indications, 2
    procedure recommendations, 108
    protocol images, 108–110, 110f, 111f
    recommendations for performance, 105, 106f
  of Asherman syndrome, 116, 117f
  color Doppler, 111f
  contraindications of, 105
  3D imaging, 111f
  for examination of uterus, 32
  pathology noted on, 116–120
    Asherman syndrome, 116, 117f
    endometrial hyperplasia, 118, 120f
    uterine adhesions, 116
    uterine myoma (fibroid), 116, 118, 119f
    uterine polyps, 116, 118f
  patient preparation for, 108
  primary focus of, 105
  and uterine myoma, 119f
Sonosalpingography. *See* Hysterosalpingo-contrast sonography (HyCoSy)
Spina bifida, 237, 241, 242f, 337–338
  clinical findings of, 338
  facts, 337–338
  sonographic findings of, 338, 338f–339f
Spine, fetal, 166, 166f, 228, 230, 231f–232f
Standard first-trimester sonography, 158–199
  AIUM recommendations for, 158–159
  anatomy and physiology of first trimester, 159–169
    abdomen and pelvis, 166–168
    chest, 166, 167f–168f
    conception, 159–160
    early gestational structures, development of, 160, 162, 162f
    extremities, 169
    fetus, development of, 162, 163f
    genitalia, 168
    gestational sac, 160, 161f
    heart activity, 162–163, 164f
    kidneys, 167
    skull, 163, 165f, 166
    spine, 166, 166f
    stomach, 166–167
    umbilical cord insertion, 167, 169f
  clinical investigation, 172–174
  common first-trimester pathology, 196–199
    anembryonic gestation, 196
    ectopic pregnancy, 196, 197f
    embryonic demise, 198
    miscarriage, 198–199
    molar pregnancy, 196–198, 198f
    subchorionic hemorrhage, 199, 199f
  equipment for, 170–171
  equipment maintenance, 172
  infection control, 171–172
  labeling of sonographic examinations, 171
  normal measurements, 194–195
  normal sonographic anatomy, 174–184
    acrania, 180, 182f
    AIUM Guidelines for Nuchal Translucency Measurements between 11 and 14 weeks, 180, 182–183, 182f–183f
    corpus luteum of pregnancy, 183, 187f
    cul-de-sacs, 183–184, 188f
    embryo/fetus less than 10 weeks, 176–177, 176f–179f
    endometrium and intradecidual sign, decidualized, 174, 174f
    fetal stomach, 183, 184f–185f
    fetus (≥10 weeks gestational age), 178, 179f

Index **353**

    gestational sac, 174, 175f
    placenta, 183, 186f
    yolk sac, 175, 175f, 176f
  patient positioning for, 171
  patient preparation for, 169–170
    transabdominal, 169–170
    transvaginal, 170
  protocol for, 184–192
  scanning tips, 192–194, 193f–194f
Standard second-/third-trimester sonography, 245–291
  AIUM recommendations for, 245–267
  abdomen, 256, 258, 259f–261f, 260
  abdominal circumference, 249, 251, 252f
  amniotic fluid volume, 247, 247f
  biometry, 248–251, 250f
  brachycephaly, 249
  cardiac activity, 245, 246f
  cardiac axis, 256
  cerebellum, 252, 254f
  cervix, 263, 266, 266f–267f
  chest, 256, 256f
  cisterna magna, 252, 254f
  dolichocephaly, 249, 251, 251f–253f
  external genitalia, 261, 262f
  extremities, 263, 265f
  femur length, 251, 253f
  fetal presentation, 245–246, 246f
  head, face, and neck, 251–252, 253f–254f
  head circumference, 249, 251f
  heart, 256, 256f
  kidneys, 258, 259f–260f
  normal foramen, 256, 257f
  nuchal fold (between 16 and 20 weeks), 252, 255f
  number, 245
  outflow tracts, 256, 257f
  placenta, 248, 248f
  spine, 262–263, 263f–265f
  stomach (presence, size, and situs), 258, 258f
  umbilical cord, 248, 249f, 258, 260f–261f
  upper lip, 252, 255f
  urinary bladder, 260, 261f
  uterus, adnexal structures, and cervix; evaluation of, 263
  ventricular septum, 256
  video clips, 245
  weight estimate, 263
  biophysical profile, 289–290, 289t
  clinical investigation, 270–272
  equipment maintenance, 270
  infection control, 269–270
    transabdominal transducers, 269
    transvaginal transducers, 270
  labeling of sonographic examinations, 269
  normal measurements, 288–289
  patient positioning for, 268–269
    transabdominal, 268
    transvaginal, 269
  patient preparation for, 268
  protocol for, 272–287, 273f–281f, 284f, 286f–287f
  scanning tips, 287
  suggested equipment for, 268
Stomach, fetal, 166–167
Subchorionic hemorrhage, 132t, 199, 199f
Supine hypotensive syndrome, 147, 147f
Syncytiotrophoblastic cells, 160

T

*T*erm, *P*reterm, *A*bortions, and *L*iving (TPAL) children, 133t
Thermal index for soft tissue (TIs), 127
Three-dimensional gynecologic sonography, 110–115
  for general pattern of polycystic ovary, 115f
  of hyperstimulated ovary after ovulation induction, 113, 115f
  for intracavitary/suspected intracavitary abnormalities, 112, 114f
  intrauterine device (IUD) on, 112, 113f
  for Mullerian duct anomalies, 111, 112f
  of submucosal fibroid, 112, 114t
  used as adjunct to routine pelvic sonogram, 111
Three-vessel trachea view, 286f
TORCH infections, 132t
TPAL, 17
Transitional cell carcinoma of bladder, 70, 71f
Trisomy, 133t
Trisomy 13, 330–332
  clinical findings of, 330
  facts, 330, 330f
  sonographic findings of, 330–332, 331f–332f
Trisomy 18, 325–330
  agenesis of corpus callosum, 325, 326f
  choroid plexus cyst, 325, 326f
  clenched hands, 326, 328f
  clinical findings of, 325
  clubfeet/rocker-bottom feet, 330
  enlarged cisterna magna, 325
  facts, 325
  fetuses with (Edwards syndrome), 239f

Trisomy (*Continued*)
  heart defects, 327–328, 329f, 330
  hypoplastic cerebellum, 325
  micrognathia, 325, 327f
  omphalocele, 326–327, 328f
  renal anomalies, 330
  single umbilical cord, 330
  small, low-set ears, 326
  sonographic findings of, 325–330, 338, 341f
  strawberry-shaped skull, 325, 327f
Trisomy 21, 321–323, 321f–324f
  absent/hypoplastic nasal bones, 321f, 322
  clinical findings of, 321
  clinodactyly, 322
  common sonographic findings of, 321f–324f, 322–323
  duodenal atresia, 322, 322f
  echogenic bowel, 323, 323f
  echogenic intracardiac focus (EIF), 322, 323f
  facial sonographic findings of, 338, 340f
  features of, 321, 321f
  macroglossia, 322, 323f
  pyelectasis, 323, 324f
  sandal gap, 325
  thickened nuchal translucency, 321f, 322
  ventricular septal defect, 322, 323f
  widened pelvic angles, 323
Turner syndrome, 335f
Twin–twin transfusion syndrome, 315, 317, 318f

U

Ultrasound artifacts, 6, 7t, 8f–10f
Umbilical cord insertion, fetal, 167, 169f
Umbilical cord S/D ratios (normal and abnormal), 281, 281f
Unicornuate uterus, 37, 38f
Urinary bladder, fetal, 168
Urine pregnancy test, 160
Uterine
  adhesions, sonohysterography, 116
  body, 34
  fibroids, sonographic findings of, 116, 118, 119f
  fundus, 34
  isthmus, 34
  leiomyoma (fibroid uterus), 60–61, 61f–62f
  polyps, sonohysterography, 116, 118f
Uterus, 44
  AIUM recommendations for sonography of, 30–32
  anatomy, 33–36
  bicornuate, 37, 38f
  cervix, 34
    abnormalities of, 32
  congenital uterine anomalies, 37, 38f
  depth, 30–31
  didelphys, 37, 38f
  endometrium, 31–32, 35–36
  layers of uterine wall, 31
  length, 30
  myometrium, 31, 35
  perimetrium, 35
  septate, 37, 38f
  sonohysterography for examination of, 32
  three-dimensional sonography for examination of, 32
  unicornuate, 37, 38f
  uterine body, 34
  uterine fundus, 34
  uterine isthmus, 34
  vagina, abnormalities of, 32
  variants in uterine position, 36–37, 36f
    anteflexion, 36f, 37
    anteversion, 36, 36f
    dextroverted, 36f, 37
    levoverted, 36f, 37
    retroflexion, 36f, 37
    retroversion, 36f, 37
  volume, 31
  width, 31

V

VACTERL association, 290, 290f
Vagina
  abnormalities of, 32
  anatomy, 37
  obstructions in pediatric female, 95, 95t

W

Work-related musculoskeletal disorders (WRMSDs), 1, 145
WRMSDs. *See* Work-related musculoskeletal disorders

Y

Yolk sac, 160, 161f, 175, 175f, 176f